Advance Praise for *Western Herbs for Martial Artists and Contact Athletes*

In this one volume you can access accurate and dependable Western herbs that are safe and effective treatments for sports injuries. Dr. Peterson has done a wonderful job of organizing the information and presenting it in an understandable and usable way. As a writer, I can only imagine the hundreds, no, thousands of hours that went into this volume.

—Carolyn Dean, M.D., N.D., *from her foreword*

Generated out of a sincere interest to assist other martial artists in making wise choices about how and when to use or not to use herbal treatments to augment their martial arts practices, the author has utilized her considerable expertise in research and her natural flair for writing to create a book destined to become an instant classic both for herbalists and martial artists.

—David H. Price, L. Ac., M.O.M., B.A., *from his foreword*

A well researched and concise treatise on the herbs used to treat trauma and sports injuries. Provides an accessible alternative to Chinese herbal medicine for the athlete and martial artist.

—Tom Bisio, L. Ac., author of *A Tooth From The Tiger's Mouth, The Essentials of Ba Gua Zhang, Zheng Gu Tui Na*

A well-researched guide that is practical, helpful and informative. This book will be especially useful for Westerners without much background in Traditional Chinese Medicine. *Western Herbs for Martial Artists and Contact Athletes* has earned a place on my bookshelf.

—Jennifer Lawler, martial artist, author of *Martial Arts for Dummies, Dojo Wisdom, The Self Defense Deck*

Such a practical, wise and well-researched guide to successfully using herbs! This book selects herbs from both Western and Easter traditions and provides information on safety, dosage, usage and all things valuable on each plant. This book will be treasured by martial artists and health professionals of all traditions. Destined to be a classic!

—Brigitte Mars, A.H.G, Professor of Herbal Medicine, brigittemars.com, author of *Rawsome!, Desktop Guide to Herbal Medicine, Beauty by Nature, Addiction Free Naturally*

Herbs can be a great way to help heal bruises, scrapes, swellings and other injuries from all kinds of contact sports. Since ancient times, martial artists in China have been using herbal treatments. Peterson's book is unusual in that it looks at herbs readily available in the West rather than Eastern remedies.

—Bruce Fratzis, Taoist lineage holder, author of *Opening the Energy Gates of Your Body, The Power of Internal Martial Arts and Chi*

While much has been written about traditional Asian remedies, many of which are challenging to come by in many parts of the world, this is the first time I have seen a treatise on Western herbs. Peterson's examination is methodical and comprehensive, documenting findings in a way that makes the subject matter highly accessible for martial artists (and athletes of any type). Specifically, readily available herbs that can help with bruises, scrapes, cuts, sprains, breaks, dislocations, breathing, adrenaline management, and other issues and ailments common to those who practice the fighting arts are discussed in detail. Her nine principles for using medicinal herbs safely set the context, while descriptions of affects, dosages, dangers, risks, and usefulness of each plant round out the information. *Western Herbs for Martial Artists and Contact Athletes* is a unique and interesting tome, a valuable contribution to the serious practitioner's bookshelf.

—Lawrence A. Kane, martial artist, author of *Surviving Armed Assaults*, *Martial Arts Instruction*, *The Little Black Book of Violence*, *The Way to Black Belt*, *The Way of Kata*

WESTERN HERBS

for Martial Artists and Contact Athletes

WESTERN HERBS

for Martial Artists and Contact Athletes

Effective Treatments for Common Sports Injuries

SUSAN LYNN PETERSON, PH.D.

YMAA Publication Center
Wolfeboro, NH, USA

YMAA Publication Center
Main Office: PO Box 480
Wolfeboro, NH 03894
1-800-669-8892 • www.ymaa.com • ymaa@aol.com

ISBN-13: 978-1-59439-197-2
ISBN-10: 1-59439-197-1

10 9 8 7 6 5 4 3 2 1

Cover design by Axie Breen
Edited by Susan Bullowa
Photos by the author unless otherwise noted.

Publisher's Cataloging in Publication

Peterson, Susan Lynn, 1957-

Western herbs for martial artists and contact athletes : effective treatments for common sports injuries / Susan Lynn Peterson. -- Wolfeboro, NH : YMAA Publication Center, c2010.

p. ; cm.

ISBN: 13-digit: 978-1-59439-197-2 ; 10-digit: 1-59439-197-1
"For bruises, sprains, strains, breathing, dislocations, adrenaline, and more"--Cover.
Includes bibliographical references and index.

1. Herbs--Therapeutic use. 2. Martial arts injuries--Alternative treatment. 3. Sports injuries--Alternative treatment. 4. Martial artists--Nutrition. 5. Athletes--Nutrition. 6. Herbals. I. Title.

RM666.H33 P48 2010 2010933226
615/.321--dc22 1009

Warning: The authors and publishers of this material are NOT RESPONSIBLE in any manner whatsoever for any injury which may occur through reading or following the instructions in this manual. The information in this book is not meant as a substitute for medical treatment or advice. This book is not written to replace your regular medical doctor or the medicine thereof, but for your knowledge and informational purposes only. The activities, recipes, recommendations, usage advice, physical or otherwise, described in this material may be too strenuous or dangerous for some people, and the reader(s) should consult a physician before engaging in them.

Printed in Canada.

To Laura Westbrooks

Table of Contents

Foreword

by Carolyn Dean M.D.

Most people treat pain and inflammation with medication. However, strong analgesics and anti-inflammatory drugs can have serious side effects, such as bleeding ulcers, fluid retention, and digestive problems. The vilified anti-inflammatories, Vioxx and Celebrex, also cause symptoms of heart disease. To offer my patients something other than drugs, I decided to learn acupuncture in medical school. I convinced a Chinese anesthesiologist to allow me to observe in his acupuncture clinic in my second year elective. I learned about all the incurable diseases in my morning class and in the afternoon I saw them cured.

I also wanted to learn about Chinese herbs for pain and inflammation. However, when I studied Chinese herbal medicine with Jeffrey Yuen in New York, I found the subject incredibly complex. The formulas used in martial arts alone required years of study to formulate and apply, a well stocked herbal formulary, and a knowledgeable herbalist to mix the ingredients. As a consumer, if you have to wade into your local Chinatown and purchase herbs without a single letter of usable English on the label, you aren't in do-it-yourself territory. I was surprised when the last wound plaster I got from a TCM practitioner contained acetylsalicylic acid (aspirin) when I read the fine print on the label.

Now, in this one volume you can access accurate and dependable Western herbs that are safe and effective treatments for sports injuries. Dr. Peterson had done a wonderful job of organizing the information and presenting it in an understandable and usable way. As a writer, I can only imagine the hundreds, no, thousands of hours that went into this volume.

As a clinician, I immediately gravitated to Chapter Four, which gives prescriptive advice for joint pain and inflammation, sprains, fractures, bruises, wounds, bleeding, puncture wounds, itchy sores, abrasions, chapped skin, old wounds, bruised lips, muscle cramps, aching muscles, scars and more. Active people suffer other symptoms besides musculoskeletal, so, Dr. Peterson also covers simple colds, anxiety, insomnia, digestion, motion sickness, and even fungal infections.

Chapter Two is a great herbal reference of over sixty herbs that answers the basic questions: What's it good for; How do you use it; How much do you use; and What should you be aware of before using it. Other chapters tackle the difficult topics of herbal side effects and herb/drug interactions. My bias, of course, is to use herbal remedies first before turning to drugs, but if you are already on a medication you need to know if a certain herb will accentuate the drug's effects or heal the condition and make the drug superfluous!

The book is called *Western Herbs for Martial Artists and Contact Athletes* but it has a much broader appeal. I'm going to recommend it to every athlete I know. Actually, to everyone I know because anyone can pull a muscle or fall and hurt himself on a curb or trip over a stone and benefit from Dr. Peterson's guidance.

Carolyn Dean, M.D., N.D. is a medical doctor, naturopath, herbalist and homeopath. She is the author and co-author of 17 books on health, an online newsletter, and online health programs at www.drcarolyndean.com.

Foreword

by David Price

Over the course of several generations, the Pacific currents that have conveyed the Asian martial arts to the West have also carried with them bits and pieces of the Chinese medical tradition used in the treatment of traumatic injuries. Occasionally, the martial artist is fortunate enough to meet a master who has firsthand knowledge of the correct application of special liniments or training formulas. A friend of mine recounts a story of just such a master who would prepare a rare elixir, an efficacious formulation with the immediate effect of loosening stiff and painful joints to allow for continued training. The same individual, however, also impressed me by casually mentioning how he had sipped White Flower Oil, a toxic external-use therapeutic rub, to eradicate colds. Obviously, in between indecipherable characters and miraculous cures, lies a chasm fraught with pitfalls for the overzealous martial arts enthusiast who yearns to explore both the combative and medicinal wisdom of the East without adequate resources and schooling.

My study and practice of Chinese herbal medicine over the past 15 years has been both arduous and humbling. Building upon a lifelong interest in herbal medicine, I began in earnest with a distance learning program followed by four years of formal training in Chinese acupuncture and herbology. A few years after receiving my diploma, I took a position teaching Chinese medical theory to graduate students. With every course in Chinese herbal medicine I teach and every formulation I craft in my private practice, I gain a little more expertise and even more appreciation for both the brilliant minds of ancient physicians and the complexity and difficulties inherent in the practice of medicine. As Ms. Peterson remarks, the skillful and safe use of Chinese herbs demands much more than passing interest and access to popular literature—Chinese medicine is a refined and erudite blend of science and art.

The present text offers one solution for the intrepid martial artist with an interest in herbal therapies. Recognizing the challenges of procuring quality Chinese materials, grasping the essence of classical Eastern diagnosis, identifying appropriate traditional formulations and modifying them, and preparing and administering treatments, the author explores instead the myriad possibilities in our own native Western traditions of herbology. The result is a delightful and scholarly addition to both the herbal and martial arts literature. Pragmatically organized, the prose is, nonetheless, lively and enjoyable, avoiding the dry language found in many older herbals and making this a wonderful read.

It is crucial to spend some time reading through the introduction and the first chapter, "Using Herbs Safely," a mandatory primer for smart herbal usage. Distilling good herbal practices into nine basic principles, Ms. Peterson has addressed many of the mistakes that lead to problems using herbs. Chapter Two, "The Herbal," introduces a wide range of common herbs with meticulously researched information. One particularly noteworthy feature is a grading scale for the properties ascribed to the herbs, allowing readers to evaluate the credibility of actions and indications associated with each substance. In the subsequent chapter, "Preparing the Herbs," detailed information is given regarding the various, and sometimes complex, preparation methods and their benefits and disadvanatages. This section takes you a bit closer to considering actually working with herbs. In "Applications and Uses," we are introduced to more sophisticated uses of herbs in synergistic mixtures. The book concludes with "Herbal Contraindications," "Further Resources," and the "Glossary," rounding out the text with clear lists featuring details on key terminology and the general properties of the herbs, as well as the best places to continue educating yourself regarding effective and appropriate herbal therapeutics.

Motivated by a sincere interest to assist other martial artists in making wise choices about how and when to use or not to use herbal treatments to augment their martial arts practices, the author has utilized her considerable expertise in research and her natural flair for writing to create a book destined to become an instant classic both for herbalists and martial artists. In fact, you need not fall into either category in order to enjoy and value this informative book. I have no doubt that you are holding in your hands a text that will quickly become a favorite for anyone fascinated by medicinal herbs, representing a step forward toward better understanding of the power, both for serious harm and for profound health and well-being, of our planet's immense and rich apothecary.

David Price, B.A., M.O.M., L. Ac. is a graduate of Pomona College with a concentration in Asian Studies. He received a Master's degree from the International Institute of Chinese Medicine and trained at the Chengdu University of TCM. He is currently Clinical Dean at the Asian Institute of Medical Studies in Tucson, Arizona, and operates White Pine Clinic of Classical Chinese Therapeutics (www.whitepineclinic.com).

Acknowledgements

Writing involves spending a surprisingly large amount of time alone in a room with stacks of books and a computer monitor. These acknowledgements are mostly of those people who were always there when I poked my nose out from my cave.

First—always first—is Gary, my husband. Without his steady support for the last twenty-nine years, I could not do what I do and probably would not be who I am.

Thanks also to: Laura Westbrooks, friend, helping hand, and moral support; the brains behind the dojo, and a good part of its heart as well. I'm glad our paths have crossed. My life is much richer because they have. Shawn Koons, friend and fix-it guy, always generous with time and resources. My mom and dad, Don and Shirley Johnson, for growing a few of the herbs for me to photograph (and for everything else as well). The folks at KoSho Karate Pantano—students and parents. You've been great company along the way. David Price, who opened my eyes to the possibilities of Chinese herbalism, and who helped patch me together after too many hours of sitting in one place looking at a computer screen. Don Brandenburgh, whose career advice and guidance have always gone above and beyond the call of duty. Krista Goering, my literary agent, for heart and head both offered in service of the project. The generous folks of Wikimedia Commons and Flickr, especially Renate Eder. Many of the illustrations in this book are available thanks to these good citizens of cyberspace.

Acknowledgements for Herbal Illustrations. Thanks to those who let me use the following illustrations in Chapter 2. I have also included the illustrations I provided.

Alan Cressler (Goldenseal, *Hydrastis candensis*); **Anne-Miek Bibbe** (Fenugreek, *Trigonella foenum-graecum*): **Badagnani** (Turmeric root, *Curcuma longa*); **Barbara Studer** (Arnica, *Arnica montana*); **Björgvin Steindórsson** (*Rhodiola rosea*); **FloraFarm GmbH Katharina Lohrie** (Ginseng, *Panax ginseng*); **Foodista** (Fennel, *Foeniculum vulgare*); **Forest and Kim Starr** (Gotu Kola, *Centella asiatica*), (Shepherd's Purse, *Capsella bursa pastoris*); **Hans-Joachim Fitting** (Flax, *Linum usitatissimum*); **Henri Pidoux** (Devil's Claw, *Harpagophyum procumbens*); Jappe Cost Budde (Tea tree, *Meleuca* genus); **Joan Simon** (Agrimony, *Agrimonia eupatoria*); **Johannes Keplinger** (Cat's Claw, *Uncaria tomentosa*); **Karduelis** (Coltsfoot, *Tussilago farfara*); **Karel Jakubec** (Evening Primrose, *Oenothera biennis*);**Laura Westbrooks** (*Echinacea purpurea*), (Horsetail, *Equisetum arvense*), (Valerian, *Valeriana officinalis*), (Yarrow, *Achillea millefolium*); **Love Krittaya** (*Ginkgo biloba*); **LuckyStarr** (A hops cone, *Humulus lupulus*); **Marcia Martínez Carvajal** (*Rosa Mosqueta, Rosa affinis rubiginosa*); **Michael Thompson** (Peppermint, *Mentha piperita*); **Ohio Department of Natural Resources** (Slippery elm bark, *Ulmus rubra*); **PDPhoto.org** (Catnip blossom, *Nepeta catarica*); **Piouswatson** (Ashwagandha, *Withania somnifera*); **Renate Eder** (European Elder, *Sambucus nigra*), (Feverfew, *Tanacetum parthenium*); (Goldenrod, *Solidago virgaurea*) (The leaves and nut of a horse chestnut, *Aesculus hippocastanum*), (Marshmallow, *Althaea officinalis*);

(Witch Hazel, *Hamamelis virginiana*); **Rob Hille** (German Chamomile, *Matricaria recutita*); **Stanislav Doronenko** (Astragalus, *Astragalus membranaceus*); **Stanislav Doronenko** (Leaves of the *Eleuthero plant, Eleutherococcus senticosus*), (St. John's wort, *Hypericum perforatum*); **Steve Hammonds** (Bilberry, *Vaccinium myrtillus*); the author **Susan Lynn Peterson** (Aloe Vera), (Anise, *Pimpinella anisum*); (Commercially prepared bromelain tablets); (An assortment of peppers of the *Capsicum* genus); (Caraway "seeds," *Carum carvi*); (True Cinnamon, *Cinnamomum zeylanicum* (left) and *Cassia Cinnmon, C. aromaticum*), (Cloves, *Syzygium aromaticum*), (Comfrey, *Symphytum officinales*), (Leaves and bark from on the the 733 species of *Eucalyptus*), (Commercially encapsulated fish oil), (Whole flax seeds), (Garlic, *Allium sativum*), (Ginger rhizome, *Zingiber officinalis*), (Horseradish root, *Armoracia rusticana*), (Lavender, *Lavandula augustifolia*), (Dried licorice root, *Glycyrrhiza glabra*), (Myrrh, *Commiphora molmol*), (Nettles, *Urtica dioica*), (Rosemary, *Rosmarinus officinalis*), (Sage, *Salvia officinalis*), (Thyme, *Thymus vulgaris*); **Teo Siyang** (Andrographis, *Andrographis paniculata*); **U.S. Department of Agriculture** (Willow bark, *Salix alba*).

Introduction

Healing with herbs has long been a tradition in the martial arts. Liniments for bruises, tonics for energy, herbal infusions to strengthen connective tissue, warm muscles, even to heal broken bones—all are part of the martial arts legacy. Most martial artists are aware of that legacy. Not all have access to it first-hand.

It bears saying right here at the beginning of the book that if you do have access to a capable professional martial herbalist, you are most fortunate. Nothing this or any other book can teach you can compare with the hands-on expertise of a medical professional trained in traditional Chinese herbal medicine. Chinese herbal medicine is both more systematic and more comprehensive than Western herbal medicine, and a good Chinese doctor can be a martial artist's greatest boon. If that medical professional is also your martial arts teacher and can teach you as well as treat you, you are twice blessed. Yet few of us are fortunate to study with teachers who understand and can teach the traditional Chinese formulas. The rest of us pick up what we can, wherever we can. This book is for the rest of us.

The Quandary

In the last fifteen years, books about healing with Eastern herbs and traditional Chinese medicines have begun to be published in English. Though tested by time, these remedies often prove impractical for Western martial artists engaged in self-teaching. Traditional Chinese remedies fit into a larger system of medicine that is very different from the Western tradition of seeing complaints as "one-problem, one-treatment." Chinese remedies tend to be systemic, treating the entire person to foster health rather than treating a symptom to fix pathology. The ingredients tend to be native to China, some being very difficult to obtain in Europe and North America. Those ingredients that do find their way across the ocean are sometimes of questionable purity.[1] Some ingredients mentioned in the traditional books—those made from animal parts (such as bear gallbladder and wingless cockroach), molds and fungi, and various other "exotic" materials—are off-putting to Westerners. Moreover, Western-style medical documentation about the safety of Eastern herbs and medicines is often sketchy. Without a teacher or other formal training in traditional Chinese medicine, many Western martial artists are left with little more than blind trust that the book in front of them is a faithful transmission of a legitimate tradition, and that the herbs they ordered online are, if not what the label says, at least not too toxic.

Western Herbs and this Book

Yet even if you are reluctant to log on to eBay and purchase and brew a packet of herbs from China, that doesn't mean you must turn your back on the martial tradition of healing with herbs. Though advances in chemistry in the nineteenth century steered Western medicine away from herbal remedies for more than a hundred years, we too have a tradition of healing with herbs. In recent years, that tradition has begun to be folded back into mainstream medicine. A new interest in alternative and complementary medicine has led to studies investigating which herbs do indeed have healing properties. We know more now about the efficacy and dangers of Western herbal medicine than at any other time in history.

The purpose of this book is to investigate those herbs that are readily available to the West. Most of the herbs in this book are either native to Europe and/or North America or have become common in these continents. For each herb I look at evidence for its effectiveness, evidence for its safety, and how specifically to use it. In short, this book is a compilation and distillation of modern evidence for a traditional Western art.

My research is a survey of the various strands of Western herbalism. That research pulls from five main sources:

- British herbalism (which had a heavy influence on North American herbalism)
- Continental European herbalism (especially from Germany's Commission E)
- Traditional Native American herbalism
- Folk uses in Europe and North America
- Standard scientific research from around the world (especially the United States)

It is a combination of tradition and new research, practical experience and scientific method, and it pulls from literally hundreds of sources in an attempt to get the "big picture" for any given herb.

Among the references regularly cited are these:

- The 1918 U.S. Dispensatory. This volume is the twentieth edition of a reference book used mainly by pharmacists back when you could still get an herbal remedy made up for you by your local pharmacist. It is the last of the dispensatories to deal in depth with herbal medicine, and it represents the best science of its time.
- "The Eclectic School" was a branch of American medicine in the late nineteenth and early twentieth century. This school believed in merging traditional herbalism with other treatment methods. Eclectic physicians reserved the right to choose whatever methods most benefited their patients, hence the name "eclectic" from the Greek *eklego*, meaning "to choose from." The last Eclectic medical school closed in Cincinnati in 1939. Two authors have passed down to us the knowledge of the Eclectic School. Harvey Wickes Felter authored *The Eclectic Materia Medica, Pharmacology and Therapeutics*. And John William Fyfe, a teaching physician in New York, authored three manuals for physicians detailing how herbs can be used to treat specific conditions. They are *The Essentials of Modern Materia Medica and Therapeutics* (a.k.a. *Fyfe's Materia Medica*), *Pocket Essentials of Modern Materia Medica and Therapeutics*, and *Specific Diagnosis and Specific Medication*.
- Commission E monographs. The Commission E monographs are analyses of various herbs, commissioned by the German government to assist in the national regulation of herbs. These monographs, written by health professionals are some-

times detailed and carefully reasoned. They sometimes read like "medicine by committee." But they do reflect a modern take on traditional European herbalism.

- *The PDR for Herbal Medicine*. The herbal counterpart to the *Physicians Desk Reference*, it is a reference book for modern mainstream physicians. It contains information on therapeutic properties and drug interactions.
- *A Modern Herbal. A Modern Herbal*, despite its name, isn't modern. The edition cited here was published in 1931 by Maud Grieve, president of the British Guild of Herb Growers. She was one of the leading experts in British traditional and folklore uses of herbs during and after World War I.

The Purpose of this Book

It is not my intent here to investigate every possible use of every herb, but to focus on those herbs that may be of particular use to martial artists. I look at herbs that may help with bruises, scrapes, and cuts, sprains, muscle strains, and breaks and dislocations. I look at those that help with breathing. I look at those that deal with management of "adrenaline" and other products of the fight-or-flight system such as anxiety and insomnia. And I look at a couple of minor issues that tend to plague martial artists: battered feet, skin chafed from gear, plantar warts, jock itch, athlete's foot, and for those who commonly kick or grapple after supper, flatulence.

Those familiar with Eastern herbs will see a couple of large gaps. I don't deal with herbs for conditioning of hands and feet or herbs for regulation of *qi* before or after martial injury. Why? Western medicine has no equivalent for these uses. The typical Westerner has no need to condition hands. As for *qi*, because its very existence is questioned by Western doctors, it's not likely to pop up in Western clinical trials. I omit these topics not because they are unimportant. I omit them because of a complete lack of available Western information about them.

Apart from those particular gaps, the research here is eclectic and wide-ranging. I have investigated insights from Europeans, North Americans, and Native Americans about what has worked for their people throughout the centuries. But I've also gone digging into the research: clinical trials, animal trials, and chemical analyses. I've gone looking for herbs that would impress not just the grandmother who learned herbal lore from her mother, but also the granddaughter training in modern biochemistry.

As for precautions, this book is full of them. Though I believe in boldness, I also believe there is another name for a beginner who would charge boldly into great risk for small reward. That other name is "fool." This herbal is a beginner's guide. It is written for people who don't have enough experience to give them instincts about which herb uses are safe and which are not. For that reason, I've included even the most conservative cautions postulated for each herb. Some trained herbalists will scoff at some of them. I include them anyway, so the beginners reading this book may have as long a view as possible of the herbal landscape and its potential dangers.

The goal is to give the martial artist enough information to make an informed choice about which Western herbs to experiment with. In terms of "acceptable risk," there are those herbs that nobody should use, those that only expert herbalists should use, those that only people with a high tolerance for risk should use, and those that just about anyone can use. The goal is to help you sort out which is which. On the other hand, there are herbs that scientific studies, herbalists, and medical doctors all agree work; herbs that only traditional herbalists acknowledge; and herbs that your Cousin Phil used once and now swears by. Again the goal is to help you sort out which is which. If you can come away from this book with a clear preliminary risk–benefit analysis for an herb that may meet a training need, the book will have met one of its main goals.

A word about my credentials and philosophy in using herbs: First of all, I am not an herbalist; I'm a researcher. My educational background, my work experience, and my writing for the last twenty years has trained me to sift through mountains of information, to pull out the useful bits, and to present them in a way that's clear and immediately useful. That's what I've tried to do here. This book rests not on my own personal ability to prescribe or use herbs, but on my ability to seek out the best of the best among those people who do. That's why the book is heavily endnoted, so you can follow the trail of my research, dig deeper if you'd like, and draw your own conclusions. Most of all, I'm not telling you what you should use; I'm telling you what I have discovered about these herbs. If you chose to use any of the herbs presented in this book, it is your responsibility to go beyond my research until you yourself are convinced of the safety and efficacy of the herb you are using. It's for that purpose that I have documented my sources and offered resources for further investigation. Any time you take a drug, supplement, or botanical, you must remember this: it is your body, your choice, your responsibility to bear the consequences. I wish you wise choices.

Throughout the book I use my own grading scale from zero, and one to five. One is "somebody, somewhere thought the herb might be useful." Five is "pretty much everybody, traditionalists and Western scientists alike, thinks it's useful." Here are the criteria I used:

◆◆◆◆◆ Universally recognized by both conventional medicine and alternative medicine as being a safe, reliable remedy. Large–scale clinical tests say this herb works. This level is the "holy grail" of herbal medicine. Few if any herbs or dietary supplements gain this kind of recognition. No remedy is a sure thing, of course, but this one has far fewer documented risks and far more documented success than the vast majority.

◇◆◆◆◆ Recognized by several scientific studies as well as by ample tradition as being a reliable remedy. This herb is well on its way toward gaining the recognition of both conventional and alternative medicine. We are also beginning to get a firm handle on the associated risks. Only a small handful of herbs have gained this level of recognition. No remedy is a sure thing, of course, but this one has more documented success than most.

Research combined with traditional evidence is promising, but more results are required to draw definitive conclusions. Some studies show that the herb might be an effective remedy. Either these studies are solely on animals, are unduplicated, or are not up to the highest standards of research; or they test not the herb but only one active ingredient of the herb. Generally, research into the herb's safety is similarly sketchy. A worthy experiment, but with some risks.

We have confirmation by more than one source of this herb's usefulness. Perhaps scientific research is unavailable, but anecdotal evidence is good. This herb has been used to treat this particular condition either throughout centuries or by at least two independent cultures. Or scientific research is preliminary, substandard, or contradictory but it agrees with some minimal anecdotal evidence. The herb might be worth an experiment, but with unknown risks.

Minimal evidence. Some anecdotal or hearsay evidence says the herb might be useful in treating this condition. We have, however, no clear pattern to usage between cultures or throughout time. If you experiment with this herb, there are no guarantees regarding efficacy, risk, or safety. Proceed with caution and a bit of skepticism.

Multiple tests indicate either that the herb does not work for this condition, or tests indicate that the herb does more harm than good for this use. Don't use this herb at all for this use without the guidance of a trained naturopath, herbalist, or savvy physician.

Chapter One

Using Herbs Safely

Why Herbs?

Why herbs? Walk the aisles of any drugstore or supermarket, and you'll see hundreds of "over-the-counter" remedies. Why not use them? And beyond that, why not rely on just what the doctor gives you? In 2006, Americans walked right past standard remedies to spend $22.3 billion on herbal supplements. They would not be spending that kind of money if they didn't see some kind of attraction. What draws people to herb use?

Gentleness

One reason people turn to herbal remedies is gentleness. Herbs are typically less refined, less distilled than standard remedies.

For example, Mormon tea contains pseudoephedrine, the same active ingredient as the over-the-counter cold remedy Sudafed®. The actions of Mormon tea aren't as harsh, however, because the plant contains less of the active ingredient than Sudafed, the plant's pseudoephedrine is buffered by other ingredients, and it hasn't been distilled to magnify the effect. Furthermore, with Mormon tea, you get the liquids that are so crucial to a cold, and you get the warmth and the steam, which soothe irritated tissues. Moreover, you *don't* get the fillers and the red dye #40. Similarly, if you compare prescription sleep aids with herbal remedies, you'll see the difference between something that knocks you out and something that helps you sleep. Even if you don't appreciate the difference in the evening, you will in the morning when you're trying to clear the residual from your system.

In short, one of the differences between herbal care and standard Western medicine can be the difference between a nudge and a shove. Mormon tea, willow bark, thyme, eucalyptus, peppermint—all these herbs have distilled, more potent counterparts in over-the-counter medicines. Using the herbal version sometimes gives you the option of taking a gentler amount of the active ingredient.

It is not true, however, that all herbal remedies are less potent than their counterparts. Some are more potent, perhaps dangerously so. If you use Listerine®, for example, you get the disinfectant properties of thymol (an active ingredient in thyme) in a well-tested form. If you decide to "go herbal" and use the essential oil of thyme or thymol straight, you could kill yourself with it if you don't take proper precautions. Though, in general, herbs are gentler than their refined counterparts, some herbs are not at all subtle in their effects. If you're going to use herbs, especially internally, you must know the difference between the two.

Complexity

Another benefit that draws people to herbal remedies is the complexity of herbs. Most prescription and over-the-counter medicines have one or two active ingredients in some kind of carrier. By contrast, herbs usually contain a blend of several chemicals, each with active properties.

What that means is that sometimes herbs are a fortunate blend of several active ingredients working in concert. For example, arnica contains not just the anti-inflammatory compounds that it's famous for, but also chemicals that function as antiseptics and anesthetics. Some herbs—hops for example—don't have a single verifiable active ingredient, but all the ingredients together have a verifiable cumulative effect, especially when blended with other herbs. In other words, one reason to use herbs is a faith—and I choose that word deliberately—in nature's benevolent complexity. A corollary of that statement of faith is the belief that when we refine an herb into a single active ingredient, we may be refining out benefit as well as "inactive" ingredients.

Is such faith warranted? Partially. To be honest, though, herbs' complexity can be either the good news or the bad news. The bad news is that you may be getting problematic ingredients with helpful ones. For example, borage oil contains a powerful anti-inflammatory, but it also contains the liver toxin pyrrolizidine. Licorice is an outstanding remedy for coughs, but it also contains glycyrrhizin, which messes up the electrolyte balance of the body. The bottom line is that some herbs have a beneficial complexity; some have hidden harmful ingredients. Only careful investigation will tell you which is which.

Novel Effects

Another reason people use herbs is to gain effects not available in standard Western medicines. If you go to your doctor and ask for something to help keep you from getting a cold this winter, chances are the doctor won't be able to help you. The herbal shop down the street, however, has echinacea, andrographis, elderberry, astragalus, and all manner of other exotic sounding herbs, each claiming to offer help in warding off a cold. Similarly, if you go into the doctor with a bruise from heavy training, the doctor will probably tell you to ice it and hope for the best. Go to the local herb shop, and the proprietor may give you arnica, bromelain, perhaps some comfrey.

For most people, money, time, or just a fear of doctors has created a line between significant ailments and ordinary ones. If annoyance with a physical problem exceeds a certain level, they'll go into the doctor. Below that threshold, however, is where they turn to herbs. Frankly, this realm of "ordinary ailments" is where herbs excel. They can help clear up minor annoyances, they can help foster health and well-being, and they can make you feel better while you're healing. An herb may not "cure" a cold, but neither will a visit to the doctor. Furthermore, a nice cup of chamomile tea will probably make you feel better than sitting for a couple of hours in a doctor's waiting room.

Herbs typically are gentler, have fewer side effects, treat not just major physical malfunctions but minor day-to-day physical annoyances, and they don't require a trip to the doctor. Perhaps that's why sales of herbs have taken off in the last decade. However, with the rise in herb use has come a rise in the number of people being careless in their use of herbs, some fatally so.

Safety with Herbs

First, let me say that this section is not for the attorneys of this world; it's for you and me. It is my attempt to nudge you in the direction of healthy attitudes toward herb use. In my research, over and over again, I've run across an appallingly cavalier attitude toward herbs. Many people put herbs in their mouths and on their skin without a single thought to their side effects or their interactions with other herbs, prescription drugs, and over-the-counter remedies. They don't bother to look into an herb's background or track record, but rather take the herb in response to the latest news report, or worse yet, magazine ad. What I offer to you here is a reality check, something to think about before you begin experimenting with the herbs in this book.

Principle Number One:

Just because it's natural doesn't mean you can be as stupid as you want with it. Some herbs are poisonous. Even those that aren't can make you quite miserable if you use them badly. A few years ago, kava was the flavor of the month. Health food magazines, television health reporters, and of course vitamin and herb stores were touting it as a near-magical stress-buster. People started taking it by the handful. Then the reports of liver failure started floating in. The numbers weren't huge, but a few otherwise healthy people damaged their liver to the point of needing a liver transplant. The FDA jumped in and issued an advisory. Herbalists replied, citing all the people using kava who don't need liver transplants. The debate continues to rage. Google "kava, liver," and you'll get an overview of the arguments, both rational and irrational. Yet one fact is not really in dispute: you can be stupid with kava. You can be stupid with any herb.

The point is this: You wouldn't pull bottles from a pharmacist's shelves and try two of these, four of those and a small handful of that. Yet you'd be surprised at how many people do something very similar with herbs. Herbs work in the body using the same mechanisms of action as drugs do. They interact like drugs do. They have safe and unsafe doses like drugs do. And they can do you a world of hurt if misused, just like drugs do. "Natural" does not mean "harmless." If you don't know where the line is between "safe" and "stupid" for any given herb, don't use it.

Principle Number Two:

Just because it looks like the herb in question doesn't mean it is the herb in question. Plants are trickier than you might think to identify in the wild. For example, comfrey and foxglove—the plants themselves as they grow in the wild—look quite alike. Moreover, the range for comfrey and the range for foxglove overlap considerably; the two can grow side-by-side. What would happen then if you decide to harvest your own comfrey and end up with foxglove by accident? Brew some comfrey tea, and it will probably clear your sinuses. Brew some foxglove tea, and it could very easily stop your heart.

Each species of herb has enough variety that only a fool tries to make an identification based on pictures in a book. If you don't have the benefit of training with a reputable herbalist, don't go collecting in the wild.

Similarly, if you want to try growing your own herbs, the wisest course is to get some training from an experienced herbalist. You want to be sure you know which of the plants you planted is the herb and which is a weed. You'll need help sorting through nurseries and seed companies, to learn which have good seeds and cuttings and which don't. Besides, without the right care and harvesting, herbs can lose potency and effectiveness. In short, if you want to start your herb use with the seed or the plant, get some hands-on training.

Principle Number Three:

Not all herb companies are reputable: Let the buyer beware. So you've decided not to go harvesting in the woods on your own and are now standing in your local herb shop surrounded by hundreds of bottles and dozens of different brands. How do you know what you're looking for?

Even herbs purchased in health food stores can be problematic. Packages of herbs from the Far East, South America, and Eastern Europe usually contain the herb stated on the label. Sometimes, though, they contain something completely different. Stories of mislabeled herbs can even be found in the U.S. and Europe, where labeling laws are stricter. The unfortunate fact is this: Though mislabeling is uncommon, all it takes is one mislabeled bottle to spoil your day completely.

Even if the packaging company has harvested the right herb and packaged it in a bottle with the right label, the herb still may not be healthy or effective. Offering herbs for sale involves far more than picking leaves and stuffing them into bottles. Potency can decline quickly with poor growing practices or sloppy handling. Label information varies widely from product to product. The "recommended daily dose" can be a very arbitrary thing (or not mentioned at all) on some of the poorer quality brands. Some herbs have been found to be contaminated with metals, prescription drugs, microorganisms, and other unhealthy ingredients.

How do you know you are getting good quality herbs? Here are a few general principles: First, countries with low levels of regulation tend to turn out the least consistent quality. The Far East, South America, and Eastern Europe are typically less reliable because of lax regulation. The U.S. has truth in labeling laws—the herb in the bottle must legally be the herb named on the label—but it has very little regulation of herb quality. Potency, therefore, is an iffy thing for some U.S. companies. Some U.S. companies turn out great herbs, some very poor herbs. It takes a bit of sleuthing to figure out which is which. European countries, most notably German and the U.K., will, in general, have tighter regulations than North and South American countries. Consequently, in general, the quality of their herbs tends to be higher.

Other indications of quality include in-house testing. A reputable company should do batch checks, and they should have strict quality control policies. If you're looking for reputable companies, check out their Web site. Those who do in-house testing tend to feature it prominently on their site.

You can also look for quality assurance seals from independent third-party certification programs on the label. One such seal is the NSF International seal. The NSF (formerly the National Sanitation Foundation) inspects both the herb itself and the manufacturing process. Those products that pass inspection are allowed to bear the NSF seal. What the seal means is that not only is the herb inside the bottle the herb on the label, but no additional herbs are present that aren't on the label. The NSF seal says nothing about potency, however, just purity of product and accuracy of labeling.

American Herbal Products Association (AHPA) members agree to abide by a code of ethics. That code includes ethical business practices, protection of endangered species of herbs, truth in labeling, disclosure of added constituents, and warnings about safety issues involved in herb use. The association relies on members to regulate themselves, but members who are found to be out of compliance can be expelled from the association.

The USP seal says a little more than that of the NSF or AHPA. "USP" stands for "United States Pharmacopeia." USP is an independent, self-sustaining, nonprofit, science-based public health organization. The USP seal on a bottle of herbs says that the label on the bottle actually contains what it claims on the label. It also says that the product doesn't contain harmful levels of specified contaminants, that the binders or capsules containing the herb will break down and release in the body, and that the company making the herbs uses good manufacturing processes. In other words, if a bottle of herbs bears the USP seal, that means that the herb is pure, uncontaminated, and potent. The seal also says that the shelf life dates are reliable and that the suggested doses on the label are reasonable. The tests and standards used by USP are recognized by the FDA. In other words, the USP seal is probably your best indication of quality in American-made herbal supplements.

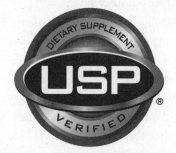

The United States Pharmacopeia seal
(Used with the permission of the United States Pharmacopeia)

Let's say that you are back in the herb shop and faced again with a choice of which herb to buy. None of the bottles carry third-party seals. You don't know anything about the brand names. How can you minimize your risks? According to one study, price seems to be a fairly reliable mark of quality.[2] If one brand is significantly cheaper than the others, be suspicious. On the other hand, if an herb is standardized to one of its active ingredients, that's a good sign. Check where the herbs were grown or harvested. If they were imported from a country with poor regulation—China, an Eastern European country, a South American country—be cautious. German, Swedish, Finnish, or British manufacturing companies tend to be more reliable. In fact, since the advent of the European Union, the quality of all European herbs is becoming more consistently regulated and consequently better. (What this tight regulation means for the availability of herbs and herbal advice is another, more complex and hotly debated issue, but regulation has made the quality of the herbs sold more reliable.)

If you plan to use herbs regularly, find a brand or a distributor who offers consistent quality and buy each time from them. What you don't want to do is to buy from hotdog_joe73 or zhangsherbs on eBay or some random Web site. Hot Dog Joe or Zhang may sell great herbs, but you have no way of telling. The material in the capsule may be the best herb you've ever used or it may be wallpaper paste.

Principle Number Four:

Never look solely at the common name for an herb. Always check the scientific name for an herb. Not only does one plant often look like another, the names of plants can be similar as well. For example, gotu kola (Centella asiatica) is not the same as kola (Cola acuminata). Gotu kola has adaptogenic and wound healing properties. Kola (kola nut or "cola") is the stimulant found in colas. "Gardenia" in the United States is a pleasant ornamental (but not medicinal) flower, composed of several species in the Gardenia genus. In China, "gardenia" refers to Fructus Gardeniae, a medicinal herb.

Quite aside from the obvious possibilities for confusion between common names is the issue of which species are most potent. For example, some species of echinacea work better than others. Do the contents of your bottle of echinacea contain one of the better species or one of the cheaper, less effective species? The only way to know is to check the scientific name.

Principle Number Five:

Homeopathy is not herbalism. Creams and other products made using homeopathic methods will often have the same name as herbal creams. The two, however, are not interchangeable. For example, homeopathy uses arnica just as herbalism does. In fact, in the U.S. most arnica cream offered for sale in herb shops is homeopathic arnica, not an herbal preparation. The two are made using very different processes. Homeopathy leaves very little of the herb in question in the final product. It also uses the resulting preparation differently. Look for either the abbreviation HPUS, or a number followed by X, e.g. 10X. That means it's a homeopathic formula, not an herbal one. It also means that this book says nothing about that particular formula, its use, or its potential effectiveness.

Principle Number Six:

If you diagnose yourself, you have only yourself to blame if you're wrong. Just because you think you know what you're treating doesn't mean you're right. Diagnosing yourself and treating yourself with herbs can delay a much-needed trip to the doctor.

That being said, we all do it. We all look at life's injuries and ailments and say, "Nah, I don't have to go in to the doctor. It's just a ___." Be aware, though, that treating symptoms can mask a larger, more serious underlying condition. Taking responsibility for your health means not just learning which herb to use when, but also when to put away the herbs and seek professional help.

Principle Number Seven:

An herb is more than just its component compounds. Just because the plant has been found to contain a compound that is helpful to you doesn't mean the whole plant will be helpful. The great advantage, and the great problem, with herbs is their complexity. On the one hand, you have all kinds of chemicals and compounds working together to achieve effects that no single compound could achieve. On the other hand, just because a single helpful compound can be isolated in the lab, that doesn't mean the herb taken in its entirety will behave like that single compound. An herb containing a known anti-inflammatory won't necessarily behave like an anti-inflammatory if other compounds buffer that action.

What does that mean in practice? It means you should be cautious about taking an herb just because you know it contains something useful. Laboratory analysis of the active ingredients of an herb can give us some idea of its healing potential, but it is no substitute for long-term, human clinical trials. How do you know an herb is safe, reliable, and effective? You know that only if it's been used on large numbers of people, studied and found to be so. Frankly, we aren't there with most herbal supplements. Large-scale clinical trials cost money—pharmaceutical-company amounts of money, not small-scale-herb-grower amounts of money. In many cases we have to supplement clinical testing with traditional and anecdotal reports of an herb's effectiveness. Sure, when researchers find a known active ingredient in an herb, that's hopeful news. But with medicinal herbs especially, the part is not the whole.

Principle Number Eight:

When you take an herb, you aren't treating just your condition but your whole body. Just because an herb is a common treatment for what ails you, that doesn't mean it's good for your overall health situation. For example, cayenne pepper can help you decongest if you have a cold, but in doing so it can also aggravate a case of high blood pressure. Herbs that work well for adults might be too strong for the young and the old. Look at herbal tests, and you'll see very few tests on children and seniors. We really don't know if herbs affect them differently or not. Many herbs are ill-advised for pregnant or nursing women. If you are taking prescription medicines, herbs might decrease their effectiveness or interact with them in a way that's dangerous. Even the caffeine in your morning coffee can interact with some herbs.

What does that mean? If you are taking medication, if you have a preexisting health problem, or if you are pregnant or trying to become pregnant, the herbal landscape changes for you. You need to talk to an herbalist, naturopath, or informed doctor or pharmacist before using herbs. If you are not fully grown or if you are over 65, you may need to adjust the dosage of herbs you take. Some herbs may be just too strong for you. In other words, experimenting with herbs demands prudence of healthy, young adults. If for some reason you don't fit into that category, it demands even more prudence of you.

Principle Number Nine:

Just because it's safe as a food doesn't mean it's safe in medicinal doses. Have you ever eaten cayenne pepper, peppermint, or licorice? They're safe, just food, right? Well, yes and no. When you used cayenne, you probably didn't steep it in alcohol first. When you used peppermint, you probably used a well-diluted extract made for cooking, not the highly concentrated essential oil. And the licorice? Well, the "licorice" you had may not have contained any actual licorice at all.

Culinary herbs are prepared to bring out the flavor. Medicinal herbs are prepared to bring out the active ingredients. They are much more potent. Even if you're using them in a way that's not more potent than you would for cooking (in other words, dried, not made into tinctures or essential oils), you're probably still taking them in larger quantities. You may be taking them in capsules, which shields your mouth from any irritating properties but not your stomach. You're probably taking them over a longer period of time. In short, medicinal doses have effects that culinary uses don't.

And, by the way, did you know that cayenne, peppermint, and licorice can all put you in an emergency room if you use them irresponsibly?

Good Herbal Habits

Are you still reading, still thinking about trying herbs? Have you decided you're willing to take responsibility for your own herb use? Then let's look at how to build some good herbal habits, habits that will help keep you safe.

Begin with Professional Help If You Can

If you can find a good herbalist, Eastern or Western, begin with one. He or she can save you a lot of trial and error. Once you get past the "chamomile tea stage" of herb use, you're looking at real medicine, and you can't learn the subtleties of real medicine by reading a book or two. If you plan on going beyond the most superficial stages of herb use, you need to find a guide to help you.

Question Everyone

It seems that herb information is everywhere—news programs, grocery store flyers, the Internet. Be aware of people's motives in telling you that a botanical supplement is good for you. Health food stores want to sell you something. Magazines and news programs want to sell ad space and air time. The traditional medicinal establishment—doctors, hospitals, drug companies—want you to stick with a system that's comfortable for them, one that they have expertise in (and one that makes them money as well). Herbalists and alternative medicine practitioners also have a bias toward what they know as well. Knowing who your information source is is critical.

Internet sites, especially those trying to sell you something, are notorious for their omissions. For example a study of herbs with toxic effects found that only three percent of the sites surveyed mentioned the toxic effects of borage oil, a drug banned in Germany because of its risks.[3] If you are getting the bulk of your herbal information from online herb stores, you have a problem.

Similarly, avoid headline chasing. You've probably seen them, the stories on the evening news about St. John's wort, echinacea, and other popular herbs. They hit big, everyone talks about them, and then they disappear. The media's herbal "flavor of the month" is often a story based on a single study. That single study is then "spun" to sell papers or air time. Once the herb hits the public and garners interests, other media outlets will jump in to capitalize on that interest. In other words, you'll learn more about an herb's *popularity* from the media than you will about its safety or efficacy. You need to make sure that if you decide an herb is safe enough to try, you do so because of a body of data, not because of the latest media blitz.

Where do you get good herbal information? Government sites tend to be good, very conservative usually, but good. Germany's Commission E monographs contain a nice blend of science and tradition. The Dietary Supplement Information Board has information about dosage and interactions. The *PDR for Herbal Medicine* does as well. Check Chapter 6, "Further Resources," in this book for more ideas about where to look.

Know Where Your Information Comes From

In addition to knowing who's telling you to use a particular herb, try to trace herb information back to the original research. Frankly, when it comes to herbs, information is patchy. Some herbs have been well researched. Others have not undergone clinical trials at all. Some herbs have a strong consensus of use from culture to culture, past to present. Others have been used for everything under the sun. The only thing that's certain is that if you are trying to get a picture of an herb's efficacy, you'll find a huge spectrum of evidence: in vitro research results, clinical studies, traditional herbalism, folk uses. You'll often need to make a decision based not on well-designed large clinical trials but on whatever you can get your hands on.

On the one end of the spectrum is the Western medical community. In the United States, the FDA has the final word about herbs and what claims an herb can and can't make. Herbs are classified as dietary supplements not herbal medicines. If an herb manufacturing company wants to be able to make medical claims, they will be held to the same standards as prescription drug manufacturers. In other words, they must prove that a discrete component in the herb treats a discrete health problem both in laboratory and clinical trials. The FDA doesn't care about history, tradition, or anecdotal evidence when it decides what claims herb companies can make about an herb. The FDA wants chemical analysis and large-scale trials. If herbs cannot pass the FDA gatekeepers, those herbs are not considered to be medicine, and they may not make any specific health claims.

Somewhere in the middle of the spectrum is Commission E. Commission E, Germany's official government collection and analysis of herbal research, is much more likely to listen to traditional use than the FDA. That's not to say they ignore research and trials. In fact, Germany is known for its herbal research. But if an herb has a strong tradition and is unlikely to hurt you when used properly, Commission E will recommend it. The translated findings of the commission are available but expensive. A more affordable summary is available in Steven B. Karch's *The Consumer's Guide to Herbal Medicine.*

On the other end of the spectrum are the traditional herbalists. Throughout time herbalists of many cultures have been using herbs, experimenting with them, watching their effects and passing that knowledge down from master to apprentice. This knowledge, of course, is only as good at the observer's ability to watch with a trained, unbiased eye. It is also only as good as the method by which the knowledge is transmitted from teacher to student.

The British approach to herbs is to make this observation and transmission process rigorous. Their National Institute of Medical Herbalists has high standards for membership. British herbalists have had the protection of the crown since Henry VIII's day, so herbalism students can not only study in small private schools like they do in the U.S. but also in herbal programs in major universities. Mentoring (essentially a sophisticated master–apprentice relationship) has been taken to the extent that students can achieve postgraduate levels of education combining supervised hands-on work and classroom training.

The FDA's end of the spectrum offers proof of herbs' effectiveness in terms that someone trained in Western medical ways of thinking can understand. Unfortunately, it doesn't offer that proof very often because rigorous testing of herbs is not very common. On the other end of the spectrum is much more experience with herbs, but by American medical standards (AMA standards) it's not very rigorous. Most articles and recommendations come from one source or another. Wise herb users learn what they can from both.

Use a Safe Dose

The advantage of prescription medicine is that it comes in a bottle with very precise instructions on the label. You know that the medicine has been formulated and tested at that standardized level. Using prescription drugs is simple. Herbs don't have that benefit. Bulk herbs and some bottled herbs have no dosage information at all. Those that do, vary from brand to brand. It's up to you to seek out information about safe dosage and to follow it.

The Dietary Supplement Information Board, for example, has online information about dosage and safety for a number of herbs. Herbs that have a USP seal on the label will also contain reliable information about dosage.

Once you find that commonly accepted dose, follow it. More is *not* better for many herbs. Some are toxic at high doses, and it doesn't take much for the dose to be "high." Sometimes as little as a drop or two can mean the difference between effective and unsafe. For example, essential oils, the essence of the plant extracted commercially using steam distillation, are *very* strong. A dose that looks like nothing could be enough to do you serious damage. Always know what preparation you're taking, how strong it is, and what the maximum dose for that particular preparation is.

Even "food" herbs can be dangerous in large doses. A little cayenne in your chili spices things up, but too much taken in capsule form can damage your liver. A little cinnamon in an apple pie is a wonderful thing; too much cinnamon or cinnamon oil can cause signs of central nervous system shutdown.[4]

With prescription medicine, you expect the drug to jerk you around, to work its effects whether the body wants to go there or not. Herbal medicines, on the other hand, are not a club to beat your body into a cure. Though some work quickly, others are a quiet support for the health that your body wants. The test of whether an herb is working is not always whether you "feel something" immediately after taking it. The test is whether you are healthier in a reasonable amount of time. How long is a "reasonable amount of time"? That depends on the herb. It also brings me to my next point.

If you are going to be taking herbs, you need to know which are short-term herbs and which are long-term herbs. Some herbs, like valerian for example, seem to work better if you take them for a while. Others like ginger or peppermint work quickly and so are typically used as short-term herbs. Some herbs are addictive or lose their effectiveness if you use them too long. Others, those that are primarily antioxidants, for example, work mainly as a health support, and don't have clear "effects" per se. You need to know which category your herb falls into before taking it.

Research Widely Before Using an Herb

Never take information from just one source (even this one). Cross-check everything for accuracy. The last thing you want to discover the hard way is that the author of some book accidentally misplaced a decimal point when recording dosage. Here are the things you want to cross check before using an herb: dosage, warning signs, contraindications, and interactions.

If you are thinking about using herbs, it's probably because you have decided to take more personal responsibility for treating your own ailments. What I'm inviting you to think about here is the place that research plays in that personal responsibility. If you use herbs, you must either find a reputable herbalist, or if you want to do it yourself, you must learn what the herbalist knows about the herb you want to use.

Purchase a modern herbal or two. Then go to reputable Web sites for the most recent updates on contraindications. Books can go out of date. Just as I'd rather be treated by a doctor who studied from twenty-first century text books rather than those from the 1850s, I'd rather use herbal information from yesterday than from the 1850s. Web resources are listed in Chapter 6.

Work with your Doctor, but Always Double-check your Doctor

Bottom line: You should always double check any drug, any supplement, any botanical that you put in your mouth. People—be they doctors, authors, herbalists, or pharmacists—all make mistakes. More than 1.5 million Americans each year experience an adverse drug event: receiving the wrong medication, the wrong dose, the wrong instructions for taking the medicine, or some other preventable error. According to the Institute of Medicine (part of the United States National Academy of Sciences), in hospitals, the problem is even worse. In hospitals, if you factor in prescribing, filling prescriptions, administering and monitoring, the error rate rises to an average of one medication error per patient per day.[5] These are statistics for prescription medicines dispensed by a system with sophisticated checks in place. Now add a self-administered herb or two into the mix, and you see why you need to take responsibility for knowing about doses and interactions.

For everything you take, you should know what it is, why you're taking it, and have a rough idea of how it works. This is true for prescription drugs, over-the-counter drugs, and botanicals. If you don't know, ask someone who does.

Check herb–medication interactions for yourself as well. (See Chapter 6, "Further Resources" for places you can check dosage and interaction of herbs.) Again if you see a problem or just have a question, talk with someone who has more training.

Always talk to your doctor and pharmacist about what you're taking. It's nice to have a doctor who is savvy about botanicals. Though most aren't familiar with botanicals and their effects, an increasing number are reconciling themselves to the fact that some patients insist on using them. Even if your doctor is a skeptic and cracks jokes about you're acting like you have a doctorate in "oregano," you still need to let him know what you are taking.

Keep a list of everything you're taking—herbal, prescription, and over-the-counter—and bring it with you to the doctor when you go. Show the list to your pharmacist as well if the doctor prescribes any prescription drugs. Recheck everything with your doctor and pharmacist every time you begin taking a new medication. If you need surgery, speak up if you are taking any botanicals. Some can cause increased bleeding and changes in heart rate and blood pressure. Your doctor has resources and can check interactions even if he was never trained in herbs in medical school.

Pay Attention

Herbs require that you be aware of what's happening in your body. It's like people and their cars. Some know every sound, every vibration, every nuance in the steering wheel and gearshift. Others are completely oblivious. They drive day in and day out without a care or a clue until a dashboard light goes on. Even then their first thought is, "How long has that been on? I wonder if I can drive this until the weekend and get it taken care of then."

If you are careless and clueless about your body, herbs aren't for you. You probably won't recognize the signs of when it's time to stop taking them. And you may not notice their effects, which can be subtle and occur over the span of weeks or months.

Even if you are well in touch with your body and its normal state of health, you still need to pay attention. Keep track of what you're taking and any reactions you have to it. Keep a record of all the supplements you take—what they are, how much you take, how often, why. Keeping a record of what did and didn't work can help you next time you want to use the supplement. If you have a bad reaction, write it down. Make sure your family (or whoever has your durable power of attorney for health care) also has a copy of the list. If you get hit by a bus, the emergency room personnel would like to know if you are taking something that affects heart rate, blood pressure, or clotting time.

Reevaluate Periodically

If your health changes, you need to reevaluate the botanicals you take. If you become pregnant or are nursing, you need to talk with your doctor before taking any herbs. Many of the entries in the herbal section of this book say "don't use this herb if you are pregnant or nursing." Frankly, we don't know the effects of most of these herbs on a fetus or a small baby. Until more information becomes available, it's probably prudent to avoid taking herbs unless specifically told to do so by your doctor. If you are beginning to feel the effects of age, or develop long-term health issues, check with your doctor. All of these factors can influence the way your body uses herbs.

Lock Everything up

If you have young children, lock up your herbs just as you would drain cleaner and paint thinner. Some essential oils and herbs can kill outright. Others can make a child much sicker than an adult taking the same amount. You might consider doing the same thing if you have pets. I once had a cat who dove head first into a wastebasket to retrieve a broken valerian capsule. Not eager to do my own personal animal testing, I took it from her, but not before she'd hauled it halfway across the bathroom floor in her mouth.

Label Everything

If you make your own preparations, label everything. Never reuse a container unless you completely remove or cover prior labels. If you carry herbs in a separate container (to the gym or dojo), label that container. If it doesn't have a label, throw it out. You don't want to guess wrong.

Get Help If You Want to Mix Herbs

Some herbs interact; some even interact in ways we are not yet aware of. A common—though not always smart—way of combining herbs is to mix several that have the properties you are looking for. In other words, you may mix up a remedy that has one herb for swelling, another for pain, another for tissue repair, another to help you sleep. The end result *might* have all those properties. Or it might be mud, with one herb's effects canceling out another's. Or it might be considerably stronger than you anticipate, with one herb's effects compounding another's. The wrong combinations can be like a junior chemistry set experiment gone bad.

In other words, mixing herbs is an advanced skill. Stick to either trusted recipes or find a good herbalist if you want to branch into combinations. Commission E also has lists of herbs that can be combined safely.

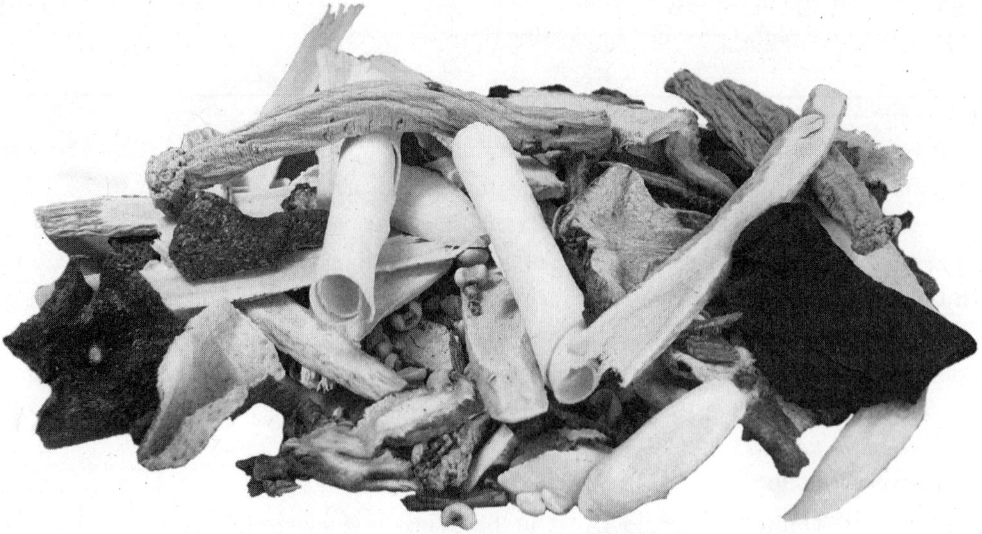

A Chinese formula containing multiple interacting herbs

For those of you used to Chinese medicine, you might be surprised at how many herbs in this book are used as simples, in other words, one herb alone, not in combination with others. Traditional Chinese medicine has an elaborate system for combining herbs. Frankly, it's much more sophisticated than any herb combining in the West. They combine herbs to compound the effect, to buffer undesirable qualities, and to treat a complex of symptoms and imbalances in the patient. Through centuries of use, they have charted not just the action of herbs but the interactions between herbs. The combinations they have arrived at are not just a cure for symptoms; they are a treatment of the patient, who has not just an injury, but also a body with various balances and imbalances. If you don't understand the basis for a particular combination, you won't know if that basis applies to a particular person and his injury.

Let me say it again: combining herbs is an advanced skill. If you aren't a trained herbalist, get help.

Start Slowly

Take a small amount, well under the therapeutic dose to start. If you buy unstandardized herbs, do this each time you get a new bottle. The potency of herbs varies tremendously. Always have someone else in the house when you're trying an herb for the first time just in case you have a bad reaction.

Find your own Personal Risk Tolerance

Experimenting with herbs entails some risk. There is no way to eliminate that risk, but you can reduce it. How much you reduce it depends on your own personal tolerance for risk. To get a rough idea of how much risk you are willing to accept, ask yourself these questions:

How much do I trust what I read in books? If you have a low tolerance for this kind of risk, the best idea is to run everything past an herbalist or naturopath. Have them supervise you the first time you try an herb. If you have a moderate tolerance for this kind of risk, try to get corroboration for what you read from another source.

How much do I want to risk interactions between herbs? If you have a low tolerance for this kind of risk, use only simples (single herbs) to reduce the chance of interaction. If you have a moderate tolerance, check the Commission E monographs for information about which herbs combine safely. For an extra margin of safety, you can run any combination in any book past someone with a sound training in combining herbs. Even if you have a high tolerance for risk, at least find some corroboration for your combinations in books or existing products before using them.

How much am I willing to risk illness from taking the wrong herb, the wrong dose, or wrong combination of herbs internally? If you have a low tolerance for this kind of risk, limit your use to topical use only. Some herbs can still hurt or even kill you when applied topically. But simply not putting an herb in your mouth lowers its chances of harming you. If you have a moderate level of tolerance for this kind of risk, check the herb and the dose in at least two sources, check to see if you are allergic to related plants, and then start with a lower dose the first time you try it. Even if you have a high tolerance for this kind of risk, you should use only herbs obtained from trusted sources for internal use.

How much am I willing to risk infection? If you can't guarantee its sterility, don't use a topical preparation on an open wound. The use of homemade ointment on open wounds has a long history. That history also includes things like loss of limbs and life to infection. If you have a low tolerance for the risk of infection, don't use any herbal remedy on an open wound. If you have a moderate tolerance, you might consider only using commercial herbal preparations on open wounds. Reputable companies probably have a better knowledge of and facility for sterile procedures than you do. Even if you have a high tolerance for this kind of risk, you should watch any wounds you treat with herbal preparations for signs of infection and get help immediately if you see anything amiss.

How much do I trust my ability to handle the most potent herbal preparations? If you don't completely trust yourself to handle the more dangerous preparations, avoid essential oils entirely or at least avoid the ones that are potentially fatal. The good news about essential oils is that they are very concentrated and powerful. The bad news is that they are very concentrated and powerful. One way to skirt the dangers of essential oils is to use them only with professional supervision, and limiting your personal experimentation to whole herbs and the preparations you make from them. In fact, the most conservative course of action is to limit yourself to only those herbs that have a history of use as food (chamomile tea, for example). If you have a higher tolerance for this kind of risk, you should at least use your strictest safe handling procedures when using essential oils. Be careful of unintended residues on utensils. Label everything that contains essential oils. Treat them with extreme respect.

Herbs have tremendous benefits for people seeking more involvement in their own health and well-being. They are not magic bullets, but they have advantages you won't find in other forms of health care. Using them, however, is a skill like any other. It takes time, effort, and care to master.

Chapter Two

The Herbal

Agrimony

Scientific name: *Agrimonia eupatoria*

Also known as church steeples, cocklebur, sticklewort, philanthropos, stickwort, liverwort, common agrimony

Agrimony is a perennial plant; some might say "weed." Various species of *Agrimonia* grow throughout the northern hemisphere, including North America, England, Scotland, and China. *Agrimonia eupatoria* is native to Europe. It grows in sunny fields and waste areas, and in hedgerows and stone walls. The aboveground parts are used medicinally. The roots are typically not.

The Greeks used it. So did the Anglo–Saxons. In the fifteenth century, it was one of the ingredients in "eau de arquebusade," which was a remedy for treating gunshot wounds on the battlefield. The Meskwaki Indians used the root of the plant of the same genus (*Agrimonia gryposepala*) as a styptic for nosebleeds.[6] Another relative of agrimony, *xian he cao* (*Agrimonia pilosa*), has been used in China as a remedy for bleeding and wounds.

Agrimony became popular as a medicinal plant for two reasons. The first is the tannins. Tannins are astringent, meaning they tighten or constrict skin. Agrimony also contains silica. Not until the late twentieth century did pharmaceutical companies began using fine silica on wound and burn dressings to heal these wounds more quickly. The silica in agrimony, however, has been used to treat wounds for centuries.

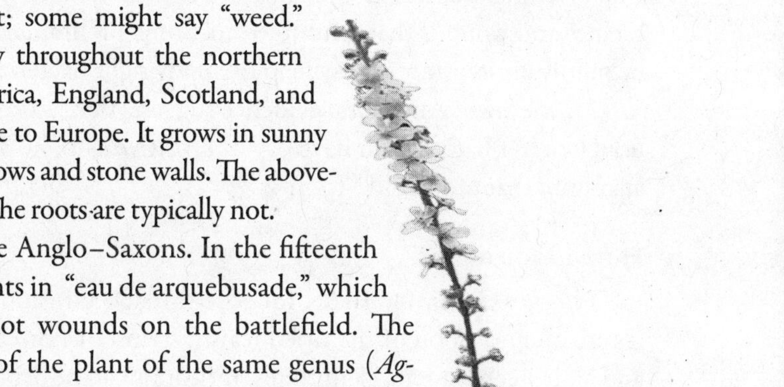

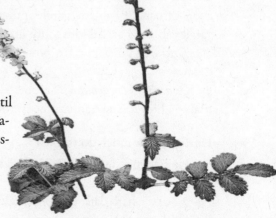

Agrimony, *Agrimonia eupatoria*

(Courtesy of Joan Simon)

What is it good for?

Much of what we know about agrimony is anecdotal. The number of studies conducted regarding its safety and efficacy can be counted on one hand. It does contain catechin tannins, an astringent. Commission E recommends it for several uses, both topical and internal. If you're looking for scientific research to tell you agrimony is safe and effective, however, you're going to have to wait because it's just not there right now. Traditional use, however, recommends it for the following:

Sore throats. We have a sound oral tradition through several cultures that says agrimony is good for sore throats and laryngitis. Used as a gargle, it can help take down swelling and relieve pain.[7] It also contains flavonoids and Vitamin C. Commission E recommends it for oral and pharyngeal inflammation.

Skin Injury or inflammation. Commission E recommends it for topical use. It can aid in the healing of wounds and bruises, and because of its astringent properties, it may help stop bleeding. Because of the silica and tannins in agrimony, it can be particularly useful for scrapes and wounds that tend to weep. Some preliminary research suggests that it may also be mildly antiseptic and may help the body fight bacteria, viruses, and fungi.[8]

Muscle aches. Anecdotal evidence suggests that agrimony is good for muscle aches when used in a hot bath. If you have dry or sensitive skin, however, the tannins in agrimony may aggravate that problem.

How do you use it?

Infusion (taken internally for sore throat). Infusion brings out the best in agrimony.[9] Infuse one teaspoon of the dried leaves, stems, or flowers in a cup (8 ounces) of hot water and let it steep for 5 to 15 minutes. Infusions can be drunk as tea or used as a gargle or rinse for sore throats or mouth wounds.

Decoction (for topical use and as a gargle). Prepare a very strong decoction and allow the mixture to cool. Soak a compress in it and apply it to the affected area several times a day. For a sore throat or laryngitis, gargle and spit the decoction up to three times a day. A decoction gargle can also be used for mouth injuries. Rinse and spit; don't swallow.

Tincture. Tinctures are possible but work somewhat less well than infusions and decoctions.

Ointment (for wounds). See method two for creams and salves in Chapter 3 for instructions on how to make an ointment from an infusion or decoction.

Dosage: How much do you use?

No scientific information is available about how much agrimony is safe. A traditional dosage is

3 g of the herb daily used internally

One cup of tea (1 teaspoon of the herb, brewed approximately 5–10 minutes) at a time, no more than three times per day

¼–½ teaspoon of the tincture, three times per day.

What should you be aware of before using it?

We don't know much about the potential risks of agrimony. It hasn't been studied much at all.

These are the precautions we do know about (or at least suspect):

If you can't insure the purity of your ingredients and the sterility of your procedures, don't use a homemade ointment on an open wound.

Agrimony is high in tannins. No high-tannin herb should be taken internally over the long term (more than a few months).[10]

Don't take it internally if you are also taking butterbur.

Don't take it internally it if you are constipated. Don't use large doses internally because they can lead to constipation.

Agrimony taken internally can affect blood sugar levels. If you are diabetic, check with your doctor before taking agrimony internally. Be cautious when using it in conjunction with herbs known or suspected to affect blood sugar levels. (See Chapter 5 for a list.)

If you are taking a diuretic (including some blood pressure medicines) check with your doctor before taking agrimony internally.

If you are prone to high blood pressure, check with your doctor before taking agrimony internally, as agrimony can raise blood pressure, especially if you take it in high doses.[11]

Be careful about sun exposure after using agrimony internally. Sun sensitivity reactions have been reported.[12]

No scientific information is available about how well agrimony is tolerated topically.

Note that though agrimony is sometimes known as "cocklebur," it is not the common cocklebur found throughout North America.

Also, be aware that the Chinese agrimony, *xian he cao* (*Agrimonia pilosa*), and *Agrimonia eupatoria* have different properties and are *not* interchangeable.

Aloe Vera

Scientific name: *Aloe vera, Aloe vulgaris,* or *Aloe barbadensis*

Also known as Barbados or Curaçao aloes

The *Aloe* genus contains at least 324 species of herbs, shrubs, and trees.[13] The most commonly used medicinal aloe is *Aloe vera*, and it is the one we'll be referring to here. *Aloe vera* is a succulent, meaning that it is a plant that stores water in fleshy leaves or stems. It grows wild in Africa and Madagascar, but because of its medicinal and decorative properties, it is now a common houseplant throughout the world. It also grows perennially outdoors in the frost-free parts of Florida, Texas, and Hawaii. Aloe leaves contain a clear gel that can be squeezed or scraped from the outer skin. It is this gel that is used medicinally.

For centuries, aloe gel has been used for burns and minor wounds. We have evidence of its use dating back to before the first century. Alexander the Great is rumored to have conquered Madagascar so his army would have an adequate supply of aloe to treat wounds. Cleopatra used it as part of her beauty regimen. Hippocrates and Arab physicians also used it. The Egyptians called aloe the "Plant of Immortality" though not because of its health benefits but because it can live for long periods of time bare-rooted, without soil.[14] In both Chinese and Ayurvedic medicine it is used, among other remedies, as a treatment for eczema.[15] In traditional Arab medicine, it's used for wound healing.[16]

What is it good for?

Minor burns. Aloe is best for first degree burns. It may also be used on small, minor second degree burns. This use has centuries of folk medicine behind it. In fact, the use of aloe on burns has good recognition not just in the popular culture, but also in segments of Western mainstream medicine as well. Animal studies show great advantage to using aloe on burns of all severities.[17] Clinical studies show that burns can heal in about two-thirds the time when treated with aloe.[18]

Minor wounds. Aloe can also be used on cuts, scrapes, and other minor wounds and skin irritations. The traditional evidence for using aloe to treat minor wounds is also strong. At the very least, aloe provides a protective barrier over the wound. That much is fairly universally agreed upon.[19] The gel also contains several active ingredients that have been isolated in the laboratory: pain relievers, anti-inflammatories, and ingredients that relieve itching and increase blood flow to an injured area. Some research suggests that it may also have antifungal, antibacterial, and antiviral properties.[20] Clin-

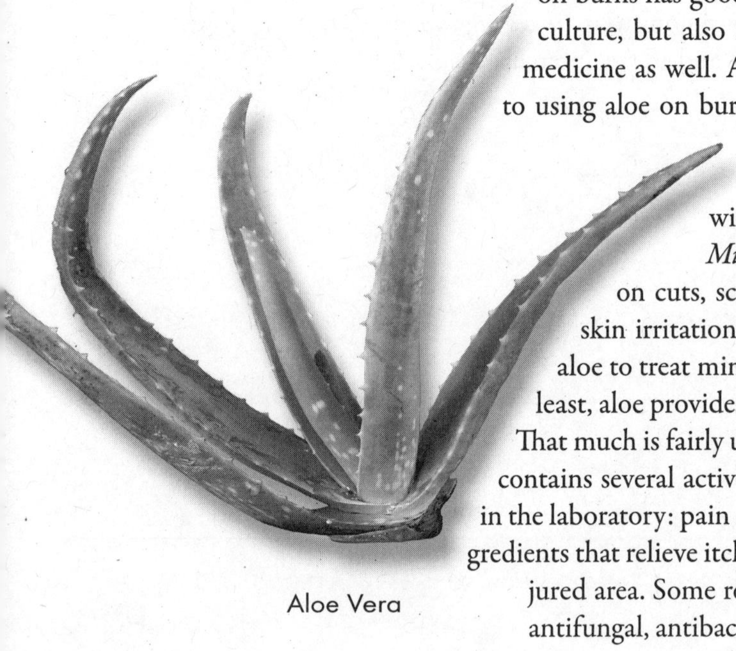

Aloe Vera

ical trials have been mostly but not completely positive.[21] In humans, aloe has been shown to speed healing from deep scrapes, canker sores, frostbite, and flash burns of the conjunctiva.[22] One study of aloe on surgical wounds, however, showed that it may actually slow wound healing time for deep or major wounds.[23] But in general the evidence for benefit in treating superficial wounds is better than for most herbal remedies.

Plantar warts. Plantar warts, warts on the soles of the feet, may respond to aloe compresses. This use is not backed by research and is mainly anecdotal, but if aloe does indeed have antiviral and immune stimulating properties, those properties may help in the elimination of plantar warts.

Major wounds. Studies using aloe for more major wounds, for example post surgical wounds, have been less impressive, showing that aloe actually slowed wound healing over a placebo.[24] Similarly, healing from dermabrasion[25] is slowed by aloe. Aloe should be used only for minor wounds.

How do you use it?

Fresh gel. Aloe is one herb that's easy to grow and is best when used fresh. If you keep an aloe plant on hand, you can remove a leaf, split it open, and either squeeze or scrape out the gel, or you can simply apply the entire split leaf directly to burns or wounds like a poultice.

Commercially processed gel. If you don't have a plant or prefer to keep gel on hand, make sure it is processed well. Improperly processed aloe can lose its medicinal effects. The International Aloe Science Council provides a seal of certification for products that have followed proper processing procedures.[26] To treat a burn, immediately cool the effected area with cool water. After the burn is thoroughly cooled, apply the aloe gel topically.

Baths. For sunburn, you can add 1–2 cups of aloe juice to a lukewarm bath.

Ointments. If you apply an aloe ointment to sunburn, make sure that ointment does not contain petroleum jelly, benzocaine, lidocaine, or butter, because these can make a sunburn worse.

Compress. For warts, apply a pea-sized amount of the gel to a compress and completely cover the wart with it. Change the compress daily.

Dosage: How much do you use?

Aloe is typically tolerated very well when used externally. If you use commercially prepared aloe, make sure that it's pure (98% or more aloe). When using aloe on sunburns, you may wish to use a diluted product. Make sure that the dilution is no more than 80%, with at least 20% of the product being aloe. For burns or scrapes, apply the aloe two to five times per day.

What should you be aware of before using it?

If a product says simply "aloe," it could be aloe vera, or it could be one of several other species of aloe. Evidence is coming in that some of the other species are carcinogenic (cause cancer).[27] Be aware of what kind of aloe you are using.

Topical use. Don't use aloe topically if you are allergic to onions or garlic. If you've never used aloe before, or if you're using aloe from a different plant, try a little bit on a small area. If you develop an irritation, discontinue use.

If you have any of the following symptoms after using aloe, call poison control or your doctor: throat swelling or breathing difficulty, severe burning or pain in the throat, nose, eyes, ears, lips, or tongue, severe abdominal pain or vomiting, severe skin irritation or rash.

Internal use. Don't use aloe internally without medical supervision. Though aloe vera has been used internally for centuries, sometimes by people who proclaim near-miraculous properties to it, modern research casts doubts on its safety. Aloe for internal use is not usually standardized and is sometimes mislabeled. The dose that works fine for you this time might be very different from the dose you get next time from the same product.

Aloe can be a violent purge. As a result, it can affect electrolyte levels.

It can also affect blood sugar, perhaps dangerously so if you are hypoglycemic, diabetic, or on blood sugar medication. Be cautious when using it in conjunction with herbs known or suspected to affect blood sugar levels. (See Chapter 5 for a list.)

If it is taken orally for diarrhea for more than a week, it can cause dependency. For these reasons, the FDA has banned the use of aloe in over-the-counter laxatives,[28] and it recommends that aloe not be taken internally.[29] If you should choose to ignore these recommendations, be sure you consult with a trained herbalist and learn about contraindications and interactions, for they are many.

Injected use. Never use injected aloe intravenously or intramuscularly. Four cases of death have been associated with *Aloe vera* injections.[30]

Be aware that though the African plant aloe and the North American plant agave, sometimes known as "American aloe," may look similar but they are very different in their medical uses. Also the word Aloes, in Latin *Lignum Aloes*, used in the Bible refers to a completely different plant, the *Aquilaria agallocha*.

Andrographis

Scientific name: *Andrographis paniculata*

Also known as chiretta, heart-thread lotus leaf, and *kariyat*, *kalmegh*, *maha-tita*, *chuan xin lian*, *yi jian xi*, and *lan he lian*, *chyun sam ling*, *senshinren*

Andrographis is a small annual shrub native to tropical Asia. The leaves and roots are used medicinally. It is very bitter.

Andrographis is sometimes called "Indian echinacea" for its use in supporting the immune system. It has been a part of Chinese and South Asian medicine for centuries. In Chinese medicine, andrographis is believed to dispel heat and it is used for conditions involving fever, inflammation, and the formation of pus.[31] In Indian medicine, it was credited with stopping the 1919 Indian flu epidemic. Combined with eleuthero, andrographis is now a major part of one of the most popular herb blends in Sweden (Kan Jang®). It is used there to treat colds and for immune support during the cold and flu season.

What is it good for?

Colds and flu. The active ingredient in andrographis is andrographolides, which are believed to have immune-stimulating, anti-inflammatory properties.[32] Several double-blind studies have shown the effectiveness of andrographis in reducing symptoms of the common cold.[33] Improvement is shown in fever, headache, muscle aches, throat symptoms, cough, nasal symptoms, general malaise, and eye symptoms.[34]

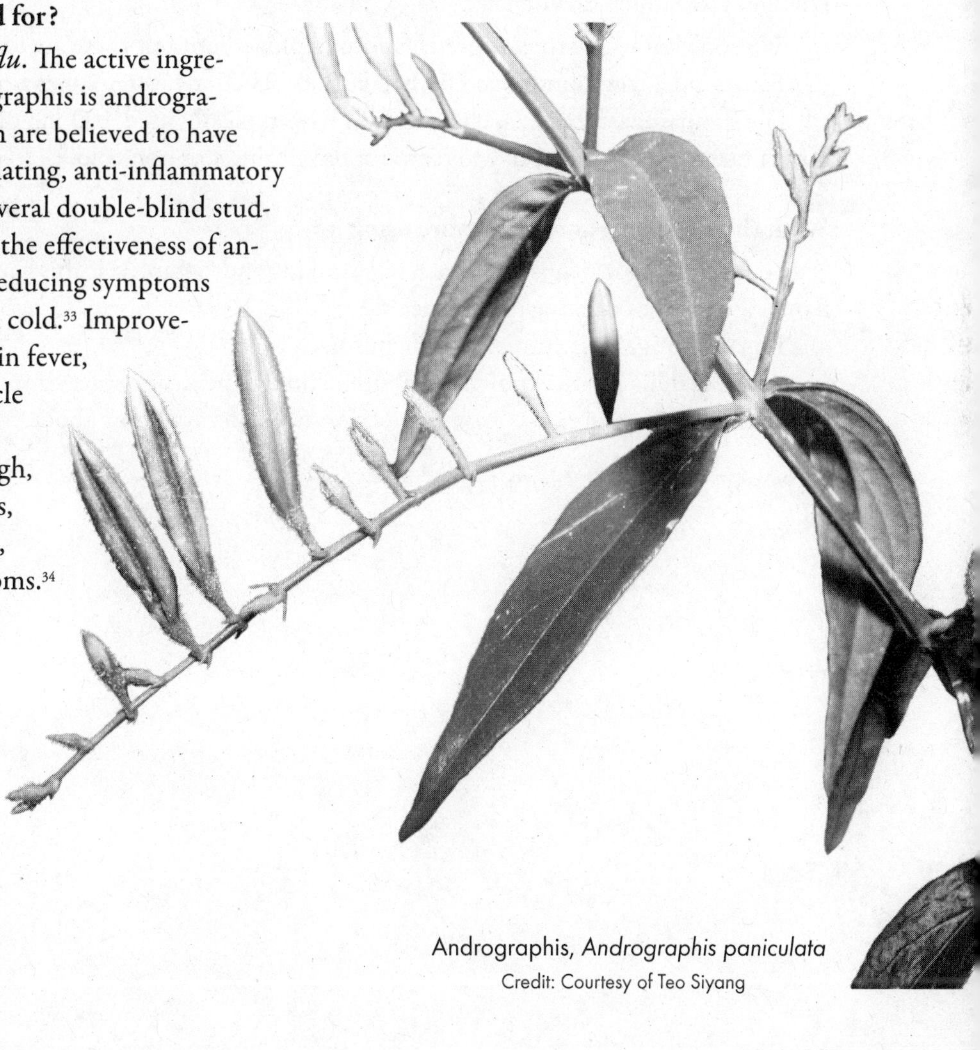

Andrographis, *Andrographis paniculata*
Credit: Courtesy of Teo Siyang

It is more effective than placebo in treating upper respiratory tract infections.[35] It helps treat

sinusitis.[36] It inhibits streptococcus bacteria in vitro.[37] According to Chinese medical tradition, it is better for flu symptoms (with fever) than for cold symptoms (with just congestion and no fever). ◊ ◊ ◆ ◆ ◆

Immune support. The hype says that andrographis stimulates the immune system[38] and reduces inflammation.[39] Though it may indeed do so, we don't have the clinical studies that prove that it does. What we have is one small-scale study of young adults which showed that andrographis cut the risk of catching a cold in half.[40] ◊ ◊ ◊ ◆ ◆

How do you use it?

Andrographis is taken internally, either as dried herb in a capsule or as a standardized extract.

Dosage: How much do you use?

We don't know exactly how much andrographis is safe, but these are typical doses:

For capsules containing dried herb, take 500–3,000 mg, three times per day.[41]

For standardized extracts, clinical trials have typically used 100 mg of a standardized extract taken two times per day to treat or prevent the common cold.[42]

What should you be aware of before using it?

Some people get an upset stomach when taking andrographis. If this happens to you, try reducing the dose or taking it with meals.

It may also aggravate ulcers or heartburn.

Andrographis has no known drug interactions. The drug, however, is new enough to Western medicine that it may have interactions we don't yet know about.

Anise

Scientific name: *Pimpinella anisum*

Also known as anise, aniseed, *jintan*, sweet cumin

Anise originally grew only in the Near East. As anise became popular as a spice, it became more widely cultivated. The ripe syncarp (fruit) is the part used medicinally. The syncarp is typically referred to as "anise seed," though it is not strictly a seed. It's the essential oil from this seed/syncarp that contains the medicinal properties.

Pimpinella anisum is the same anise that is used in foods, especially candy and bakery goods, throughout Europe and the Middle East. It is also a flavoring in ouzo and root beer. Its medicinal use goes back to both ancient Rome and ancient Egypt. Hippocrates used it as a cough remedy. The ancient Chinese used it for digestive problems. In other cultures, it has been used, with varying degrees of success, for everything from colic, to cancer, to warding off the evil eye.

What is it good for?

Coughs. Anise is used for the treatment of coughs. The Cherokee Indians used an infusion in hot water as a respiratory aid for catarrh.[43] Commission E recommends it for "catarrhs of the respiratory tract." The 1918 U.S. Dispensatory mentions an expectorant effect. The *PDR for Herbal Medicine* describes it as "antibacterial," though this effect appears to be mild. Use as a cough remedy has ample anecdotal evidence, but no known clinical trials support it. Laboratory research, however, is hopeful. One study suggests that an ingredient in the oil increases the movement of the cilia in the bronchial passages of animals. Both infusion and tincture of anise also helped dilate the bronchial passages of pigs.[44] If the same is true in humans, anise might have a measurable expectorant effect.[45]

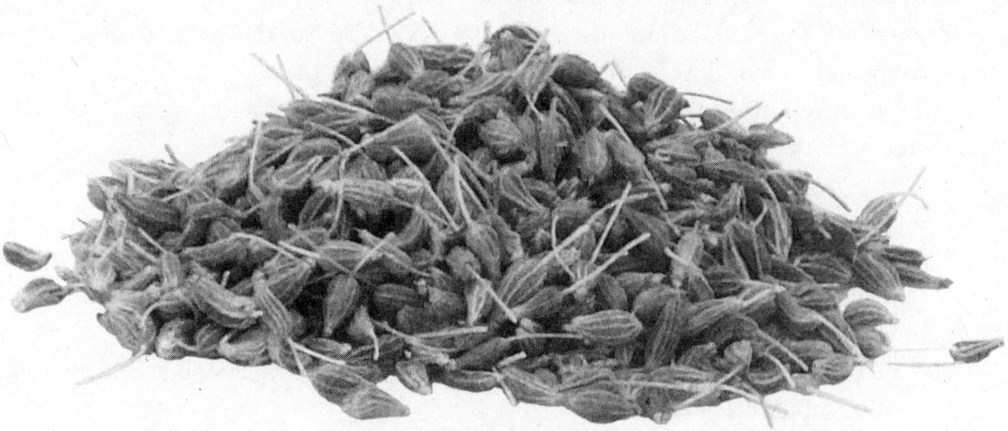

Anise, *Pimpinella anisum*

Antimicrobial. Preliminary test-tube studies show that the essential oil of anise seed may have an anti-fungal effect.[46] Anise may also have a very mild antibacterial effect, but studies seem to show that it's not significant.[47]

Flatulence. A Modern Herbal and Eclectic school both recommended it for flatulence and gas pains. Though use as a carminative is widespread and common, this use has no known scientific backing.

How do you use it?

The essential oil seems to be the part of the plant that has the most active ingredients. Some herbalists, however, prefer to use the whole seed, both for convenience's sake and to avoid the dangers of overdosing on the essential oil. If you choose to use the whole seed, grind it fresh just prior to use.

Infusion. Infusion brings out the best in anise.[48] Gently crush the seed just before infusing to release the volatile oils. Boil one cup of water, let it cool until it drops back off the boil, and then pour it over 1–2 teaspoonfuls of the seeds. Let it stand covered for 5 to 10 minutes.[49] Avoid boiling anise, as doing so tends to boil off the essential oils. Infusions can be used either topically or internally.

Tincture. The 1928 U.S. Dispensatory notes that anise's essential oils are dissolved well by alcohol, so tinctures are also a possibility for topical or internal use. Anise-flavored liqueurs are available and have been used for many of the same purposes as anise tea.

Essential oil. When using the essential oil externally, dilute it to no more than 10% in a carrier oil. Be very careful when using the essential oil internally. Dilute it well and don't exceed the recommended dosage.

Dosage: How much do you use?

Seed: A typical dosage is three g of seeds daily.[50]

Essential oil: You can take internally up to 0.3 g (12 drops) of the essential oil per day.[51] The recommended single dose is .1 g or roughly four drops of the oil.[52]

Infusions: If you are using infusions, you can drink one cup containing up to 1 g of seeds, up to three times daily.[53]

What should you be aware of before using it?

The FDA has anise on its list of "substances generally recognized as safe" for use as a spice.[54] That does not necessarily mean, however, that it is safe in large medicinal doses. In Germany and Canada, it is recognized as an over-the-counter drug.

The 1970s saw some concern that anise oil might be carcinogenic, but evidence was never found to support that claim.[55]

Some people are allergic to anise. If you are taking anise for the first time, take appropriate precautions. If you are allergic to any other member of the *Umbelliferae* family (which includes caraway, carrot, celery, dill, and parsley), be especially cautious the first time using anise.

Be cautious when using the essential oil. Too much can be toxic.[56] It can cause nausea and vomiting.

Anise essential oil has been shown to influence glucose absorption in rats.[57] If you have blood sugar issues, check with your doctor before using anise seed oil internally. Be cautious when using it in conjunction with herbs known or suspected to affect blood sugar levels. (See Chapter 5 for a list.)

Anise contains anethole, an active estrogenic agent. Traditionally, it was used to promote menstruation and facilitate birth. Avoid medicinal quantities of anise while pregnant.[58] Be cautious about using it if you are prone to hormone imbalances or estrogen-induced migraines.

Theoretically, anise may increase the risk of bruising or bleeding, though this effect has not been observed in clinical studies. If you plan to have surgery, tell your surgeon you have been taking anise and discontinue use. Be cautious when using it in conjunction with other herbs that may increase the risk of bleeding. (See Chapter 5 for a list.)

The Chinese star anise (Chinese name: *ba-jiao,* scientific name: *Illicium verum*) has a similar flavor, but it is unrelated and has different medicinal effects. Japanese star anise (*Illicium anisatum*) is toxic and used only for incense.[59]

Arnica

Scientific name: *Arnica montana*

Also known as mountain arnica, mountain tobacco, leopard's bane, wolfsbane, European arnica, Arnica flos (dried flower head)

The most commonly used medicinal species of arnica (*A. montana*) is native to the mountains of Europe, though several arnica species grow in the Americas as well. *Arnica chamissonis*, which has some of the same properties as *Arnica montana*, is native to the western United States. The flowers are the most commonly used part of the plant, though the rhizomes (underground stems) are used on rare occasion.[60]

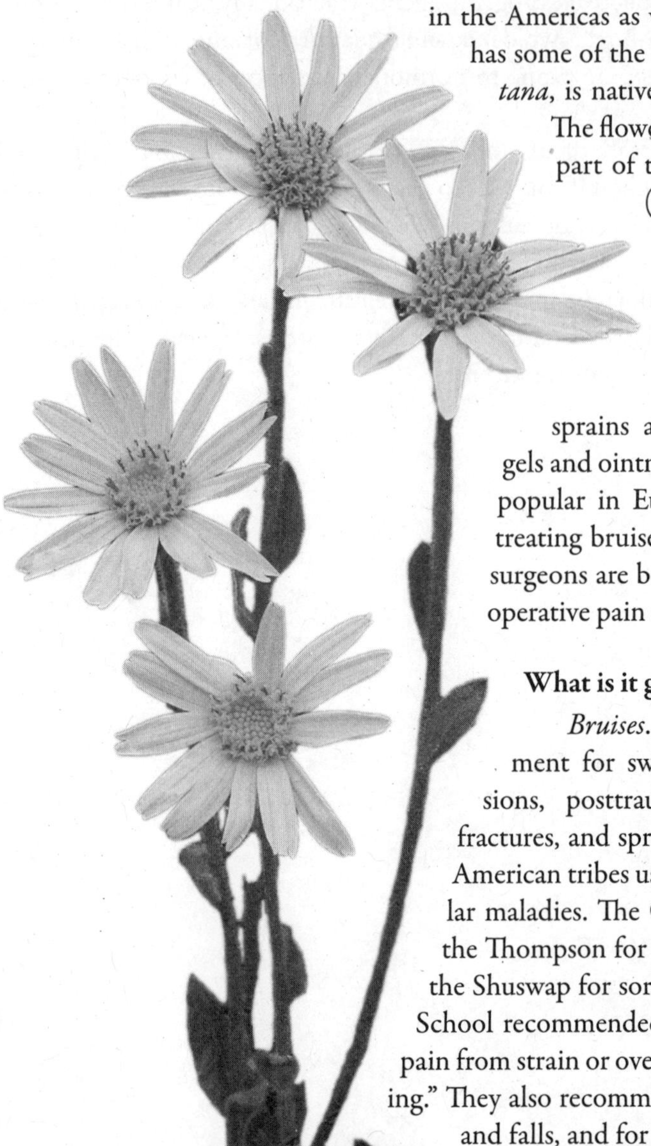

Arnica, *Arnica montana*

Courtesy of Barbara Studer

We can trace the use of arnica flowers as medicine back to the Middle Ages when they were used in Europe for sprains and bruises. In modern times, gels and ointments containing arnica are very popular in Europe, especially Germany, for treating bruises. Even some American plastic surgeons are beginning to use arnica for postoperative pain and swelling.[61]

What is it good for?

Bruises. Arnica is best known as a treatment for swelling due to bruising, contusions, posttraumatic edema, joint injuries, fractures, and sprains. In North America, Native American tribes used New-World species for similar maladies. The Catawba used it for back pain; the Thompson for swellings, bruises and cuts; and the Shuswap for sore eyes.[62] Doctors of the Eclectic School recommended it for "muscular soreness and pain from strain or overexertion" and for "bruised feeling." They also recommended it for bruises from blows and falls, and for strains. In short, the traditional evidence for effectiveness is strong.

From a clinical standpoint, we are now beginning to learn why arnica seems to work on bruises. Arnica contains a mild anesthetic.[63] It also contains thymol, an antiseptic. Perhaps most importantly, it contains helenalin, an anti-inflammatory agent. Helenalin works using a different mechanism from aspirin or other anti-inflammatories in the Western pharmacopeia. Helenalin's exact mechanism is still not understood, but the literature contains consensus that it does work. Clinical tests of non-homeopathic arnica are sparse, however. Two studies have showed some improvement in postoperative bruising in facelift patients who used arnica cream,[64] the benefit being mainly reduction in swelling, not reduction in the "black and blue" discoloration.[65] Another cosmetic surgery study, however, showed no improvement.[66] ◊ ◆ ◆ ◆

Osteoarthritis. One study showed that arnica helped with pain and stiffness due to osteoarthritis of the knee.[67] Another study found arnica tincture to be comparable to topical ibuprofen in treating osteoarthritis pain in the hands.[68] ◊ ◊ ◊ ◆ ◆

Mouth injuries. A study in the mid-1980s used arnica to treat individuals recovering from removal of impacted wisdom teeth. The study found that patients taking arnica suffered more pain than those who received antibiotics and those receiving a placebo.[69] Using arnica as a mouth rinse increases the chances of swallowing it, something that is ill-advised. Moreover, arnica can irritate mucous membranes. ◊ ◊ ◊ ◊ ◊

How do you use it?

Don't take arnica internally. It can be fatal. When making arnica preparations, follow safe handling practices: Keep it away from foodstuffs. Wear a mask and gloves when crushing it or handling crushed flowers. Be careful that anything that may have a residue on it (pots, strainers, spoons, etc.) doesn't come in contact with food. Label all preparations as "external use only."

Tincture. Studies show that the active ingredients in arnica reach the affected tissue when applied by means of a tincture.[70] You can make a tincture by pouring a pint of 70% alcohol over 50 g (two ounces) of freshly picked flowers or half that quantity of dried flowers. Let it stand for at least a week in a warm place.[71] For use on a compress, dilute the tincture. The strongest the diluted tincture should be is 1 part tincture to 5 parts water. If you have sensitive skin, dilute it more, as much as 1:10. The tincture and water mixture can also be used for hand and foot soaks.

Salves and creams. You can make your own cream or ointment. Make the infused oil by the hot infusion method, heating one ounce of flowers to one ounce of oil for several hours.[72] Strain and use the oil to make a salve (using method one, four, or five for creams and salves; see Chapter 3). Apply salves every 3–4 hours.[73]

Commercially produced arnica creams are available but are more widely available in Europe than North America. Be aware that some arnica creams are not herbal creams but rather homeopathic creams made with a very different method from herbal preparations.

Infusions. Use 2 g of arnica to ½ cup of water.[74] Use it as a soak or a compress.

Dosage: How much do you use?

According to Commission E, ointments should not contain more than 15% arnica oil or 20–25% arnica tincture. Dilute the tincture no less than 1:5 (tincture to water). Stronger formulations can irritate skin.

What should you be aware of before using it?

Don't use arnica on open wounds or broken skin. Arnica can suppress the mechanism by which the body fights off infection. Because of helenalin's unique anti-inflammatory properties, arnica is best used on injuries that involve swelling or inflammation, but that offer little or no chance of infection.

Internal use of arnica is hazardous. Because helenalin interacts with the body's enzyme systems,[75] even small doses can be dangerous, causing elevated blood pressure, shortness of breath, and heart damage. An overdose can be fatal. The FDA classes arnica as an unsafe herb.[76] Though internal use of arnica was not unheard of in less-knowledgeable times, almost everyone today agrees that the dangers far outweigh the benefits. Topical use of arnica does not appear to have the same toxic effects as internal use, though research into the hazardous effects of topical use is not as comprehensive as we would like.

Don't use arnica near eyes, nose, or mouth.

Arnica can cause allergic dermatitis in some people.[77] The likelihood of your reacting to arnica depends of a number of factors: how much helenalin is in the product, what other ingredients are used and whether they enhance or mitigate the effect of the helenalin, how sensitive your skin is, and whether you are allergic to the *Compositae* family of plants (a common allergy to the family that contains ragweed). If you have other contact allergies, try a small amount of arnica on a healthy patch of skin before using it more extensively. Limit the amount of arnica you use to recommended amounts, or less than recommended amounts if you have sensitive skin. Avoid long-term use. If the area seems to be getting redder and more swollen, discontinue use.[78]

Don't use arnica during pregnancy.

Arnica is one of the herbs used in homeopathic medicine. Because homeopathy dilutes its ingredients (using its own distinctive process), homeopathic arnica may be safe for internal use. The effectiveness of homeopathic arnica, however, is still in dispute. It is widely used, perhaps more so than herbal arnica. Yet several studies show homeopathic arnica cream to be no more effective than placebo for bruising.[79] For our purposes here, suffice it to say that if you use homeopathic arnica, you will be getting a different dose of arnica than if you use an herbal preparation. Therefore, these assessments and warnings do not necessarily apply.

Though the American arnica, *Arnica chamissonis*, has some of the same properties as *Arnica montana*, it has not been nearly as extensively tested. We don't know much about its properties or dangers.

Ashwagandha

Scientific name: *Withania somnifera*

Also known as winter cherry, *varaha karni*, Indian ginseng, and *ajagandha*

Ashwagandha is a member of the *Solanaceae* or nightshade family. Various species of the plant can be found in India, Africa, and the Mediterranean. The root is the most common medicinal part, though the berries are used in India and North Africa to coagulate milk to make cheese.

Conventional wisdom has it that ashwagandha gets its name because its roots smell like a horse. (*Ashwa* means "horse" and *gandha* "odor.") The use of ashwagandha goes back so far that we can't begin to guess when it was first used. For more than 2000 years, it has been used as a part of the Ayurvedic system of natural healing in India. Though the tradition is long, it has been mostly limited to one branch of Indian medicine. The effects have been documented, but they are linked more to ashwagandha in combination with other herbs than to ashwagandha alone. Moreover, the toxic effects of ashwagandha are not well known. Some scientists insist that the leaves are toxic. Others cite their long usage, supposedly without ill effects. Nobody seems to be offering hard evidence either way. If ashwagandha does what the Ayurvedic practitioners and herb salespeople says it does, it could be a very valuable herb indeed. Right now, however, we can't say for sure that the reality is as strong as the reputation.

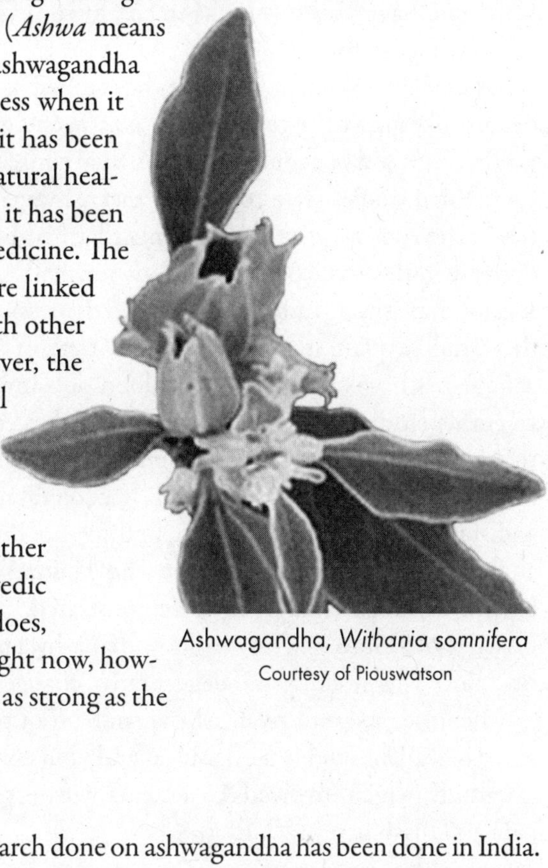

Ashwagandha, *Withania somnifera*
Courtesy of Piouswatson

What is it good for?

Endurance and energy. Most of the research done on ashwagandha has been done in India. Animal and test-tube studies abound, as do studies that mix ashwagandha with other traditional ingredients. Well-designed, focused human studies, however, are scarce.[80] Studies with rats show that the rats can swim farther in cold water when given ashwagandha. Rats stressed by exercise showed less stress response to that exercise as well.[81] However, we don't really understand why ashwagandha should boost endurance in rats, and no comparable studies have been done with people.[82] We do know that rats fed ashwagandha over the course of four weeks had heavier livers than the controls, something researchers attributed to increased glycogen.[83] We also know that ashwagandha contains many steroids and glucocorticoids known to enhance liver glycogen stores, which in turn may have an impact on endurance. ◊ ◊ ◆ ◆ ◆

As for clinical studies, however, we only have a couple. A study in which Indian children given powdered ashwagandha in milk for sixty days showed slight increases in the following areas: hemoglobin, packed cell volume, mean corpuscular volume, serum iron, body weight, and hand grip. The children also showed significant increases in mean corpuscular hemoglobin and total proteins.[84] In another study 101 normal healthy men, 50–59 years old, were given three grams per day of the powder for one year. All subjects showed significantly increased hemoglobin and red blood cell count and decreased SED rate (a marker of inflammation in the body).[85] In short, research has given us several pieces that might indicate that ashwagandha has some value as an energy tonic, but we can't yet say that it increases energy or endurance in humans.

Adaptogen. Western herbalists have taken to calling ashwagandha "Ayurvedic ginseng" because like ginseng, its primary use is as an energy tonic.[86] Ashwagandha is especially useful for tiredness and burnout that has a sexual consequence (impotence, lack of libido). At least two animal studies seem to suggest that ashwagandha may have anti-inflammatory properties.[87] The root powder given to rats that had been made to swim to exhaustion caused a decrease in the waste products a body normally puts out when it is stressed.[88] Some studies suggest that ashwagandha causes a mild depression of the central nervous system—an effect that would explain its use as an anti-anxiety or anti-burnout agent. An alkaloid in ashwagandha has been shown to lower blood pressure, heart rate, and respiration rate in dogs.[89] But other studies didn't find any effect on the central nervous system.[90] One study suggests that it might have an antioxidant effect on the brain (again in rats).[91] Compounds isolated from ashwagandha had a beneficial effect on rat immune systems and boosted their memory and ability to learn.[92] All of these findings are hopeful, but again, a rat is not a person, and an ingredient in an herb is not the whole herb. Whether ashwagandha is useful as an adaptogenic in humans has yet to be demonstrated.

Arthritis. Studies with rats show that ashwagandha may be beneficial for treating arthritis.[93] Both paw swelling and degenerative changes were reduced in rats with induced arthritis when the rats were given ashwagandha root powder for fifteen days.[94] Only one human study is available and it used ashwagandha in conjunction with zinc and two other herbs.[95] The study, which involved 42 patients with osteoarthritis, found significant reduction of pain and disability.

How do you use it?

Ashwagandha is commonly used in powdered form, which is made from the root. Commercially prepared powders, both in and out of capsules are available. Buy from a reputable company and follow label directions. Take it with a meal and/or a full glass of water.

Dosage: How much do you use?

Commercial preparations: Capsules are often standardized to 2–5 mg with anolides, one of the active ingredients. For these standardized capsules, a dose of 150–300 mg is typical.

Root powder: For the root powder, 2–3 g taken three times a day (up to 9 g per day) is a typical Ayurvedic dose.[96] Western herbalists most commonly recommend somewhat less, roughly 3–6 g per day[97] Experiments on rats suggests that a single dose (25 or 50 mg/kg taken orally) taken an hour before anticipated stress may help ameliorate some of the physical consequences of that stress.[98]

What should you be aware of before using it?

We know little or nothing about the consequences of long-term use.

Many members of the nightshade family are toxic. Ashwagandha roots have been used for thousands of years. If the dangers were obvious, they would have received much wider attention than they have. That, however, does not guarantee that it is completely safe.

The plant can make some people drowsy, so you should be cautious about driving and engaging in dangerous activities that require quick reaction time until you figure out how much this particular side effect affects you. Taking ashwagandha with other herbs with a sedative effect can compound the sedative effect. Be cautious about mixing it with melatonin or herbs that make you drowsy. (See Chapter 5 for a list.)

If you have thyroid problems, check with your doctor before using ashwagandha. Thyrotoxicosis has been reported in humans and increased blood levels of thyroid hormones have been reported in animals.[99]

If you have immune system issues, discuss ashwagandha with your doctor before taking it. Studies show that it may have an immunosuppressant effect.[100]

There is some question as to whether it is safe to use ashwagandha during pregnancy. The Western literature says no. Ayurvedic practitioners have used it as a pregnancy tonic for years. However, one of its other traditional uses is as an abortifacient. Prudence dictates that you not use it during pregnancy, at least not without professional supervision.

One article suggests that it causes kidney lesion in rats.[101]

One study showed that high levels of ashwagandha (3000 mg/kg per day for a week) hampered sexual desire and function in male rats.[102] But it has a reputation for having the opposite effect in humans.

Another study demonstrated that it's possible to kill a rat if you give it enough ashwagandha.[103] More is not better. Stay within recommended doses.

Ashwagandha contains some nicotine. If you have a problem with cigarette addiction, you may want to be a bit cautious about using it.

Astragalus

Scientific name: *Astragalus membranaceus*

Also known as *huang-qi* or *huang-qui*, milk vetch, tragacanth, goat's horn, goat's thorn, green dragon, gum dragon, hog gum, locoweed

Astragalus is a hairy-stemmed perennial plant, mainly grown in China. It is, however, becoming ever more common in the West. It is a relative of licorice. The dried root is used medicinally.

The Chinese have been using astragalus for more than a thousand years. It is used mainly as a tonic to enhance and balance vital energy, especially among the elderly. It is also used topically as a vasodilator to speed healing. Though use in the Western world dates back to the 1800s when it was included in various tonics, only in the last twenty-five years or so has astragalus become common. What boosted astragalus sales the most was when herb sellers began touting its alleged anti-cancer properties. The media picked up the story, and astragalus became

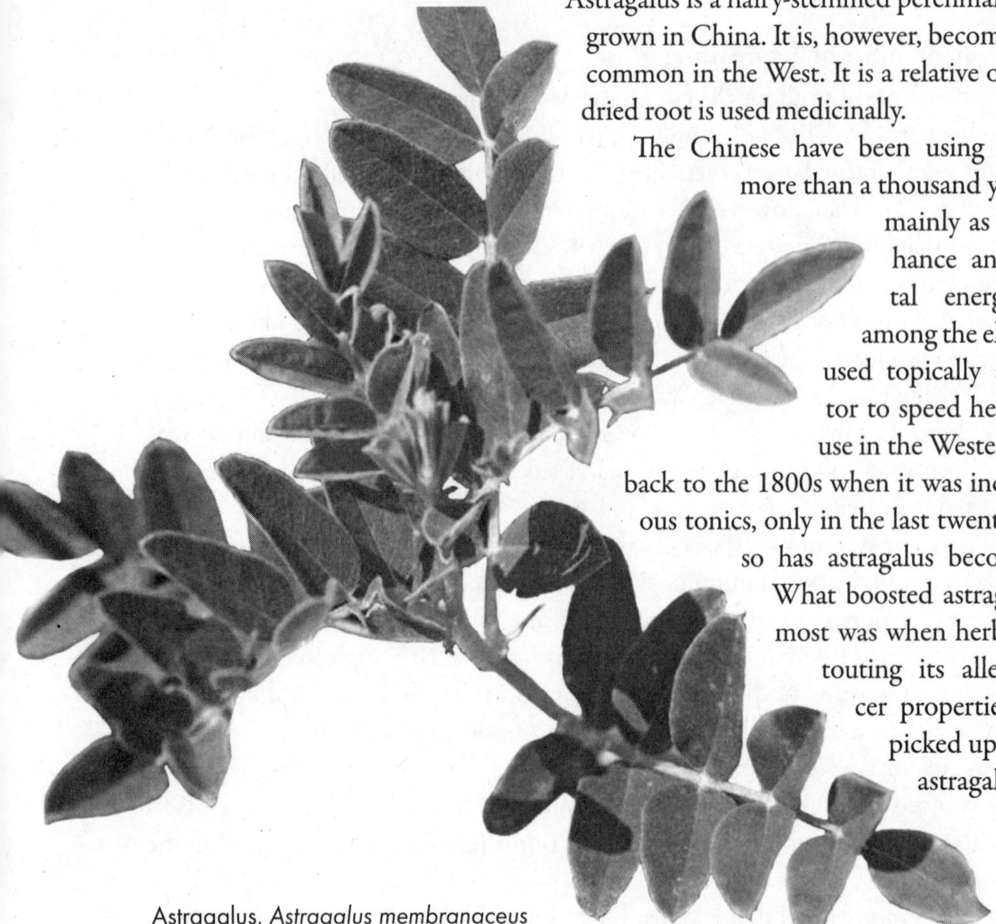

Astragalus, *Astragalus membranaceus*
Courtesy of Stanislva Doronenko

widely available. Since then it has come to be used most commonly to help ward off viral and bacterial infections. Tests of the herb's effectiveness and safety, however, are also fairly new. The herb, nonetheless, shows great promise. Once Westerners become more familiar and comfortable with its use, it may join echinacea and vitamin C as common treatment for colds and flu.

What is it good for?

Immune support. The most common use for astragalus in the West is as a cold-and flu fighter. Surprisingly, the clinical evidence for that use is slim. What we do know is this:

Extracts contain COX and LOX inhibitors, suggesting that astragalus may have anti-inflammatory properties.[104] In the laboratory, extracts of the drug were able to protect liver cells from environmental toxins.[105] Astragalus appears to stimulate the production of interferon, a protein produced by the body to hamper the ability of viruses to multiply.[106] It may also stimulate the body's killer cells and white blood cells, both of which protect the body against invading organisms.[107] Note, however, the qualifiers: it *may* stimulate interferon and it *may* stimulate killer cells. These studies have been of extracts of the herb, which may or may not behave like the whole herb. So far, all the studies have been preliminary and unconfirmed. Some limited human research has examined the use of astragalus for viral infections. In a clinical study, 1,000 people experienced fewer colds and less severe colds while taking astragalus.[108] However, most human studies have been small, poorly designed, and unduplicated.[109]

Energy and endurance. The anecdotal evidence for this use is strong in China, where astragalus is used especially by young people as a tonic to promote muscle growth and increase stamina.[110] Animal tests show preliminary support for this use. Mice that were fed astragalus could swim longer in cold water.[111] However, clinical studies have yet to show this effect in healthy adults. A couple of studies have shown that it can improve heart function in patients with heart disease.[112] Another study suggests that it can improve breathing in patients with asthma.[113] To date, however, we have no evidence that it can improve circulation, respiration, energy levels, or endurance in healthy athletes.

How do you use it?

Decoctions work best for astragalus. Use 1 teaspoonful of the root per cup of water, bring to boil and simmer for 10–15 minutes.[114]

Commercially prepared capsules containing extracts of the roots are available. Good ones are standardized to 0.5% glucosides and 70% polysaccharides.

Tinctures tend not to work very well for astragalus. Instead, make a strong decoction and preserve it with 22% grain alcohol[115]

In China, the root is sometimes cured with honey. Conventional wisdom says that the cured root has more energizing properties.[116]

Dosage: How much do you use?

No safe dose has been determined by Western herbalists or regulatory agencies. The probable effective daily dose of the root is 2–6 g.[117] In China, however, typical doses can be quite large, as much as 8–15 g, or higher, per day.[118]

If you are using the standardized extract, take 200–500 mg standardized extract four times a day for an acute condition, at the onset of a cold, for example.[119] For ongoing use, take 200–500 mg once a day.[120] Of course, if you get a preparation that's standardized to a different level of glucosides and polysaccharides than the one mentioned above, read and follow label directions.

What should you be aware of before using it?

One of the few dangers in using astragalus is that we Westerners aren't really sure what it is and what it does. Western studies are sparse. Commission E has no recommendations or guidelines. The FDA says little about it. The tradition of use in the West is short. It has been used in China and Japan for centuries with little ill effect and possible benefit, but those uses are different from a Western style of using herbs. What we do know is that as astragalus makes its way into the mainstream of Western society, it hasn't been accompanied by any reports of toxicity, indicating that it is a relatively safe herb.[121]

Based on theoretical considerations, the following dangers are possible:[122]

Immunosuppressant (in high doses).[123]

Neurological dysfunction due to selenium content.[124] Pigs fed high doses of a selenium-rich species (*A. bisulcatus)* developed weight loss and severe neurologic toxicity, including paralysis within five days.[125] We have no studies on the effects of *Astragalus membranaceus*' lower selenium content. Nonetheless, it is wise to avoid taking more than recommended doses.

It may increase the effects of antithrombotic drugs.[126] It may also increase the risk of bleeding and/or bruising. If you plan to have surgery, tell your surgeon you have been taking astragalus and discontinue use. Be cautious when using it in conjunction with other herbs known or suspected of increasing the risk of bleeding. (See Chapter 5 for a list.)

It may increase or decrease the affects of immunosuppressants.[127]

Be cautious if you are taking drugs that act as a diuretic, as astragalus can compound that effect. Be cautious when taking it in conjunction with other herbs with diuretic properties.[128] (See Chapter 5 for a list.)

We don't know enough about astragalus to know whether it's safe for children.[129]

Related species are harmful to pregnancies, but we don't know if this species of astragalus is.[130]

Astragalus may lower blood pressure, especially at high doses. Be cautious when using it in conjunction with other herbs known to have blood pressure lowering properties. [131] (See Chapter 5 for a list.)

People with diabetes or hypoglycemia, and those taking drugs that affect blood sugar, should talk to their doctor before using astragalus.[132] Be cautious when using it in conjunction with herbs known or suspected to affect blood sugar levels. (See Chapter 5 for a list.)

Also be aware that not all species of astragalus can be used medicinally. Some are inactive, and some are toxic.[133] For example, the American astragalus, typically known as locoweed (*Astragalus mollissimus* of the American Southwest and Rocky Mountain states) is toxic. Be sure to check that you are getting the correct species.

Bilberry Fruit

Scientific name: *Vaccinium myrtillus*

Also known as huckleberry, blackberry, blaeberry, bog berry, whortleberry, dwarf bilberry, whinberry, myrtill, burren myrtle, dyeberry, false huckleberry, hurtleberry, whinberry, and wineberry

Bilberry is native to North America. It grows on low bushes in acidic soils, in forests and moors in the Rockies of the United States, as well as Europe and Western Asia. The bilberry is very similar to the cranberry and the cowberry (*V. vitisidaea*), both of which are close relatives and both which have many of the same properties. Though typically harvested wild, some bilberries are cultivated commercially. The ripe fruit is used, both fresh and dried.

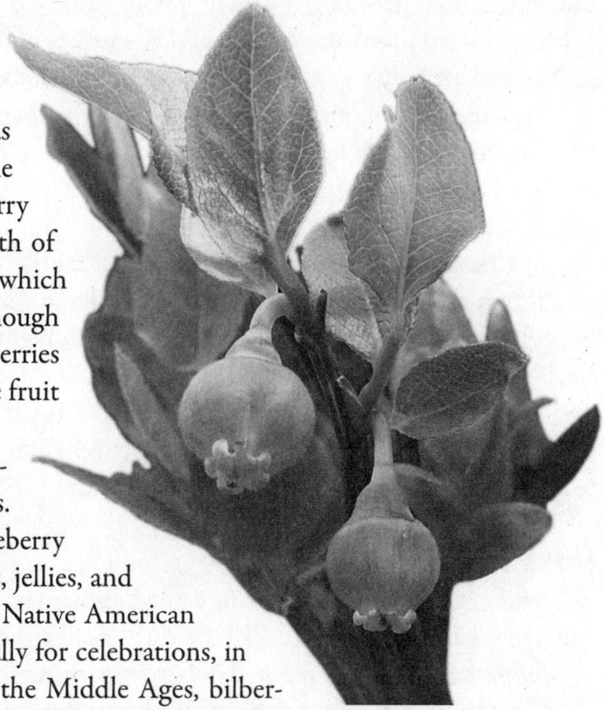

Bilberry, *Vaccinium myrtillus*
Courtesy of Steve Hammonds

Bilberries are one of the few medicinal botanicals that are delicious. They taste like a cross between a blueberry and a cranberry and are used in jams, jellies, and juices in Europe. In the U.S., several Native American tribes used the berry as food, especially for celebrations, in addition to using it medicinally. In the Middle Ages, bilberries were an effective treatment for scurvy because of their high vitamin C content. They also contain higher levels of antioxidants than commercial North American blueberries.[134] The deep blue color has been used as a dye and an ink.[135]

What is it good for?

Improvement of night vision. RAF pilots during World War II used bilberry to help improve night vision. At least four subsequent studies showed improvement in night vision and the ability of the eyes to adapt to darkness after exposure to bright light.[136] However, recent studies done by the U.S. Air Force failed to find the effect.[137] ◊ ◊ ◆ ◆ ◆

Protection against eye diseases. Preliminary research suggests that bilberry may reduce or reverse effects of degenerative eye disorders such as macular degeneration, cataracts, and glaucoma.[138] ◊ ◊ ◆ ◆ ◆

Bruising. In one Italian study, bilberry's anthocyanosides relaxed and dilated arteries, fostering blood circulation.[139] In another human study, 47 adults with circulatory problems (atherosclerosis, a tendency to bruise easily, hemorrhoids and varicose veins) were given bilberry extracts. A statistically significant number reported reduced symptoms.[140] These studies, however, are very preliminary and more useful as a direction for future research than as a guide to treatment of any particular condition. ◊ ◊ ◊ ◆ ◆

Adaptogen. An adaptogen is an herb that helps the body successfully deal with the physical consequences of stress. Because stress is such a complex phenomenon, it's hard to measure just how an herb might benefit a body under stress, but preliminary research into the effects of bilberry look promising. In rats, extracts of bilberry, specifically the chemical that makes the berry blue, helped protect the body against the effects of toxins.[141] The berry is also a good source of quercetin, an anti-inflammatory.[142] Moreover, the flavonoids have an antioxidant effect that might help prevent hardening of the arteries.[143] Though none of this research is conclusive, it does suggest that bilberry might indeed have adaptogenic properties. ◊ ◊ ◊ ◆ ◆

Sore throat and diarrhea. We have significantly less evidence that bilberry helps treat sore throat and diarrhea. Folk wisdom says that dried bilberries are good for these conditions. Bilberry does contain a pigment that is thought to inhibit the growth of bacteria. A small-scale study showed that it may help the body ward off bacterial infections.[144] Moreover, it does contain tannins, which have had some traditional use as an astringent to treat diarrhea and sore throat. We have no direct scientific evidence, however, to support its effectiveness against either sore throat or diarrhea. ◊ ◊ ◊ ◊ ◆

How do you use it?

Fresh or Dried. If you can't find fresh bilberries, you may be able to find them dried (though it's almost certain that they won't be cheap when you do find them).

Infusion. Simmer the mashed bilberries in water for 10 minutes and then strain.

Commercially prepared extracts. Both standardized and not, bilberries are available in capsules, extracts, and tablets. Most of the standardized extracts are European. The best European preparations are high-quality, pharmaceutical-grade bilberry extract from whole, dried, ripe fruit. Standardization to 23% to 37% bilberry anthocyanosides is typical.[145]

Dosage: How much do you use?

Dried. The dried ripe berries are used in a dose of 20 to 60 g daily, eaten whole or prepared as a tea (infusion), divided into three doses.

Extracts. Standardized products with 25% anthocyanosides can be taken at a dose of 120 to 320 mg per day, divided into two or three doses.[146]

What should you be aware of before using it?

Bilberries have been used as a food for centuries and have no known toxicity. However, large quantities of the fresh fruit can have a laxative effect. In fact, that is also one of the traditional medicinal uses. Be cautious when using bilberries in conjunction with herbs known or suspected to have a laxative effect. (See Chapter 5 for a list.)

If you are diabetic, hypoglycemic, or are taking insulin, glyburide, or a related drug, check with your doctor before using bilberries. Preliminary research indicates they may affect blood sugar levels.[147] Be cautious when using it in conjunction with herbs known or suspected to affect blood sugar levels. (See Chapter 5 for a list.)

If you are taking antithrombotic agents, check with your doctor before taking bilberries.[148] Bilberries may retard clotting and increase the chance of bruising. If you plan to have surgery, tell your surgeon you have been taking bilberries and discontinue use. Be cautious when using it in conjunction with other herbs known or suspected of increasing the risk of bleeding. (See Chapter 5 for a list.)

It is probably best to avoid the leaves. Though they have some traditional uses, including the ability to lower blood sugar levels, their safety is in question. Oral tradition among herbalists says the leaves may be dangerous. Not enough research exists to evaluate how great or precisely what that danger may be.[149]

Bilberries contain ferulic acid, a known uterosedative. Though no reports of problems for pregnancy have been reported in the literature, it's probably safest to avoid medicinal bilberry while pregnant until its safety has been better examined.

Though bilberries are sometimes called huckleberry, they should not be confused with members of the *Gaylussacia* genus, also called huckleberries, which are an entirely different berry. They should also not be confused with the berry more commonly called "blackberry," *Rosoideae rubus*.

Borage Oil

Scientific name: *Borago officinalis*

Also known as burrage, starflower, bugloss, borage oil, starflower oil

An annual plant with bristly stems and blue star-shaped flowers, borage is native to the Mediterranean region and to central and eastern Europe. It has, however, become a common herb in western European herbal gardens, where it is also ornamental and attractive to bees. It grows wild as an introduced species in the northern states of the United States. Borage oil is extracted from the seeds. The dry leaves can be made into a tea or a tincture, or the fresh leaves can be juiced.

An old saying goes like this: "*ego borago gaudia semper ago.*" ("I, borage, always bring courage.")[150] In old England, the leaves and flowers were added to wine to "drive away sadness, dullness, and melancholy."[151] John Evelyn, writing at the close of the seventeenth century, described how sprigs of borage helped students hold up under arduous studying.[152] A modern take on the theme is that borage contains an essential fatty acid with possible adaptogenic properties.

Borage oil contains gamma-linolenic acid (GLA), an omega-6 fatty acid, which may have anti-inflammatory properties. Though other plants, most notably evening primrose and black currant, also contain GLA, borage oil contains it in higher concentrations.[153] GLA is converted in the body into a hormone-like substance that helps regulate inflammation.[154]

What is it good for?

Arthritis. A small-scale 1993 study showed improvement in people with rheumatoid arthritis who took borage seed oil for twenty-four weeks.[155] Another showed that it reduced damage to joint tissue in the rheumatoid arthritis sufferers who took very large doses.[156] Animal studies show similar improvements for various inflammatory conditions.[157]

Stress. One study suggests that the GLA in borage oil helps the body deal with stress. In a small study, ten men who had been taking borage oil for 28 days had a statistically lower blood pressure and decreased heart rate when faced with experimental stress. Performing better than olive oil and fish oil (the controls), borage oil

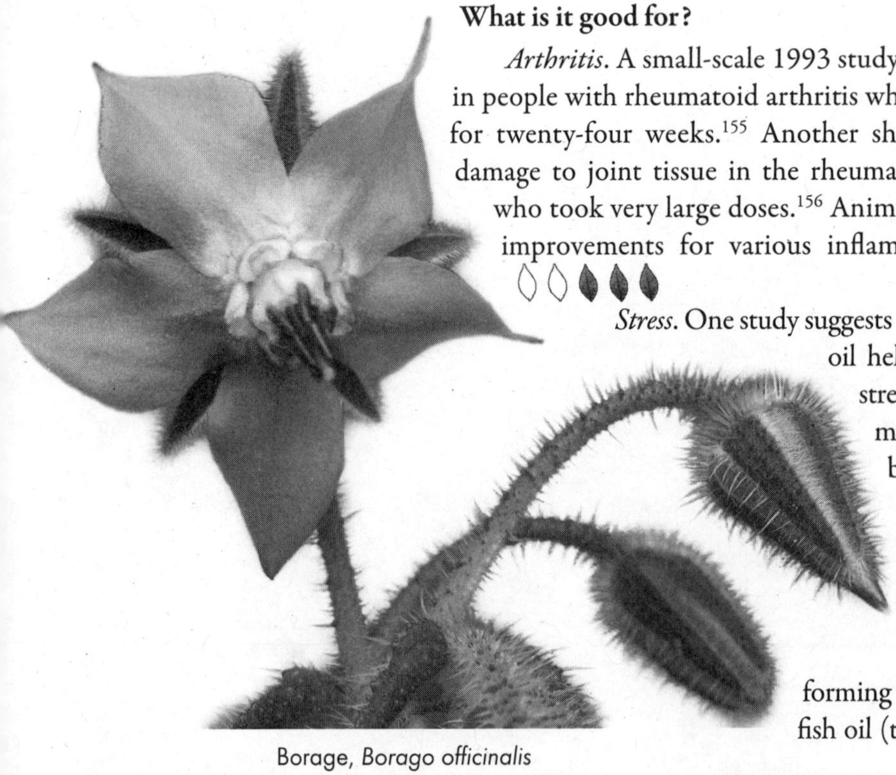

Borage, *Borago officinalis*

not only decreased the stress reaction but increased performance of the men while under stress.[158] The study, however, was very small and not duplicated. Furthermore, the anecdotal evidence for borage oil as an antidote to stress is slim. One study and almost nonexistent tradition are together probably not enough to warrant taking borage oil to deal with stress.

Eczema. Herbalists sometimes prescribe borage oil (taken orally) for eczema. We have some evidence that it is the GLA in borage oil that is helpful for this condition. People with eczema tend to have abnormal levels of linoleic acid in their blood. GLA taken regularly may help restore normal levels.[159] The evidence for this effect, however, is slim and equivocal, and many conventional doctors are still doubtful.[160]

Adrenal support. A popular claim of supplement stores is that borage leaf tea stimulates the adrenal glands. The old saying that borage gives courage would seem to support this claim. Modern research, though admittedly slim, doesn't show any adrenal connection. Given that borage leaves have significant safety issues, it's probably wise to leave them alone and to find your courage elsewhere.

How do you use it?

Oil is available in commercially prepared capsule form.

Dosage: How much do you use?

Recommended daily doses of the oil range widely, from 300–500 mg[161] to 1,000–1,300 mg.[162] If the oil you're taking is standardized, look for roughly 240 to 300 mg of GLA.[163] Studies tend to use very high doses of borage seed oil. While high doses don't seem to have any adverse short-term effects, we still aren't sure what pyrrolizidine in that amount is doing to the liver. (See the "What should you be aware of" section for more information on pyrrolizidine.)

What should you be aware of before using it?

The German government no longer permits the sale of borage. The plant contains small amounts of the liver toxin pyrrolizidine.[164] Some herbalists suggest that the German government's decision was an overreaction, citing the fact that borage has been used safely for centuries both as a food and as a medicine, and other legal herbs have more pyrrolizidine than borage. For safety's sake, it's probably best to avoid borage leaves entirely. Most of the uses for the leaves do not go beyond local, anecdotal tradition. Clinical evidence of benefit is lacking.[165] As for the oil, if you can't wait for studies to verify its safety, strongly consider either using it only short-term or having long-term use overseen by a physician.

Another alternative is to try refined gamma-linolenic acid (GLA). GLA is the main (but not only) active oil in borage oil. Because it's been extracted from the rest of the borage oil, it doesn't contain pyrrolizidine. One thousand to 1,300 mg of borage oil contains 240 to 300 mg of GLA. Nearly equivalent doses of GLA can also be found in 3,000 mg of evening primrose oil or 1,500 mg of black currant seed oil.[166]

If you want to take borage oil, find a qualified herbalist, naturopath, or physician to supervise you. It's not a good do-it-yourself herb.

Borage oil may cause loose stools and/or stomach upset.[167] If you experience stomach upset, discontinue taking borage oil immediately. Stomach upset is an early symptom of pyrrolizidine alkaloids poisoning. The disease, however, can be doing damage before any symptoms manifest themselves.[168]

People with liver problems should not take borage oil.[169] Even healthy people should not take it in conjunction with any other herb or drug known to affect liver function. (See Chapter 5 for a list.)

Pregnant women and nursing mothers should avoid using borage oil supplements.[170]

Those with seizure disorders should avoid using borage oil.[171] Those taking phenothiazine drugs are at increased seizure risk if they take borage concurrently.[172]

Furthermore, high doses (24 g per day) of borage oil can increase spontaneous clotting of the blood.[173] If you plan to have surgery, tell your surgeon you have been taking borage oil and discontinue use.

Bromelain

Scientific name: Sulphydryl proteolytic enzyme, cysteine-proteinase

Bromelain is an enzyme obtained from pineapple. Though bromelain can be derived from both the fruit and the stem, most commercial preparations come from the stem.

Bromelain, discovered in 1957, is not strictly an herb, but rather is an enzyme. A treatment for bruises and inflammation, it works by breaking down fibrin, a blood-clotting protein. Once the protein is broken down, circulation increases and tissues drain better. Bromelain is also an anti-inflammatory agent.[174]

What is it good for?

Bruises to skin and muscle (the attendant pain and inflammation). The most carefully controlled study was one conducted on rabbits. When bromelain was applied to a skeletal muscle and then the muscle was injured, the bromelain helped protect the muscle (as compared to similarly injured rabbits not treated with bromelain).[175] The human studies so far also show promise. In a small human study that used bromelain to treat blunt injuries to muscles, subjects receiving bromelain in addition to standard care by an orthopedist had a significant reduction in swelling, tenderness, and pain at rest and during movement as compared with those who just received standard care.[176] In another study of boxers, bruises healed significantly quicker in those who took bromelain.[177] Test-tube studies have found that bromelain contains anti-inflammatory properties, which may explain these results.[178]

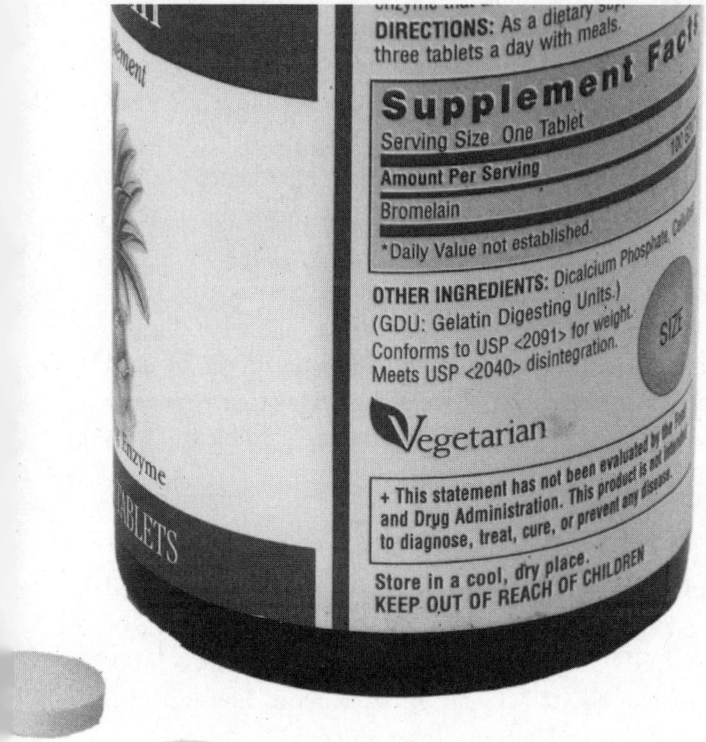

Commercially prepared bromelain tablets

Reducing joint pain, especially knee pain. Bromelain has shown some anti-inflammatory and analgesic properties in a small study. Researchers put otherwise healthy subjects, who were experiencing mild yet acute knee pain (less than three months' duration) on 200–400 mg of bromelain per day. At the higher dose, subjects experienced a reduction in overall symptoms, including stiffness, and had improved function.[179]

Arthritis. Studies investigating bromelain as a treatment for the symptoms of osteoarthritis have been promising. A least ten preliminary studies have been conducted investigating its use for treating pain and stiffness of arthritis. Though not unequivocal, evidence is strong that it can be useful.[180]

Repairing ligament and tendon damage. A German study, conducted in 1995 gave bromelain to people with torn ligaments. After one to three weeks of taking the supplements, swelling, tenderness and pain were comparable to people taking NSAIDs such as aspirin.[181]

Asthma and allergies. Preliminary studies show that bromelain may help reduce the symptoms of asthma and allergic airway disorders.[182]

Delayed onset muscle soreness. Bromelain's benefits seem to be limited to pain and swelling due to injury (either accidental or surgical). Studies into delayed onset muscle soreness (in other words, muscle soreness not resulting from injury but from strenuous exercise) show mixed results. One found no help from either bromelain or ibuprofen.[183] Another found some help from protease tablets containing bromelain and other ingredients, but it is not clear that the benefit came from bromelain and not from another one of the ingredients.[184]

How do you use it?

Bromelain comes in commercially prepared tablets or capsules. Bromelain can be used after trauma to aid healing. If, however, you anticipate a particularly grueling tournament or other event, you can also begin to take bromelain 72 hours before the event and it will help mitigate trauma. Take bromelain on an empty stomach.[185]

Dosage: How much do you use?

It is difficult to tell how much of the active ingredient you are getting as compared to the bromelain used in studies. Standardized bromelain can be measured in any one of several methods. The most common are GDUs (gelatin dissolving units) or MCUs (milk clotting units). One GDU equals approximately 1.5 MCU.[186] Bromelain can, however, also be standardized to FIP units, Bromelain Tyrosine Units, or Rorer units.

A dose of 3,000 MCU, three times per day for several days, followed by 2,000 MCU three times per day is about the highest dose found in the literature.[187] Most of the studies used smaller amounts, roughly 500 MCU taken four times per day.[188] Doses above 460 mg can begin to cause troubling side effects (increased heart rate, heart palpitations, and raised blood pressure) in some people.[189]

What should you be aware of before using it?

Bromelain is thought to have fairly low toxicity. Studies where high doses were given daily to dogs showed no ill effects after six months.[190]

Bromelain is a natural blood thinner in that it prevents platelets from sticking together.[191] Don't take bromelain if you are taking anticoagulants. In other words, choose between bromelain and aspirin or ibuprofen; don't take them both together. If you plan to have surgery, tell your surgeon you have been taking bromelain and discontinue use. Be cautious when using it in conjunction with other herbs known or suspected of increasing the risk of bleeding. (See Chapter 5 for a list.)

Bromelain may interfere with the absorption of some antibiotics.[192]

Bromelain may compound the effects of some sedatives.[193]

Don't take more than 460 mg per day if you have a history of heart palpitation.[194]

Be very conservative using it if you are prone to menorrhagia.

Occasionally gastric disturbances or diarrhea occur, especially with higher dose. If you have an ulcer or gastritis, check with your doctor before taking bromelain.[195]

Allergic reactions are possible,[196] but they are more common when the bromelain powder is inhaled than they are when it is taken orally. Be especially cautious if you are allergic to pineapple, horseradish, or olive tree pollen.[197]

Calendula

Scientific name: *Calendula officinalis*

Also known as garden marigold, pot marigold, goldblood, holligold, kingscup, maravilla, marybud, Scotch marigold, mary-bud, goldbloom

A relative of the sunflower, calendula grows to one or two feet in height. The daisy-like flowers range from a deep orange-yellow to almost red. A member of the aster (*Compositae*) family, it is a native of the Mediterranean but grows wild (as an introduced species) throughout the northeastern states of the United States. The whole flowers are used medicinally.

Calendula is one of those plants with a long history of medicinal use. It was used in ancient Greece, Rome, Arabia, and India not just for healing but also for dye, and as food.[198] Its use in Europe dates back at least to the Middle Ages, where it was used medicinally and also as a dye for cheese. Today it is not just a medicinal plant but a decorative one, adorning parks and gardens in Europe and throughout the world. Plants sold in your local gardening center under the name "marigold" are not typically calendula, however.

What is it good for?

Soothing wounds, especially abrasions, cuts, sunburn. The traditional evidence for calendula's use as a treatment for wounds is strong. It has been used for centuries, first in the ancient Near East, eventually in Europe and North America for wounds, especially those that

required a treatment with soothing properties (for example, irritations, eczema, scrapes, and insect bites). Italian folk medicine used it as an anti-inflammatory.[199] The Eclectic School cites its use as a vulnerary for ulcers, and burns. ◊ ◊ ◆ ◆ ◆

Laboratory analysis reveals possible bacteria-fighting chemicals,[200] antiviral chemicals,[201] and triterpenoids,[202] which are anti-inflammatory compounds that have been shown to speed wound healing in animal studies.[203] A very preliminary, poorly controlled, 2004 study showed that women receiving radiation treatment for breast cancer experienced less severe dermatitis (skin irritation, redness and pain due to radiation burns) when they were treated with calendula cream twice

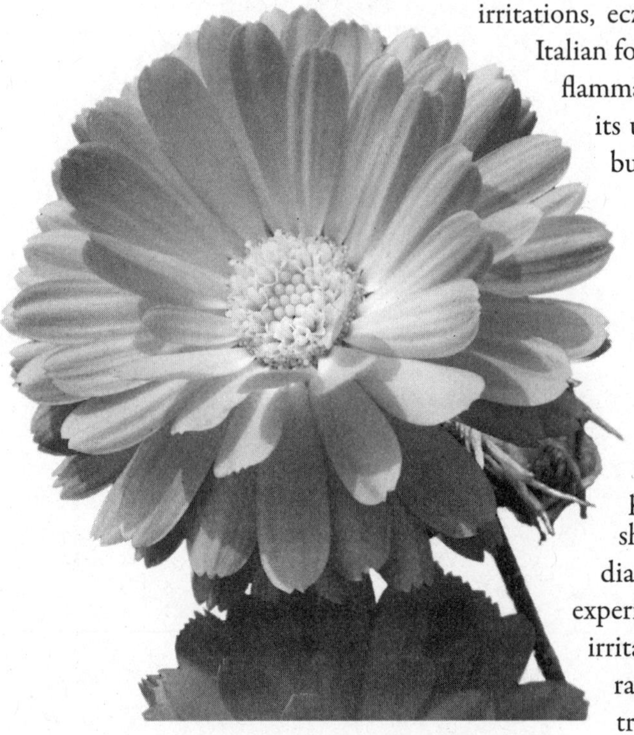

Calendula, *Calendula officinalis*

a day.[204] A second study with five volunteers found that artificially induced abrasions healed more quickly when treated with calendula.[205] A third showed accelerated healing of venous leg ulcers that were treated with calendula.[206] Though human trials are still small scale and poorly controlled, the tradition combined with the laboratory and animal evidence is strong enough that Germany's Commission E recommends it for wound healing, especially slow healing wounds.[207]

Fungal infections. Reports of calendula's anti-fungal properties are mixed. We have no experimental evidence for anti-fungal properties.[208] The tradition as a treatment for fungal infections is not as strong as that for wounds. However, the soothing properties of calendula may be a welcome relief from an itchy fungal infection.

Warts. European tradition says that a poultice of crushed stems and leaves can help soften warts and make them easily removable. Calendula may also have some antiviral properties, though we don't know that it kills wart virus. In short, we have no scientific or cross-cultural corroboration for this use.

How do you use it?

Infusion. Make an infusion for use as a wash or compress. Pour 1 cup of boiling water over ½ teaspoon of dried flowers and infuse for 10 minutes.[209]

Infused oil. Infused oil can be made by adding 3 ounces fresh ground calendula petals to 10 ounces oil. The oil is made using the hot infusion method.[210]

Tincture. Two options are possible for calendula tincture: 1:5 tincture in 90% alcohol[211] or 1:9 in 20% alcohol.[212] Dilute the tincture at least 1:3 with freshly boiled water for topical use[213] or use two droppers full of the tincture to a cup of water to make a mouth rinse good for canker sores.

Ointment. Powdered calendula can be mixed into a carrier ointment for topical use.[214] Commercial preparations are also available.

Dosage: How much do you use?

No toxic reactions have been reported for calendula.[215] A probable effective dosage is one gram of the whole flower, 1–2.5 teaspoons (5–12 ml) of the tincture per day, split into three doses. The ointment or tincture can be applied topically several times per day.[216] A 2–5% preparation has been deemed safe by the German Commission E and the European Scientific Cooperative on Phytotherapy (ESCOP).[217]

What should you be aware of before using it?

Evidence for effective topical use is much stronger than the evidence for effective internal use. Though tradition has it that internal use of calendula is safe,[218] the long-term effects of internal use have not been studied. Using calendula topically only is a conservative, but reasonable course of action.

Though calendula has a largely safe reputation, adverse reactions, including skin and eye irritation, have been reported.[219] In one study, 2% of the people using topical calendula had an allergic reaction to it. Calendula can also magnify allergic reaction to other substances used in conjunction with it (fragrances, other herbs, etc.).[220]

If you are allergic to ragweed or any other plant in the *Aster/Compositae* family, you are likely to be allergic to calendula as well. Allergies to calendula can be severe. At least one case of anaphylactic shock is on the books.[221]

Some herbalists advise against using calendula during pregnancy.[222] We don't know enough to know whether it's safe or not.

Calendula may lower blood pressure when taken internally. Use caution when combining it with other drugs or herbs that also lower blood pressure. (See Chapter 5 for a list.)

We don't know enough about calendula to know if it's safe for children.[223]

Calendula is also used in homeopathic medicines. If you buy calendula cream, be aware of whether the cream is prepared as an herbal remedy or a homeopathic remedy because the two preparations are very different.

Calendula is only one of several plants in the *Asteraceae* family that bear the name "marigold." Other marigolds—corn marigolds, desert marigolds, and the French marigolds commonly seen in the lawn and garden section of home improvement stores—do not have the same medicinal properties.

Capsicum

Scientific name: *Capsicum* spp., especially *Capsicum frutescens*

Also known as capsicum, chilies, chili peppers, Tabasco pepper, paprika, cayenne, peppers

Capsicum, the pepper genus, contains at least fifty varieties. Among the best known are *Capsicum annuum*, which includes bell peppers, jalapeños, paprika, and the chiltepin; *Capsicum frutescens*, which includes the cayenne and Tabasco peppers; *Capsicum chinense*, which includes the mouth-searing habanero and Scotch bonnet peppers; and *Capsicum pubescens* and *Capsicum baccatum*, lesser known South American peppers. Originally native to South America, peppers are now grown throughout the world both for medicinal and culinary purposes. It is the fruit of this plant, the whole red peppers, that contain the medicinal compound. They are picked when fully ripe, dried, and often ground to a powder.

The substance that gives chili peppers their medicinal value is also what gives them their heat. This compound, capsaicin (8-methyl-N-vanillyl-6-nonenamide), is an irritant that serves to protect the pepper from herbivores. Plants with more capsaicin were less

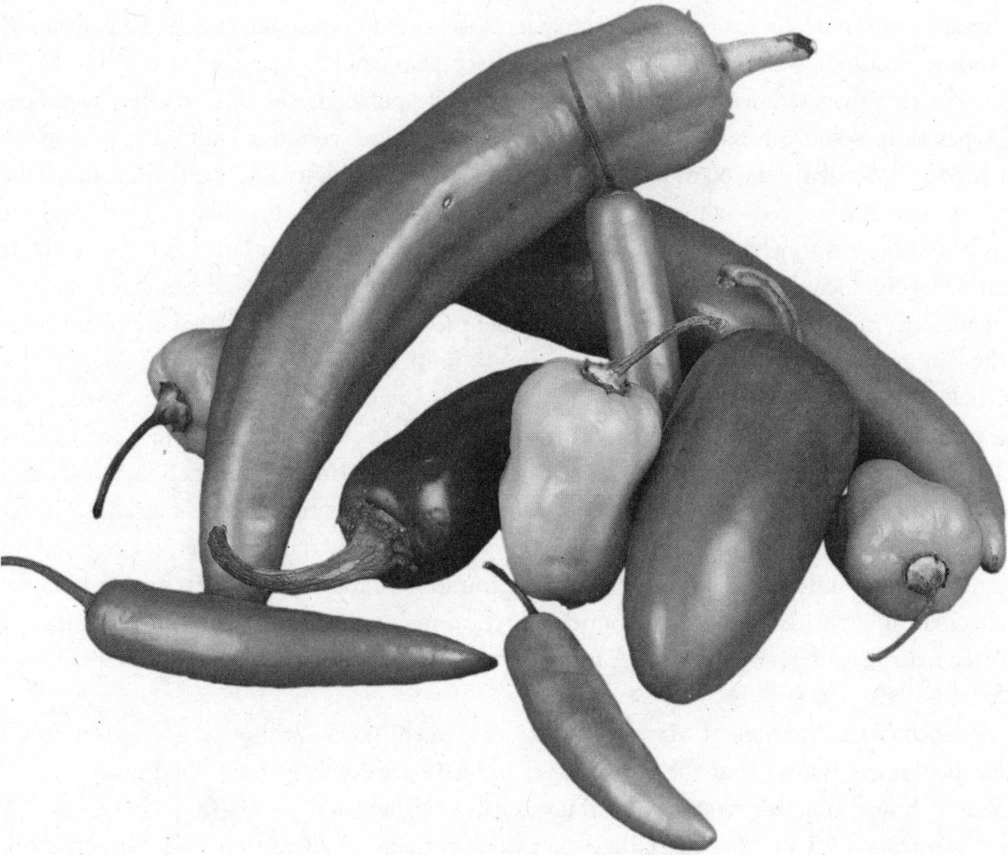

An assortment of peppers of the *Capsicum* genus

likely to be eaten and so were more likely to reproduce. Over the generations, that process naturally selected for ever hotter peppers. Capsaicin is also what gives self-defense pepper sprays their punch.

What is it good for?

Muscle aches. The Eclectic School recommended peppers for "muscular rheumatism." Tradition has it that capsicum is especially effective on painful muscle spasms in areas of shoulder, arm and spine. The mechanism by which capsaicin relieves pain is now beginning to be understood. Some of its effects are merely diversionary.[224] The sensations on the skin take the mind away from pain deeper in the body. But the effects go beyond diversion to the neurological. When the body is continually exposed to capsaicin, sensory neurons are depleted of neurotransmitters. The cause of the pain remains, but the pain signal no longer reaches the brain because of the lack of neurotransmitters. The result is a reduction in sensation of pain. When the exposure is discontinued, the neurons recover and the pain returns if the cause of the pain is still present.[225]

Clinical studies have demonstrated this pain-relieving effect. In a study of low back pain, capsaicin cream decreased pain and increased mobility significantly better than a placebo.[226] Another study showed similar benefits to low back pain from a capsaicin plaster.[227] In 2007, surgeons began experimenting with an ultrastrong, ultrapurified (to avoid infection) capsaicin preparation. Volunteers had capsaicin introduced to surgical wounds to minimize postoperative pain.[228] Similarly, the National Institutes of Health is experimenting with capsaicin for the severe pain of advanced cancer sufferers. Both of the 2007 studies are still in progress, and the jury is still out as to whether they will show benefit, but the fact that large-scale experiments are being conducted by major medical organizations shows a beginning acceptance on the part of Western medicine of capsaicin's pain relieving properties.[229] The FDA has approved over-the-counter capsaicin preparations for this use.

Relieving joint pain caused by injury or arthritis. The mechanism by which capsaicin alleviates joint pain when applied topically is the same as the way it relieves muscle pain. The 1918 U.S. Dispensatory recommends capsicum ointment (made from peppers, lard, and paraffin) as a counterirritant for sprains, bruises, and rheumatism. Topical application reduces pain and swelling from arthritis in rats.[230] In a human trial, however, it provided no pain relief for sufferers of TMJ.[231] One study found help for osteoarthritis but no help for rheumatoid arthritis.[232] Another found reduction in knee pain for both rheumatoid and osteoarthritis sufferers.[233] The FDA has approved over-the-counter capsaicin preparations for this use.

Antibiotics. The ancient Mayans used extracts of chilies as antibiotics. Modern research has begun to discover that the pepper does indeed have some antimicrobial properties.[234] Exactly how those properties can be of use is still unknown.

Treating colds and flu. The Cherokee used it for colds.[235] The 1918 U.S. Dispensatory recommended capsicum tincture for "sluggish conditions of the throat." It also has been used traditionally to help sweat out a fever.[236] Capsaicin irritates mucus membranes causing the nose to run. In that way, it can help with colds that clog the nose and sinuses, but it is unlikely to benefit colds where the primary symptom is already a runny nose. A study of a nasal spray containing capsaicin found that though it was quite painful, it did reduce nasal obstruction and nasal secretion in patients with vasomotor rhinitis (a chronic runny nose not caused by a virus or allergies) over the course of a month.[237] Such a nasal spray would probably be ill advised for colds, however, because the treatment reached its full benefit over the course of a month, long after a typical cold would be over. Capsicum has been tried with some success against tonsillitis, but this study was not very large or well controlled, so it's not sure what exactly the benefits might be.[238]

Increasing athletic performance. One study found that adding 10 g of red pepper to men's diet increased the carbohydrate oxidation without increasing total energy expenditure for 150 minutes after the meal.[239] In other words, it increased the ability of the body to burn carbohydrates for fuel without increasing the need for that fuel. A similar study found that 10 g of red pepper added to breakfast increased carbohydrate oxidation in male long distance runners both at rest and during exercise.[240] A third study of Japanese women, on the other hand, found that adding red pepper to a meal actually decreased carbohydrate oxidation. Though theoretically increasing carbohydrate oxidation could make more fuel available for athletic performance, it is by no means certain that (1) A direct link exists between carbohydrate oxidation and improved performance, and (2) capsaicin does indeed increase carbohydrate oxidation in all athletes.

Slowing bleeding. One traditional use is to take a couple of capsules or drink a half-teaspoon of capsicum in a glass of water to slow bleeding. We have no scientific backing or cross-cultural attestation for this use.

How do you use it?

Commercial preparations. By far, the safest way to use capsaicin topically is to use it in a commercial preparation. It is really the only way to control the amount of capsaicin you are putting on your skin. Too little won't give you the relief you seek; too much can damage your skin.

Infusions. Make an infusion using ½ teaspoon of dried peppers to one cup of boiling water. Stir and let the mixture sit for ten minutes. If you wish, you can strain it at this time, or you can use it without straining. Use 1 tablespoon of this infusion with a cup of water to make tea. The tea can be used to help unplug the nose during a cold. It can also be applied to a compress and used for sprains, bruising, and joint pain.[241]

Infused oil. Add 25 g of powder to two cups sunflower oil and heat in a double boiler for two hours. This infused oil is good as a massage oil for joint pain. Don't use it with additional heat (such as a heating pad, hot water bottle or warm flannel), however, because this increases the chance of irritation and blistering. If you want to take a hot bath or shower, do so first, and then let the skin cool before applying capsaicin.[242]

Tincture. 95% alcohol 1:5 (pepper to alcohol)[243] Dilute the tincture 1:10 to use as a liniment.[244]

A vinegar tincture can be made by boiling 1 tablespoon of pepper with 1 pint of cider vinegar. While the vinegar is still hot, pour it into a clean bottle without straining out the pepper.[245]

Muscle rubs: A muscle rub can be made by adding ¼ teaspoon powdered capsicum to 1 cup grain alcohol. Of course, you should use this rub topically only.[246]

Dosage: How much do you use?

The safety of chilis depends largely on how strong they are. The "heat" of the various peppers in the capsicum genus varies from nonexistent to extremely dangerous. The unit of measurement for chili "heat" is the Scoville unit. Pure capsaicin rates at 15,000,000 Scoville units; bell peppers rate at 0 Scoville units. Cayenne peppers of the species *frutescens* rate at 30,000–50,000 units.[247] If you use stronger peppers, you must adjust the dose appropriately. It cannot be stressed enough: some varieties of peppers can cause blisters and burns bad enough to strip the skin right off you. Know what you have in your hand before trying to use it medicinally.

If you are buying your capsicum preparations over the counter, Commission E recommends liquid preparations not contain more than .01% pure capsaicin.

Topical preparations. Poultices and compresses should deliver no more than 40 g of capsaicinoids per square centimeter.[248] Creams containing .025% and .075% capsaicin are available over the counter in both the United States and Canada. Stronger "back-alley" creams can be found, but are unadvisable. Don't use topical preparations for longer than 2 days; 14 days must pass before a new application can be used in the same location.[249] Generally, the preparation will penetrate the skin in thirty minutes.[250] If you'd like, you can wash the rest off the surface at that time, for example, to avoid spreading it to undesirable areas while you sleep. Warm soapy water or a mild vinegar solution will wash capsicum from the skin.[251]

Oral preparations. Be *very* cautious when using capsicum in capsules. The benefits of oral capsicum supplementation (beyond normal use as a spice) are questionable.[252] The danger to liver and digestion are, however, well documented. The main problem with capsicum in capsules is that your mouth will not be able to give you feedback about the amount of irritation your stomach and liver will have to endure. It is safe to say that making and consuming your own capsicum capsules contains more risk than reward. If, however, you insist on making your own oral preparations, use no more than 30–120 mg of dried *Capsicum frutescens* per day, taken with a cup of water.[253]

What should you be aware of before using it?

Be very cautious using any preparation that isn't standardized. Too much capsaicin can cause blistering, burns, hypersensitivity, skin ulcers, dermatitis, and temporary and permanent nerve damage.[254]

Don't use topical preparations for longer than 2 days; 14 days must pass before a new application can be used in the same location.[255]

Don't use capsicum on or near open wounds.[256]

Be very careful if you are taking capsicum as a capsule. Too much is hard on the liver and the lining of the gastrointestinal system. If you eat the peppers, the heat is self limiting, but if you take them as a capsule, you don't have that feedback. Too much can cause diarrhea, stomach pain, and a burning sensation during bowel movements.[257] It is possible to die from too much capsicum.[258]

If you have high blood pressure, check with a doctor before using capsicum medicinally.[259]

Don't take capsicum orally if you have inflammation of mucous membranes or excessive mucus, because it can aggravate these conditions. Don't use it without consulting a doctor first if you are prone to gastrointestinal problems.[260]

Too much capsicum can cause gastroesophageal reflux (GER) symptoms.[261] Contrary to popular belief, capsicum does *not* aggravate hemorrhoid symptoms.[262] It may even help protect the lining of the stomach against aspirin.[263]

Don't leave a capsicum compress on for a long time, and don't use it if you are likely to fall asleep while it's on. Too much exposure can cause irritation and even blistering. If you have fair or sensitive skin, try a little of the infusion or oil on a small area before using. Keep it out of your eyes and mucous membranes. Don't apply to broken skin.

Handle capsicum with respect. If you're grinding dried capsicum, wear a mask. If working with fresh peppers, either avoid touching the pepper directly or wear gloves. After handling peppers, never touch your eyes, nose, ears, or groin without washing your hands thoroughly. Don't use the seeds because they tend to be stronger.

Be careful training with your muscles and joints under the influence of capsicum. When you use capsicum you are masking pain signals that may be your body's way of trying to tell you something. Masking pain can lead to further injury.

Capsicum can be used topically on adults, and on school-aged children if appropriate caution is observed. It shouldn't be used on children younger than school-aged.

Capsicum may interfere with MAO inhibitors and antihypertensive therapy, and may increase hepatic metabolism of drugs.[264]

If you tend to be anemic, be careful about taking capsicum internally because it can interfere with iron absorption.[265]

Caraway

Scientific name: *Carum carvi*

Also known as *Apium carvi,* Persian cumin

Caraway is a member of the carrot family; the relationship is best seen in the shape of its feathery leaves. It is native to Europe and Asia Minor, but is now cultivated throughout the world. In some parts of the United States, wild caraway is now considered a noxious weed. The part of the plant that's used medicinally is commonly called the "seed," though it is actually a small ribbed fruit. When dried, this fruit looks like a small, crescent-shaped seed.

The smell, similar to anise, comes from carvone and limonene, essential oils in the seeds. Carvone is an antiseptic. Limonene is an antiseptic and antispasmodic.

What is it good for?

Digestion. Caraway is best known as an aid to help expel trapped gas in the intestines. It is also good for a jumpy stomach. The 1918 U.S. Dispensatory cites its use as a stomachic and carminative. The Eclectic School also cites its use as a carminative. Commission E recommends it for flatulence. Its use as a digestive aid, however, is largely untested and a matter of some dispute.[266] Only one preliminary, less than rigorous study has been done on caraway's value in treating dyspepsia. It showed that caraway appeared to help mild non-ulcer dyspepsia, but the effect may have been attributable to nothing more than time.[267] A combination study—caraway and peppermint taken together—showed that the combination worked as well at treating dyspepsia as Cisapride® (a prescription medication for dyspepsia, subsequently taken off the market due to troubling side effects).[268]

Kills bacteria. In an in vitro study, caraway's essential oils worked well against several bacteria.[269] The implications of these results for human use, however, are not clear.

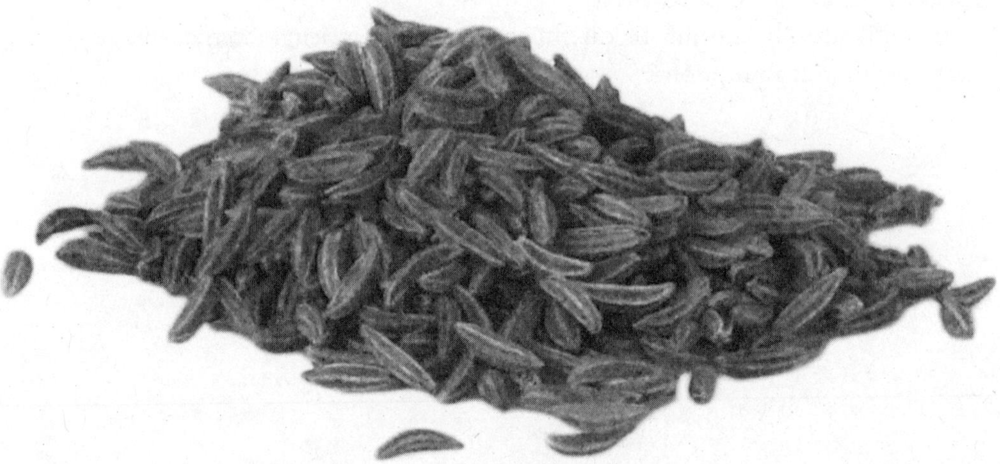

Caraway "seeds," *Carum carvi*

How do you use it?

Store caraway seeds between 40 and 75 degrees Fahrenheit (2–35 degrees Centigrade). Temperatures above 75 will degrade the essential oils.

Essential Oil. The seeds are dried before being used medicinally. The essential oil is derived from the seed by commercial steam distillation. Caraway oil is one of the few essential oils that can be taken internally in small doses. The traditional way to take it is to put a couple drops on a sugar cube.

Infusion. A tea can be made from the seeds to drink after meals. One traditional remedy involves one ounce of seed cold infused in a pint of water.[270] "Bruise" or slightly crush the seeds before making the infusion. Alternatively, the seeds can be chewed and swallowed.

Tincture. Scandinavians have a traditional "digestive" liquor made by adding the essential oil of caraway to a vodka-like distillation. Tradition says it helps digestion of rich meals. Evidence for this property is not found outside of tradition, however.

Dosage: How much do you use?

No upper dose has been set, as caraway seems relatively safe at most sane doses. A typical dose is 1–2 cups of the infusion daily for an adult.[271] Or 2–3 drops of the essential oil on a sugar cube for no more than six drops per day.[272]

What should you be aware of before using it?

Caraway is on the FDA's list of substances generally recognized as safe.[273] However, long-term intake of larger doses of the essential oil can cause kidney and liver damage.[274]

The essential oil of caraway is an irritant. It especially irritates mucous membranes and can cause contact dermatitis.

Some herbalists recommend that women avoid medicinal doses of caraway while pregnant, though this recommendation is based on conjecture from caraway's antispasmodic properties, not from any reports of miscarriage.[275]

If you are allergic to *dong quai*, anise, carrot, celery, dill, or parsley you have an increased chance of being allergic to caraway.

Catnip

Scientific name: *Nepeta cataria*

Also known as catmint, catwort, field balm, catrup

Catnip is a perennial herb—some would say "weed"—of the mint family. It grows wild throughout the United States and Canada. The leaf and flower are used medicinally.

It makes cats a bit crazy, but it will help you settle yourself. This is a good herb for those days when you have something on your mind that's giving you a headache, making your stomach do flip flops, and keeping you from sleeping. Tradition says that catnip is good for all three of these problems.

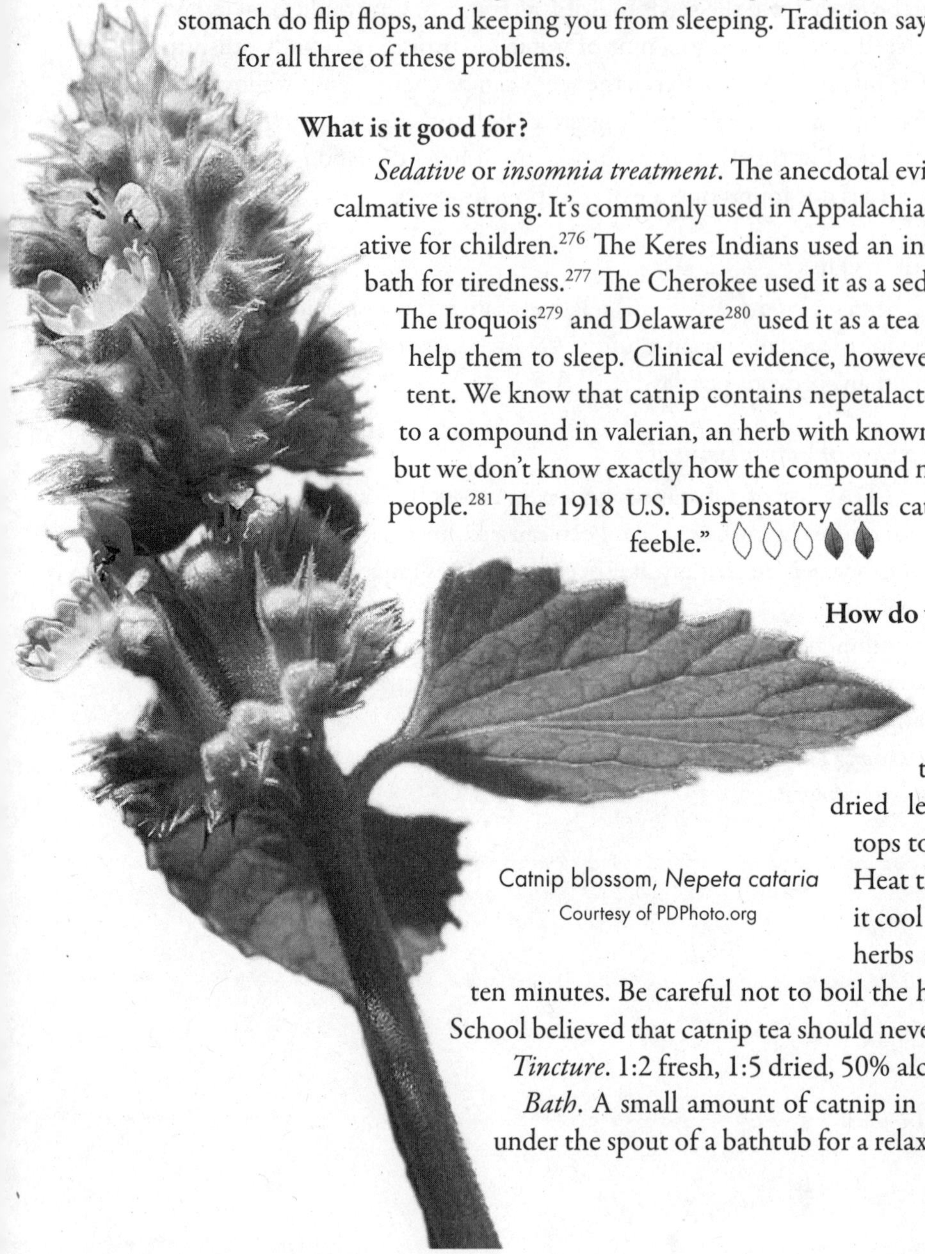

Catnip blossom, *Nepeta cataria*
Courtesy of PDPhoto.org

What is it good for?

Sedative or *insomnia treatment*. The anecdotal evidence for catnip as a calmative is strong. It's commonly used in Appalachia, especially as a calmative for children.[276] The Keres Indians used an infusion of catnip in a bath for tiredness.[277] The Cherokee used it as a sedative for hysterics.[278] The Iroquois[279] and Delaware[280] used it as a tea to soothe babies and help them to sleep. Clinical evidence, however, is all but nonexistent. We know that catnip contains nepetalactone, which is similar to a compound in valerian, an herb with known sedative properties, but we don't know exactly how the compound nepetalactione affects people.[281] The 1918 U.S. Dispensatory calls catnip "therapeutically feeble."

How do you use it?

Infusion. To relax before bed, brew a cup of tea using two teaspoons of the dried leaves and flowering tops to one cup of water.[282] Heat the water to a boil, let it cool slightly, then add the herbs and steep for about ten minutes. Be careful not to boil the herbs.[283] The Eclectic School believed that catnip tea should never be sweetened.

Tincture. 1:2 fresh, 1:5 dried, 50% alcohol.[284]

Bath. A small amount of catnip in a sack can be placed under the spout of a bathtub for a relaxing bath.

Dosage: How much do you use?

Commercial preparations will include dosage information.

If using an infusion, limit yourself to six teaspoons of the dry herb per day split between three cups of tea. If using a tincture, the dose is one teaspoon, three times per day.[285] These doses are the absolute most you'll want to take, and then only on an occasional basis. Catnip causes nasty symptoms in some people—headaches, drowsiness, and stomach irritation. It also contains tannins, which are hard on the body in high or frequent doses. Consequently, if you want a more conservative dose, that dose is one cup of tea per day, before bedtime, for occasional use only.[286] No matter which dose you decide on, you should avoid using catnip long-term.

What should you be aware of before using it?

Catnip gives some people headaches.

Some people report becoming draggy or even punchy from catnip. Make sure you know its effects on you before you try driving or training with it in your system. It may compound the effect of other sedative herbs. (See Chapter 5 for a list.)

One case of central nervous system depression has been reported in a toddler who swallowed a large amount of catnip.[287]

Too much will cause vomiting.[288]

Catnip agents are tannin substances.[289] Tannins shouldn't be used internally over the long term. Animal studies indicated that catnip might have negative side effects after long-term usage. Limit use to occasional use only.[290]

Catnip tea can have a diuretic effect.[291]

Don't use it during pregnancy.

Cat's Claw

Scientific name: *Uncaria tomentosa*

Also known as *una de gato*

Cat's claw comes from the inside of the bark of a South American rainforest vine. The name comes from the hook-like thorns it uses to climb trees.

The indigenous people of Peru's rain forests use the cat's claw for a number of purposes including arthritis, bone aches, and deep cuts.[292] Its first introduction to Western herbal medicine was in the 1970s. Since the 1990s, its use has been on the rise in Europe and North America. Fifteen years later, that use is still largely in the experimental stage. Doctors and herbalists are still investigating its ability to treat conditions as different as AIDS and ulcers, Crohn's disease and cancer.[293] Yet cat's claw is not on the Commission E recommended list because at this point we don't know enough about it to know about its dangers, and we don't have enough experience either clinical or anecdotal to predict what it might be effective for.

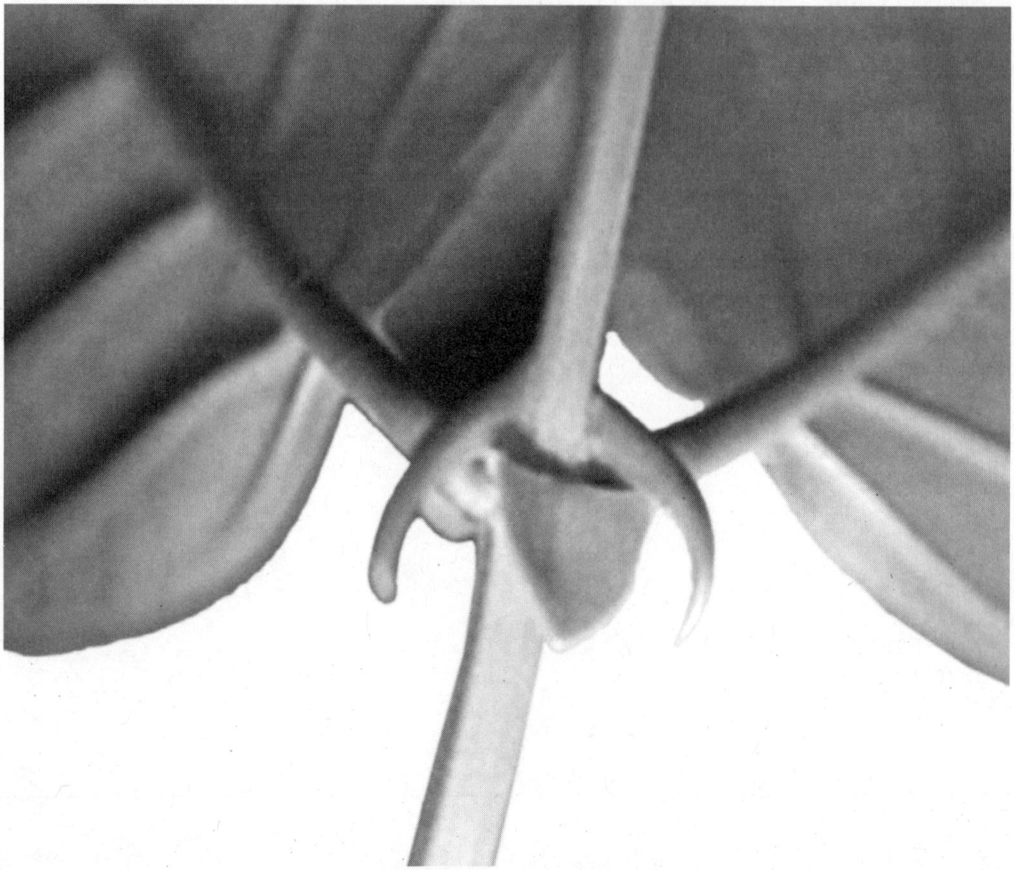

Cat's Claw, *Uncaria tomentosa*

Courtesy of Johannes Keplinger

What is it good for?

Arthritis and other joint pain. The Asháninka people of Peru have traditionally used the herb for joint pain. Research suggests a good scientific basis for this use. The beta-sitosterol and carboxyl alkyl esters in cat's claw are anti-inflammatories. In rat-paw studies, cat's claw was shown to have anti-inflammatory effects.[294] Preliminary clinical trials for rheumatoid arthritis show modest benefits.[295] Preliminary research for osteoarthritis show significant benefits.[296] Though evidence for this use is still small-scale, it is promising.

Immune stimulant. Cat's claw contains carboxyl alkyl esters, which are thought to be an immune stimulant. It is sometimes prescribed in Europe for this purpose.[297] In mouse studies cat's claw shows some immune stimulation effect.[298] However, research is very slim and not backed by clinical trials. Some anecdotal evidence for this use can be found, but it, too, is lacking.

How do you use it?

Commercially prepared capsules. Cat's claw is typically taken internally. The most common preparation is the commercially prepared capsules containing dried, powdered cat's claw.

Decoction. If you can get a hold of the bark, you can make a standard decoction, adding about a half teaspoon of lemon juice or vinegar to each cup of water to help extract more of the active ingredients.[299] Take cat's claw between meals.[300]

Dosage: How much do you use?

The bottom line is that we don't know what a good dose is. A typical dose is 3–5 g daily of the powdered vine or ½–1 cup of a decoction once a day.[301] However, the largest commercial source of cat's claw is rural Peru, and that presents a problem. Because the amount of active ingredient in the preparation varies with the age of the tree and how it is harvested, and because Latin America is yet to establish a reputation for consistency in its preparation of herbs, one cannot be quite sure how much active ingredient is contained in any given preparation.[302] In Germany and Austria, cat's claw has been standardized, but it is available only by physician's prescription.[303]

What should you be aware of before using it?

Preliminary research shows a no negative effects on either blood or liver and no significant side effects with short-term use.[304] Animal trials show a relatively low level of toxicity, but we don't know how people are going to react if they take the herb long-term.[305]

Cat's claw may cause low blood pressure.[306]

It may have an additive effect if you are taking anticoagulants.[307] If you plan to have surgery, tell your surgeon you have been taking cat's claw and discontinue use. Be cautious when using it in conjunction with other herbs known or suspected of increasing the risk of bleeding. (See Chapter 5 for a list.)

It may have immunostimulant properties and should not be taken by anyone with an overactive immune system.

It may have some antifertility properties. That was one of the traditional uses by the Peruvian Indians; however, we don't know how effective it is as a contraceptive. It should not be relied on as such.[308]

The molecular structure of some of the alkaloids in cat's claw is similar to morphine.[309] Know how the herb affects you before driving or training under its influence.

If stomach upset or diarrhea is severe or lasts longer than three or four days, discontinue use.[310]

If you are allergic to coffee, be careful taking cat's claw because they are members of the same family.

A related species, *Uncaria guianensis*, is more common in Europe. South Americans consider the two to be interchangeable.[311] However recent research has shown important differences not only between the species, but between subspecies of *Uncaria tomentosa*.[312] This section applies to *Uncaria tomentosa*, with the proviso that we may soon find that the research results don't apply to the entire species.

It is *not* the same as cat claw acacia (*Acacia greggii*) of the American Southwest. Cat claw acacia can be poisonous. It is also not interchangeable with the other twelve species in Peru that are also called *una de gato*. Make sure the cat claw you get has the species name on it.

Cayenne

(See Capsicum)

Chamomile

Scientific name: *Chamaemelum nobile, Matricaria recutita*

Also known as babuna, camamila, ground apple, manzanilla, may-then, nervine, pin heads, whig-plant

Chamomile is a small annual plant native to Eastern Europe and Western Asia. Because of its usefulness, it is now grown throughout Europe, Australia, and North America. Chamomile consists of two completely different species. *Chamaemelum nobile,* Roman Chamomile, is otherwise known as *Anthemis nobilis. Matricaria recutita* is commonly known as German chamomile. The medicinal properties of the two are reputed to be very similar, but the chemical breakdown shows profound differences.[313] Modern research has focused on *M. recutita,* German or "true" chamomile, which appears to be slightly stronger.[314] The flower is used for infusions, tinctures, as well as for the essential oil, which can be quite expensive.

Chamomile is one of the most popular herbal remedies in Europe. Since Roman times, it's been used for a wide variety of ailments. The Germans refer to it as *alles zutraut*, which means "capable of anything."[315] In Germany it's used by adults and children for medicine, cosmetics, and beverage; and for conditions as varied as colds, ulcers, wounds, and insomnia. A gentle sedative, also good for relieving indigestion, it's known as an after-dinner tea. It also contains several compounds (chamazulene, a-bisabolol, chrysoplenin, chrysoplenol, jaceidin) which have an anti-inflammatory effect.[316]

What is it good for?

Insomnia from anxiety. The herb has strong traditional use. The Eclectic School prescribed chamomile for nervous unrest. It contains apigenin, which binds to benzodiazepine receptors in the brain. This mechanism causes a mild sedative effect that affects anxiety levels but does not slow muscle function.[317] Studies in mice show that chamomile reduces anxiety and promotes sleep.[318]

Sores. Chamomile wash has traditionally been used for sores, particularly itchy and oozing ones. One traditional use of chamomile is for sunburns that blister and ooze. A related species, *Matricaria discoidea* DC., was used in North America by the Native Americans for sores. European oral tradition says that rinsing the mouth with cooled chamomile tea helps with mouth inflammation or injury.

The exact mechanism by which chamomile aids in the healing of wounds is un-

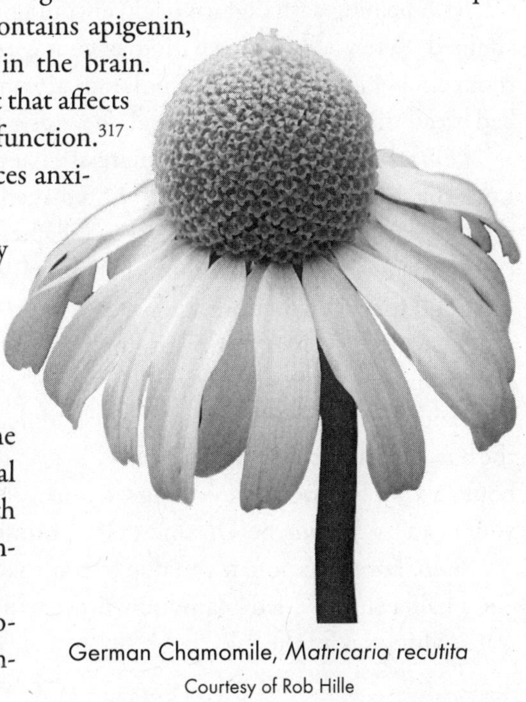

German Chamomile, *Matricaria recutita*

Courtesy of Rob Hille

known, but evidence suggests that it promotes tissue granulation and regeneration. In other words, it attracts the cells that build new tissue.[319] Several compounds in chamomile have anti-inflammatory properties,[320] and the benefits of those properties are well documented in animals.[321] It may also have some minor antibacterial properties.[322] It contains important flavonoids, including quercimeritin, which is involved in the reduction of capillary fragility.[323] The clinical research for this use, however, is still sketchy. One study found that mice with induced itching were helped by oral chamomile extracts.[324] A study of people healing after dermabrasion to remove tattoos showed that chamomile extract helped dry oozing sores and so promoted healing.[325]

Colds. This use dates back to Roman times. Roman physicians prescribed chamomile for colds, flu, and fever. In Germany it is one of the most popular herbs for cold treatment as well. We don't, however, have nearly as much research as one might expect for this use. A single 1990 study showed that people who inhaled steam containing chamomile extract during a cold reported a decrease in symptoms.[326]

How do you use it?

Infusion. Infusion is the most common way of using chamomile despite the fact that the essential oils in chamomile are not very water-soluble. Only 10–15% of chamomile's essential oil is extracted into an infusion.[327] Still people throughout the centuries have used it in this way. To make an infusion of chamomile, use the standard infusion method. Use ½ to 2 teaspoons of dried flowers for each 8 ounces of water. Pour very hot (not boiling) water over the flowers, cover, steep for 5 minutes, and then strain.[328] It makes a good after dinner tea, both helping with digestion and encouraging sleep. You can also add a quart or so of the strained tea to your evening bath to encourage sleep. Or you can use the strained infusion at room temperature as a rinse for inflammation or injuries to the mouth. It may also help with bad breath if the problem is an oral one, not a digestive one.

Ointment for wounds. Commercial chamomile ointments and lotions are available. Look for at least 3% chamomile.[329] Or you can make your own from the essential oil (using method seven for creams and salves in Chapter 3).

Essential oil. Put a few drops of chamomile essential oil in a half ounce of carrier oil.[330] It is good for skin irritations.

Tincture. 1:5, 50% (for dried flowers). For colds, use a tincture of chamomile (2–3 tablespoons) in a quart of hot water. Heat the water until steaming, add the chamomile tincture, and then inhale the steam slowly and deeply for ten minutes, keeping your head and the bowl of water covered with a towel to trap the steam. The effects peak after around a half hour and last for two to three hours. If you feel a bit dizzy while inhaling the steam, uncover your head for a moment. Dizziness is less pronounced with lower doses of chamomile.[331]

Bath. For relaxation, if you don't want to drink chamomile tea, you can use it in a bath. Tie a half a cup of dried chamomile flowers in some cheesecloth. Lay it under the running water while you fill the tub.[332]

Dosage: How much do you use?

Chamomile is on the FDA list of herbs that are generally recognized as safe (GRAS). Though higher doses have been used for specific, medically supervised treatments (e.g. ulcers), the following are common doses for internal uses:

Tincture. Use 1/8 to 1 teaspoon three times a day is a typical internal dose.[333]

Tea or infusion. Use one cup (8 ounces) of tea, three to four times per day.

Commercially prepared capsules. 400 to 1,600 mg taken by mouth daily in divided doses is a typical dose.[334] Products that are standardized are typically standardized to 1% apigenin.[335]

Bath. No more than 50 g per one quart of water.[336]

What should you be aware of before using it?

Chamomile is safe for long-term use if you use it at recommended doses. At large doses it can cause vomiting.[337]

Don't take it if you are taking warfarin or other anti-coagulants.[338] If you plan to have surgery, tell your surgeon you have been taking chamomile and discontinue use. Be cautious when using it in conjunction with other herbs known or suspected of increasing the risk of bleeding. (See Chapter 5 for a list.)

Don't use the essential oil if you are pregnant as it is a uterine stimulant.

Allergic reactions are not unheard of. At least one case of anaphylactic shock has been reported.[339] If you are allergic to members of the *Compositae* family (ragweed, daisies, aster, etc.) you have a greater chance of being allergic to chamomile. Some people are sensitive to topical chamomile. If you're prone to dermatitis, try a little before using chamomile more extensively. Some people will get headaches from drinking the tea.

Avoid skin contact with the undiluted essential oil. Be careful not to get it into your nose or eyes. It is very strong.

Chamomile is *supposed to* make you drowsy. Don't use it if you plan to drink alcohol—alcohol compounds its effects—or if you need to be alert. It may compound the effect of other sedative herbs. (See Chapter 5 for a list.)

Impurities (adulterants) in chamomile products are common. Get your chamomile from a reputable source.[340]

Though other members of the chamomile genus are thought to have medicinal properties, we don't know much about them, their benefits, or their dangers. Traditional herbalists believe that some are damaging to the lining of the stomach and intestine.[341] It is safest when using chamomile to stick with *Chamaemelum nobile* (*Anthemis nobilis*) and *Matricaria recutita*, because they have a known track record.

Note that wild chamomile, sometimes called dog chamomile or cotula, is a completely different plant with completely different properties.

Chilis

(See Capsicum)

Cinnamon Bark

Scientific name: *Cinnamomum zeylanicum, Cinnamomum verum*

Also known as true cinnamon, cinnamon

Native to Sri Lanka and Southern India, the cinnamon tree grows from twenty to thirty feet tall. To process it, the thin, inner bark is stripped from the tree. This bark curls as it dries into "cinnamon sticks" or quills. Cinnamon is sold in quills or is ground for use as a spice or medicine. The medicinal properties of cinnamon come from the essential oil. This oil is prepared by crushing the bark, macerating it in sea-water, and then distilling out the oil. The essential oil of cinnamon bark is about 90% cinnamaldehyde, a yellow, oily liquid. Cinnamaldehyde, which has antibacterial and anti-inflammatory properties, also contains a very concentrated smell and flavor of cinnamon.

The name cinnamon means "sweet wood." This sweet wood has been a highly prized spice for millennia. Records of it date back to 2800 B.C.E. in China. Before modern refrigeration it was used to preserve meat. As a potent antimicrobial, it helped retard spoilage, and the distinctive taste helped mask the taste of meat that had started to turn.

Two common species of cinnamon are sold in grocery stores in the United States: *Cinnamomum aromaticum* and *Cinnamomum zeylanicum*. *C. aromaticum*, sometimes called cassia cinnamon or just cassia, is a different species from the same genus as true cinnamon. The two have somewhat different but

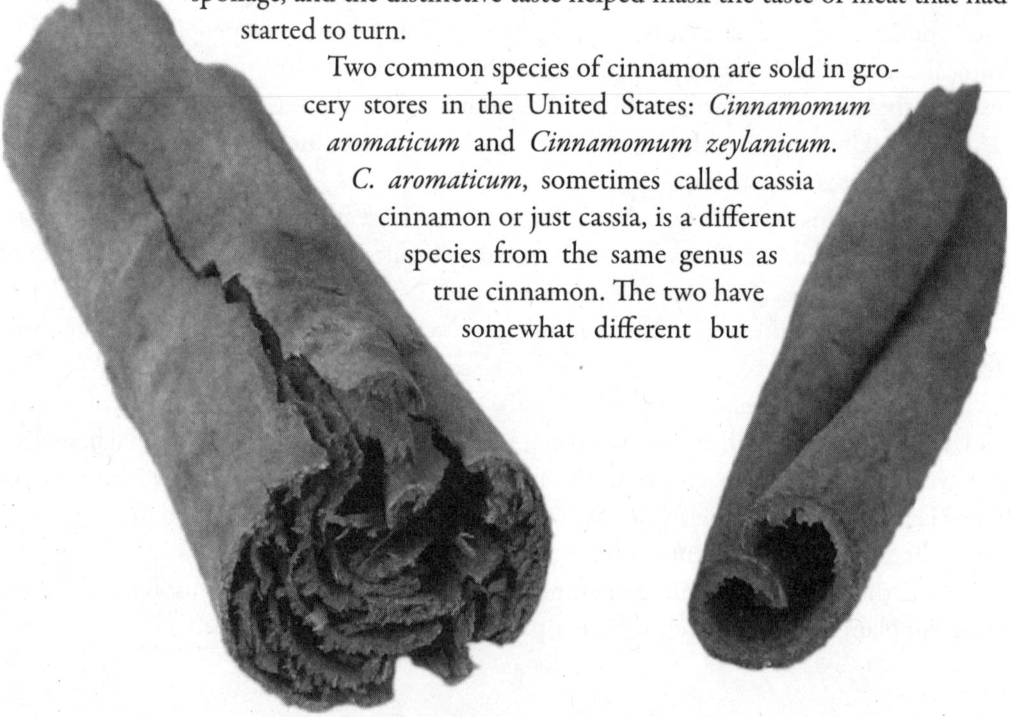

True Cinnamon, *Cinnamomum zeylanicum* (Left) and Cassia Cinnamon, *C. aromaticum*

overlapping medicinal properties. Cassia cinnamon, called *ròu gùi* in Chinese, is one of the fifty fundamental herbs of traditional Chinese medicine. In a typical grocery store, they will both be sold as simply "cinnamon," but you can tell the difference by looking at the quills. True cinnamon sticks (*C. zeylanicum*) curl into a tube, while cassia sticks curl inward from both sides, like a scroll. In some studies, little or no difference was found between the effects of cassia and true cinnamon.[342] In others, slight differences were found.[343] Here we look at the medicinal effects of the *Cinnamomum* genus in general.

What is it good for?

One of the traditional uses for cinnamon is as a treatment for infection, particularly for fungal infections such as athlete's foot. Honey and cinnamon together are a traditional remedy for fungal infections. The 1918 U.S. Dispensatory, for example, notes the powerful germicidal effects of cinnamon oil. Since 1918, laboratory research has amassed considerable evidence of these antimicrobial properties. One in vitro experiment demonstrated that the essential oil kills the fungi most likely to infect the respiratory tract of people.[344] The essential oil also inhibits candida.[345] Cinnamon has an antimicrobial effect, killing *E. coli*, when added as a preservative to food.[346] It inhibits the growth of listeria.[347] It has a broad antibacterial effect.[348] It is also an antioxidant.[349] The implications of these properties for healing infection, however, have not been tested. 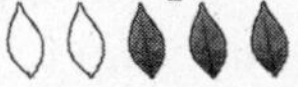

Blood sugar control. Researchers are beginning to study the effects of cinnamon on blood sugar in people with type 2 diabetes. In test-tube studies, one of cinnamon's most active compounds, methylhydroxy chalcone polymer (MHCP) increases glucose metabolism twenty-fold.[350] Similarly, in a study of rats given *Cinnamomum* bark or extracts, a decrease in blood glucose levels was observed in a glucose tolerance test. Similar effects have been observed in human studies though results in people are mixed. A small study of sixty patients with type 2 diabetes in Pakistan found that one gram of cinnamon per day (split between two doses) lowered fasting glucose by 18–29%.[351] Another study, however, found that fasting blood sugar levels did not change for postmenopausal diabetic women who took 1.5 g of cinnamon per day for six weeks.[352] In the studies that found some effect, cassia cinnamon seemed to work a bit better than true cinnamon.[353] 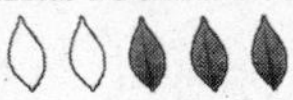

Lowers blood pressure. This effect is seen in rat studies. Supplementing the diet with cinnamon lowered the systolic blood pressure both in spontaneously hypertensive rats and in rats whose blood pressure had been artificially elevated by feeding them sugar.[354] The study was limited to lab animals and hasn't been repeated, but the results are consistent with the fact that cinnamon contains oligomeric proanthocyanidin, which helps improve circulation.[355] 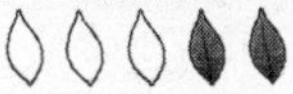

Cholesterol. The same Pakistani study that looked at blood sugar also found that as little as one gram per day of cinnamon lowered triglycerides by 23 to 30%, LDL cholesterol by 7 to 27%, and total cholesterol by 12 to 26% in people with type 2 diabetes.[356] 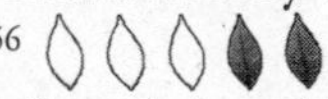

Alertness. A study conducted by a team at Wheeling Jesuit University found that the smell of cinnamon increased alertness and decreased frustration in drivers.[357] 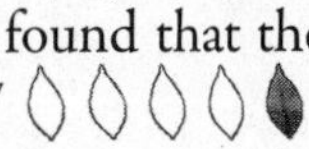

How do you use it?

Decoction. A strong decoction brings out the best in cinnamon bark. Combine the herb with water at a 1:32 ratio. Bring the mixture to a boil slowly, boil for ten minutes, cool until warm, and strain. Pour additional water through the herb to return the volume to 32.[358] MHCP, the compound that helps lower blood sugar and proanthocyanidin, an antioxidant, are both water soluble. Cinnamaldehyde, the essential oil in cinnamon that's an irritant, and coumarin, a toxic component, are significantly less so. For that reason, the best cinnamon preparation for internal use is a decoction.[359] You can also use the decoction on a pad for a compress.

Infused oil. The cinnamaldehyde in the essential oil contains the fungicidal properties of cinnamon. Cinnamaldehyde can only be extracted using oils. Powdered cinnamon infuses well in almond oil. Add the oil to the cinnamon to cover by roughly a half inch. Allow it to infuse in a warm place for fourteen days. Avoid taking oil infusions internally.[360] Be cautious when using infused oils externally because they contain the more dangerous compounds in cinnamon. Try the infused oils on a small patch of skin before using them more widely.

Essential oil. Use the smell of the essential oil as an aid to alertness. Don't inhale it directly from a bottle or diffuser, however, because it is a powerful irritant.

If you are going to use essential oil topically, you must dilute it. A dilution of 1:12 in a carrier oil is the absolute strongest you'd want to use on toenails. For use on skin, you'd want to dilute it much more than that, to roughly 1:50. Even then, patch test it on tough skin (like the heels of your feet) before using it anywhere else, and never use it on your face or other sensitive areas.

The risks of taking cinnamon oil internally vastly outweigh the benefits.

Dosage: How much do you use?

Less than 2 ounces of the essential oil can cause a serious toxic reaction.[361] Too much can kill you. The risks of taking the essential oil internally outweigh the benefits. If, however, you do decide to take it, find yourself professional supervision, and don't take more than .05 to .2 g per day.[362]

One gram (roughly ¼ to ½ teaspoon) of powdered cinnamon per day, split between two doses is enough to yield an effect on blood sugar.[363] Don't take more than 4 g per day.[364]

What should you be aware of before using it?

Cinnamon is on the FDA's generally-recognized-as-safe list.[365] But, again, this list assumes cinnamon in the kind and quantity used in cooking, not the essential oil, and not used in medicinal quantities.

Cinnamon oil is an irritant, particularly to mucous membranes.[366] Cinnamon oil taken internally (sucked from a toothpick or finger) can cause local burning, nausea, and abdominal pain.[367] The 1918 U.S. Dispensatory records an experiment in which a medium-sized dog was killed by six drachms (less than one ounce) of cinnamon oil. The dog apparently died from erosion of the lining of the gastrointestinal system.[368]

Take only water-extracted preparations internally. Oil extracted preparations contain cinnamaldehyde, which is an irritant, and coumarin, which causes cancer and liver damage.[369]

Allergic reactions are possible,[370] as is contact dermatitis.[371] It is possible to become sensitized to cinnamon over time.

Inhaling too much cinnamon dust has caused bronchitis in lab animals.[372]

Avoid medical quantities of cinnamon if you are pregnant. Pregnant lab animals fed cinnamon essential oil showed changes in the embryo.[373]

Decoctions of cinnamon have an effect on blood sugar. If you are diabetic, hypoglycemic, or have other blood sugar issues, check with your doctor before using cinnamon in medicinal quantities.[374]

Cinnamon flower is on the Commission E "Unapproved, Potentially Dangerous Herbs" list because of its likelihood to cause allergic reactions.[375]

Cloves

Scientific name: *Syzygium aromaticum*

Also known as *Eugenia caryophyllata, Caryophyllus aromaticus, Eugenia aromatica*, cinnamon nails, clove bud, *ding heung, ding xiang, dinh huong, dok chan*, eugenia bud, tropical myrtle

Cloves are native to Indonesia. The dried bud, which grows on an evergreen tree, is the part most often used medicinally. The buds are dried and sometimes ground into a powder before shipping. The essential oil is derived from either the leaves or the bud through a steam distillation process.[376]

Cloves' aroma comes from its active ingredient, eugenol. Eugenol is also the active ingredient in clove essential oil, which can be comprised of as much as 95% eugenol.[377] Commercial derivatives of eugenol have been used in analgesics and antiseptics. Eugenol is also, irrelevantly enough, an aphrodisiac for mice.[378]

What is it good for?

Mouth injuries. The Eclectic School recommended clove oil for this purpose. The 1918 U.S. Dispensatory notes that it is often used for toothache.[379] Commission E recommends it as a topical antiseptic and anesthetic for mouth pain. The eugenol and salicylic acid in cloves

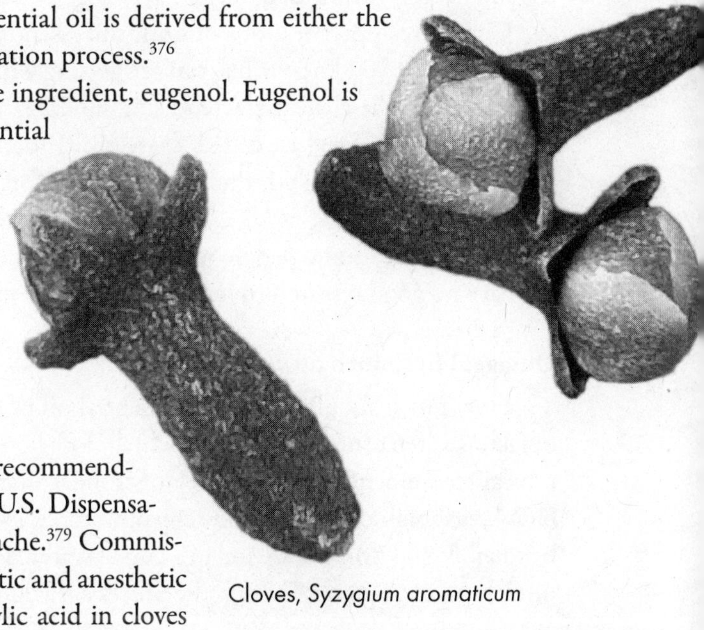

Cloves, *Syzygium aromaticum*

have become commonly accepted treatments for mouth pain, not just among herbalists, but among Western dentists as well.[380] This use is not surprising. Eugenol has antiseptic, anti-inflammatory, and anesthetic properties.[381] Test-tube studies have found that eugenol fights bacteria, viruses, and fungi, including some of the most common causes of skin infections.[382] It is also an anesthetic, depressing the sensory receptors that perceive pain[383] by means of a compound called beta-caryophyllene.[384] Cloves also contain salicylic acid, a plant hormone and the active ingredient in aspirin.[385] It is for this reason that dentists often use clove oil in fillings and dry socket preparations. Clinical research regarding cloves' effectiveness and safety in dental uses is, however, surprisingly sparse. One study showed that clove oil worked as well as benzocaine for numbing a small area before injections.[386] Other studies suggest the possibility of irritation. Beyond those few studies, we have mostly just lots of use.

Helps improve memory. It is said that the smell of clove oil can help improve alertness and strengthen memory. This use is, however, merely anecdotal at this point.

How do you use it?

Essential oil. There is no good reason to take clove oil internally and lots of good reasons not to (irritation, stomach upset, possible cytotoxicity). If you use clove for mouth injuries, spit; don't swallow. Pure essential clove oil can be as much as 72–90% eugenol.[387] Eugenol is an irritant. You should, therefore, dilute the oil with water to a 1 to 5% solution before using it as a mouth rinse.[388] Store the oil in a dark bottle in a cool place.

Decoctions. Eugenol isn't soluble in water, so decoctions are not your best bet.

Infused oil. Soak whole cloves in olive oil.[389] Infused oil tends to be less irritating than essential oil. The problem is that you can't be quite sure just how much of the active ingredient you have in the infused oil.

Commercial preparations of both the essential oil and other "clove oils" are available. Make sure that you know what you are getting when you buy clove oil. True clove oil is the essential oil of the clove extracted using superheated steam. Many preparations are diluted with other oils and still are called "clove oil." The amount of dilution will tell you how much you need to further dilute the preparation before using it. You want no more than a 5% solution.

Whole clove. Some people just hold the whole clove in their mouth near the injury.[390] We have no good research to help assess the benefits or risks of doing so.

Dosage: How much do you use?

How much should you dilute essential oil of clove before using it as a rinse? In point of fact, we aren't sure at this point which dose best balances effectiveness with prudence. A typical recommendation is to use no stronger than a 5% solution.[391] A 5% dilution would be 2.4 teaspoons of the oil in one cup of water. A more conservative dilution,[392] .06%, would be roughly 2–3 drops of the oil in a cup of water. Some people use the full strength clove oil directly on their gums. Though the practice is widespread, evidence is beginning to come in that says that this old practice may not be advisable. (See the "What should you be aware of before using it" section below for more information.)

What should you be aware of before using it?

Cloves used as a spice are generally regarded as safe. The problems occur when using clove oil or cloves in medicinal quantities.

Most of the documented problems are irritations caused by ingesting too much of the oil.[393] Anything more than minute amounts can cause stomach irritation.[394] Children are more sensitive to cloves effects than adults.[395]

Recent in vitro (test-tube) research shows that the eugenol in cloves might be cytotoxic.[396] The study has not yet been replicated, nor have the effects seen in the study been observed in human trials. Furthermore, after centuries of clove oil use, we have few or no documented cases of toxicity in adults. Even the FDA approves its use in small concentrations.[397] The cytotoxicity demonstrated in the recent study, however, should probably not be completely ignored. Until more data comes in, you might consider avoiding undiluted clove oil applied directly. Instead, use diluted clove oil as a mouthwash: clove oil diluted to somewhere between .06 and 5% (depending on your tolerance for risk) rinse and spit.

Oil of cloves can be irritating to skin and mucous membranes. Diluting the oil can help reduce irritation.

Some people are allergic to cloves. Rashes, hives, shortness of breath, and anaphylaxis have been reported.[398] If you experience any of these symptoms, discontinue use. If you experience breathing problems, get medical help immediately.

Don't use it if you are taking antithrombotic drugs because cloves may increase their effect.[399] If you plan to have surgery, tell your surgeon you have been taking cloves and discontinue use. Be cautious when using it in conjunction with other herbs known or suspected of increasing the risk of bleeding. (See Chapter 5 for a list.)

Coltsfoot

Scientific name: *Tussilago farfara*

Also known as horseweed, horsebalm, ox balm, bullsfoot, hallfoot, fieldhove, pilewort, stone root, coughwort, cough plant, and horse-hoof, *kuan dong hua*.

Coltsfoot, a perennial originally from Europe, now grows wild throughout the northeastern and midwestern United States, as well as southern Canada. It is part of the *Compositae* family, a large family that also contains daisies, asters, sunflowers, zinnia, dandelions, and even thistles and ragweed. The flowers are the principle part used, but the leaves also have medicinal value.

Coltsfoot has a long history of being used for coughs. In fact, the scientific name, *Tussilago*, comes from the Latin word for cough. Some traditions say coltsfoot is best for conditions with lots of mucus; others recommend it for dry coughs. Though they may not agree on the particulars, people on at least four continents for at least twenty centuries have been saying that coltsfoot works for throat ailments. Many European cough remedies feature coltsfoot. The Iroquois used an infusion of the roots as a cough remedy.[400] Greek physicians recommended smoking coltsfoot for asthma, advice that is now considered highly ill-advised. In France in the eighteenth century, apothecaries would paint a picture of a colt's foot on a shingle and hang it outside when they had coltsfoot cough remedies for sale.[401] In China, it's called *kuan dong hua*, and it's used for chronic coughs with lots of phlegm. It is said to force rising lung *qi* to descend.

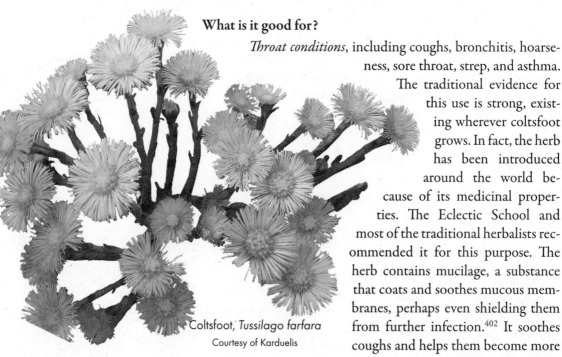

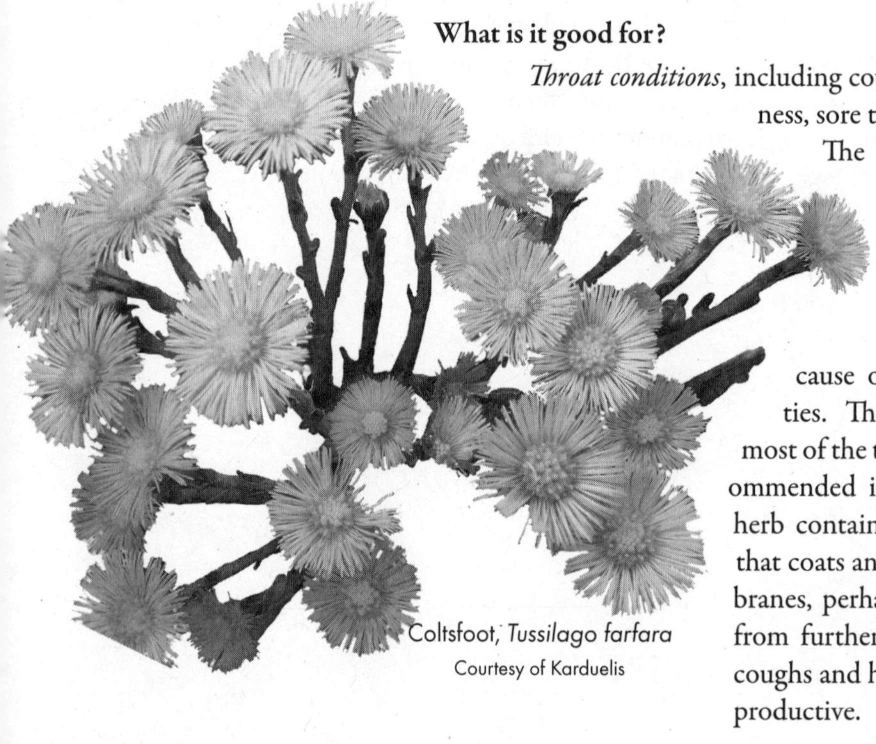

Coltsfoot, *Tussilago farfara*
Courtesy of Karduelis

What is it good for?

Throat conditions, including coughs, bronchitis, hoarseness, sore throat, strep, and asthma. The traditional evidence for this use is strong, existing wherever coltsfoot grows. In fact, the herb has been introduced around the world because of its medicinal properties. The Eclectic School and most of the traditional herbalists recommended it for this purpose. The herb contains mucilage, a substance that coats and soothes mucous membranes, perhaps even shielding them from further infection.[402] It soothes coughs and helps them become more productive. The active ingredients have antioxidative,[403] anti-inflammatory, and neuroprotective properties.[404] Test-tube analysis shows that coltsfoot has antimicrobial properties and is effective against *Staphylococcus aureus*,[405] a cause of pneumonia and other upper respiratory infections.[406] Clinical trials and human studies, even animal studies, are almost nonexistent, however.

Skin inflammations. A poultice of coltsfoot leaves is sometimes used for skin inflammations, including insect bites and burns.[407] This tradition doesn't have nearly the attestation that the throat remedies do, but given that initial research shows anti-inflammatory and neuroprotective properties, the use may not be totally unfounded.[408] The leaves of coltsfoot also contain tannins.

How do you use it?

Infusions. Coltsfoot is typically prepared as either an infusion or decoction of either the flowers or the leaves. Consult a professional for more information about how to minimize the dangers of using coltsfoot. (See the "What should you be aware of before using it" section for more information.)

Tinctures. Tinctures aren't recommended if you want the mucilage of the herb to remain intact.[409] Smoking coltsfoot, a traditional way of using the herb, also destroys mucilage.[410] Inhaling the steam doesn't work either.

Dosage: How much do you use?

Don't use coltsfoot longer than 4–6 weeks per year[411] Consult a professional for guidance in finding a proper dosage of coltsfoot. (See the "What should you be aware of before using it" section below for more information.)

What should you be aware of before using it?

One would think that an herb that had centuries of history of use would have centuries of history of contraindications as well. That's not true with coltsfoot. For centuries, it was used without restriction. Only recently have scientists discovered that coltsfoot contains pyrrolizidine alkaloids (PAs), which can cause liver cancer and liver failure.[412] So far most of the evidence has come from animal research and studies of other herbs that contain PAs, but those studies are conclusive enough that regulatory agencies are beginning to take notice. The problem is that PAs cause damage that only shows up in a liver biopsy or autopsy. By the time you have your first symptom, significant harm has already been done. The FDA has classified coltsfoot as an herb of "undefined safety." Canadian and Australian authorities have banned the herb outright.[413] Germany has set up a web of restrictions that greatly limits its use.[414]

The risk may be able to be mitigated somewhat through proper preparation of the herb and careful dosage. It may also be mitigated by using coltsfoot as a gargle rather than a tea. The wisest course of action, however, is to seek professional guidance if you want to take coltsfoot.

Don't take coltsfoot at all if :

You have any kind of liver disorder, take several kinds of medication (which are cleared through the liver), or if you drink heavily.[415] Also you shouldn't take it in conjunction with any other herb or drug known to affect liver function.[416] (See Chapter 5 for a list.)

You have heart problems.[417]

You are pregnant, nursing, or trying to conceive.[418] One baby has died because her mother drank coltsfoot tea during pregnancy.[419]

You are taking cardiac drugs (because it may decrease the effects of these drugs).[420]

You are taking high blood pressure medicine (because it may decrease the effects of the medicine).[421]

You are allergic to ragweed or other member of the *Compositae* family.

Comfrey

Scientific name: *Symphytum officinale*

Also known as ass ear, black root, black wort, knit bone, slippery root, wall wort, symphytum, healing herb, knitback, back wort, bruisewort, gum plant. Symphyti radix is comfrey root

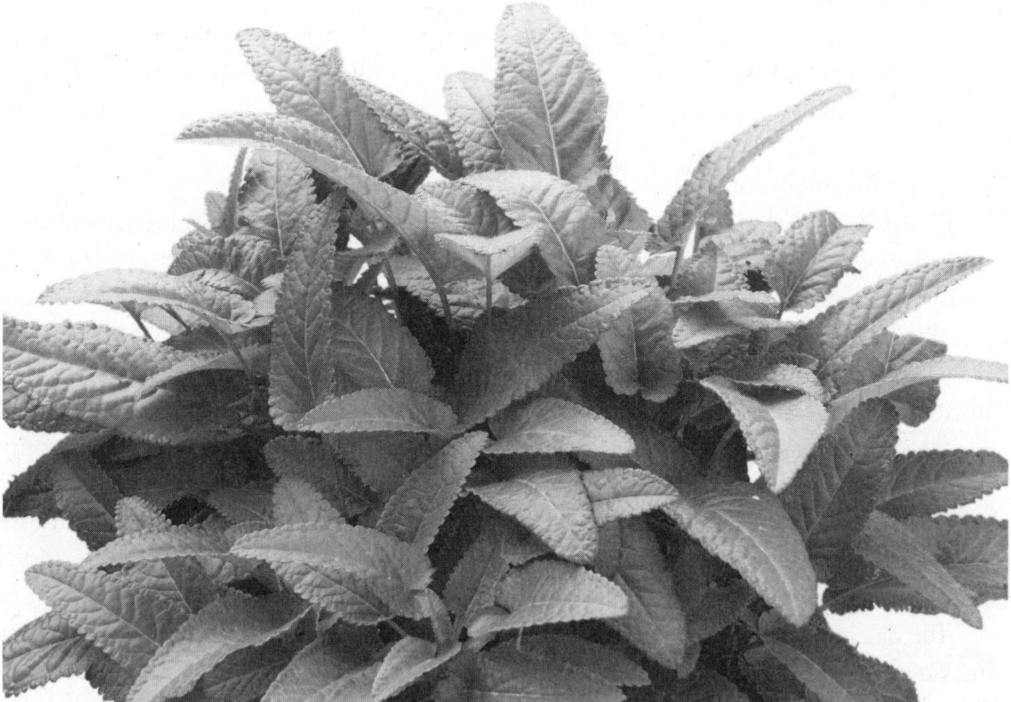

Comfrey, *Symphytum officinales*

Comfrey is native to Europe and Asia. Wild comfrey was brought to the Americas by English immigrants, who used it medicinally. It now grows wild as an introduced species in many of the northern states of the U.S. The above-ground parts and roots are both used medicinally.

The popular name for comfrey was "knit bone." In fact, the word comfrey means "grow together." The use of this herb goes back thousands of years. The Greeks and Romans used it to heal wounds and broken bones. The active ingredient is allantoin, a compound also found in mother's milk. Allantoin promotes healthy tissue growth. When applied to a closed wound, such as a bruise, sprain, or contusion, allantoin is absorbed through the skin.[422] Researchers aren't sure how it works, but the mechanism may have something to do with proliferation of white blood cells.[423] Comfrey also helps soften and protect skin.

What is it good for?

Sprains. We have considerable traditional evidence—mostly from the European and American herbal traditions—that comfrey is useful in healing sprains. Commission E recommends it for the purpose as well as for bruises and strains. The herb contains allantoin, which stimulates cell proliferation.[424] It also contains rosmarinic acid, which has antioxidant, anti-inflammatory, and antimicrobial activities.[425] Comfrey is one of the few herbs that has some solid clinical evidence behind its use. A study of 142 men with ankle sprains shows a clear superiority of comfrey over the placebo. An ointment of comfrey extract reduced both pain and ankle edema.[426] In a second study, a 10% active ingredient cream was shown to be superior to a 1% cream. The stronger cream was also tolerated well. It improved pain on active motion, pain at rest, and functional impairment significantly; and overall efficacy was judged good to excellent in 85.6% of cases.[427] In a third study, more than two-thirds of sprain patients were able to reduce or discontinue pain and anti-inflammatory medication upon using comfrey preparations.[428] In a fourth, which investigated 164 cases of sprained ankle, comfrey extract was shown to be the equal of, or perhaps even slightly superior to, Diclofenac® gel, a conventional pharmaceutical used on sprains.[429] ◊◆◆◆◆

Myalgia. Commission E recommends comfrey for muscle strains. A single study confirms the efficacy of comfrey cream in treating muscle pain. The study had good results with 104 people with back pain. Some anecdotal evidence supports this use as well. ◊◊◊◆◆

Healing bone fractures. Tradition says that comfrey speeds healing of broken bones. In fact, it was call "knit bone" during the Middle Ages. In modern times, it is mostly used for minor fractures—those not typically casted—such as fractures of ribs, toes, and hairline fractures in larger bones. We do know that comfrey contains allantoin, which encourages bone, cartilage, and muscle cells to grow. Though the traditional evidence for this use is strong, clinical evidence is lacking. The Eclectic School called the notion that comfrey can heal bones "a myth." In short, you may get some help from it for fractures, but don't expect miracles. ◊◊◊◆◆

How do you use it?

Poultice. Use a poultice of pureed leaves only on minor fractures, those not typically casted, like ribs, toes and hairline fractures in larger bones.

Decoction. Use a decoction made from the roots on sprains. The roots contain more allantoin, so it's better for deep injuries.[430] The leaves contain more tannins and are better for surface injuries where skin tightening is an issue.[431] For sprained fingers, toes, or ankles, you can use the decoction as a soak, submerging the entire joint. For larger joints, you can use a compress soaked in the decoction.

Bath. For those times when you have whole-body, fallen-down-a-flight-of-stairs style injuries, you can add the decoction to a bath. Avoid using comfrey in a bath, however, if you have any broken skin on your body.

Salve or cream. Studies show that a 10% active ingredient cream, made from 25 g of fresh herb per 100 g of cream is very effective for sprains.[432] Commercial formulations are available. Look for a 0.4% allantoin solution. Homemade salves are possible, but the concentration of allantoin in them is more unpredictable. Use method two for creams and salves in Chapter 3 for making the salve.

Infused oil. Infused oil made by the hot infusion method can be used for arthritic joints, bruises, sprains, and traumatic injuries. The oil is especially good as a massage oil while sprains are in the recovery stage. (Don't massage injuries that are still in the inflammation stage.)

Store comfrey in a cool, dry place in a sealed container.

Dosage: How much do you use?

A 5–20% ointment can be used several times per day.[433] Commission E recommends it not be used more than four to six weeks per year. Some herbalists suggest less than that, recommending three weeks at the most.[434]

What should you be aware of before using it?

Don't use comfrey internally. The herb contains liver-toxic pyrrolizidine alkaloids (PAs). These PAs are concentrated mostly in the roots and new leaves, but they are present throughout the plant. In mature dried leaves, the concentration is the lowest of any part of the plant. In fact, two studies have failed to find them in mature dried leaves.[435] The main liver injury caused by comfrey is veno-occlusive disease, blockage of the small veins of the liver, leading to cirrhosis and eventually liver failure.[436] This injury is well documented in not just lab animals but also thousands of people, some of whom took comfrey medicinally, but most of whom accidentally ate grains contaminated by comfrey.[437] (Note, however, that these reports don't distinguish between *Symphytum officinale* and the more toxic *Symphytum uplandicum* and *Symphytum asperum*. All three, however, contain PAs.) Some herbalists suggest that comfrey has gotten a worse reputation than it deserves, and that a healthy, nonpregnant person with no liver problems can get away with three weeks of comfrey taken internally.[438] If you do choose to take comfrey internally, do so under the supervision of a trained professional.

A safer route is to use comfrey externally only. All of the known deaths due to comfrey were due to taking comfrey internally. Though comfrey extracts injected beneath the skin of lab animals produced lesions, applying it to unbroken skin carries no known risk to the liver.[439] Australia, New Zealand, Canada, and Germany have chosen this safer route: use in all those countries is restricted to topical only.

Don't take it in conjunction with any other herb or drug known to affect liver function.[440] (See Chapter 5 for a list.)

Never use it on dirty wounds because it tends to cause rapid surface healing that can trap dirt or pus. Commission E recommends it not be used on broken skin or open wounds at all. Given that lab animals developed lesions when comfrey was injected beneath the skin,[441] Commission E's recommendation would seem to be prudent.

Avoid use if you are pregnant or nursing.[442]

Children should not use comfrey.[443]

Russian comfrey (*Symphytum uplandicum*) and prickly comfrey (*Symphytum asperum*) should not be used medicinally as they are even more toxic than *Symphytum officinale.*

Devil's Claw

Scientific name: *Harpagophytum procumbens*

Also known as grapple plant, wood spider, Windhoek's root

Devil's claw is native to southern Africa. It was brought from there to Europe by colonists who saw the medicinal potential of the herb. The secondary roots, also known as the storage tubers, are the only part of the plant that appears to have any medicinal value.[444] They are cut into pieces or pulverized and then dried. Devil's claw is cultivated in places in North America, but does not grow wild on this continent.

Devil's claw was introduced to Europe and North America in the 1950s and 1960s. Like many herbs, it went through a period when it was regarded

Devil's Claw, *Harpagophyum procumbens*
Courtesy of Henri Pidoux

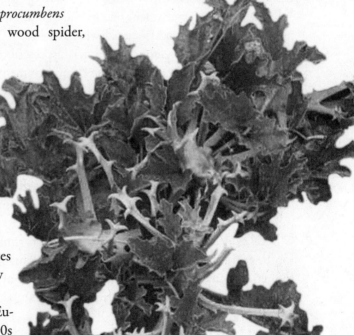

as a wonder drug—able to treat headache, loss of appetite, fever, blood disorders, and even cancer.[445] With time, as the research began trickling in, the focus has narrowed so that now devil's claw is primarily used for arthritis pain and swelling, and for back pain. In 1998, Commission E was not convinced of the efficacy of devil's claw, and did not recommend it for any purpose in their last monographs. In 2003, an article in Phytomedicine echoed Commission E's concerns about the quality of studies that showed devil's claw's analgesic and anti-inflammatory properties.[446] Since that time, however, new studies have been released, and some of them (none a large, definitive study, however) have suggested that the traditional use of devil's claw for back pain and arthritis is not entirely without foundation.

What is it good for?

Back pain. Because devil's claw is native to some fairly remote areas of Africa and is relatively new to the West, we don't have as much information about its traditional uses as we do with other herbs. Though it is used widely throughout Europe for mild joint pain,[447] Commission E does not recommend devil's claw for this use because of this lack of knowledge. Experiments on rats show that devil's claw has both pain-relieving and anti-inflammatory properties.[448] Two human trials examined its effects on back pain. They found strong evidence that doses standardized to 50 mg or 100 mg harpagoside were better than placebo for short-term improvements in pain.[449] A study testing devil's claw for mild muscle pain and stiffness of the back, shoulder, and neck found similar positive results: less stiffness and better blood supply to the muscles.[450] ◊ ◊ ◆ ◆ ◆

Arthritis. One experiment on rats shows that devil's claw might be helpful for both the pain and inflammation associated with arthritis.[451] Another shows no use at all.[452] In an open clinical study in Germany, physicians prescribing devil's claw to their patients for arthritis of the hip or knee found a 45.5% improvement for pain on palpation, 35% improvement for limitation of mobility. and 25.4% improvement for joint crepitus (creaking or grinding in the joints).[453] But again Commission E does not recommend devil's claw for arthritis. ◊ ◊ ◆ ◆ ◆

How do you use it?

Traditionally, devil's claw is taken orally as a decoction or infusion. One teaspoon of the finely chopped or powdered root is added to 1–¼ cup boiling water, and then steeped for eight hours.[454] The potency of devil's claw, however, varies quite a bit from plant to plant. Clinical evidence shows that a daily dose of approximately 50 mg of harpagoside is necessary for the anti-inflammatory effect.[455] Unless you obtain your roots from a supplier who tests the active ingredients in each tuber it ships, the only sure way to get this dose is through standardized commercial preparations (capsules).

Dosage: How much do you use?

Based on tradition, a probable effective dosage is a tea made from 4.5 g daily.[456] The tea can be taken up to three times a day.[457] If you prefer to take a standardized commercial preparation, you'll want to take around 50 mg of harpagoside per day.[458] Experiments using 25 mg show markedly less effect.[459] Short term studies have shown that people can tolerate 100 mg.[460] One well-tested standardized preparation is Doloteffin®, which is produced by Ardeypharm, a German company.

What should you be aware of before using it?

If you are taking devil's claw regularly, consult a doctor if you want to use it longer than two to three weeks. Studies have not been conducted to demonstrate its safety beyond three to four months.[461]

Possible side effects include stomach upset, low blood pressure, and increased heart rate.[462]

Don't take devil's claw if you have ulcers.[463]

Don't take it if you have biliary stones.[464]

Don't take it if you are pregnant or nursing.[465]

Don't take it if you are taking antithrombotic drugs because it may increase the effects.[466] If you plan to have surgery, tell your surgeon you have been taking devil's claw and discontinue use. Be cautious when using it in conjunction with other herbs known or suspected of increasing the risk of bleeding. (See Chapter 5 for a list.)

If you are diabetic or have blood sugar problems, consult with your doctor before taking devil's claw. Animal experiments suggest that it may affect blood sugar.[467] Be cautious when using it in conjunction with herbs known or suspected to affect blood sugar levels. (See Chapter 5 for a list.)

If you have heart problems, consult with your doctor before taking devil's claw because experiments on animals show that it does seem to have some effect on the heart.[468] Don't use it in conjunction with other herbs that have an effect on heart function. (See Chapter 5 for a list.)

Echinacea

Scientific name: *Echinacea* spp.

Also known as purple coneflower, black Sampson, black Susan, cock-up-hat, combflower, snakeroot, hedgehog, Indian head, Kansas snake root, red sunflower, scurvy root, solhat, sun hat

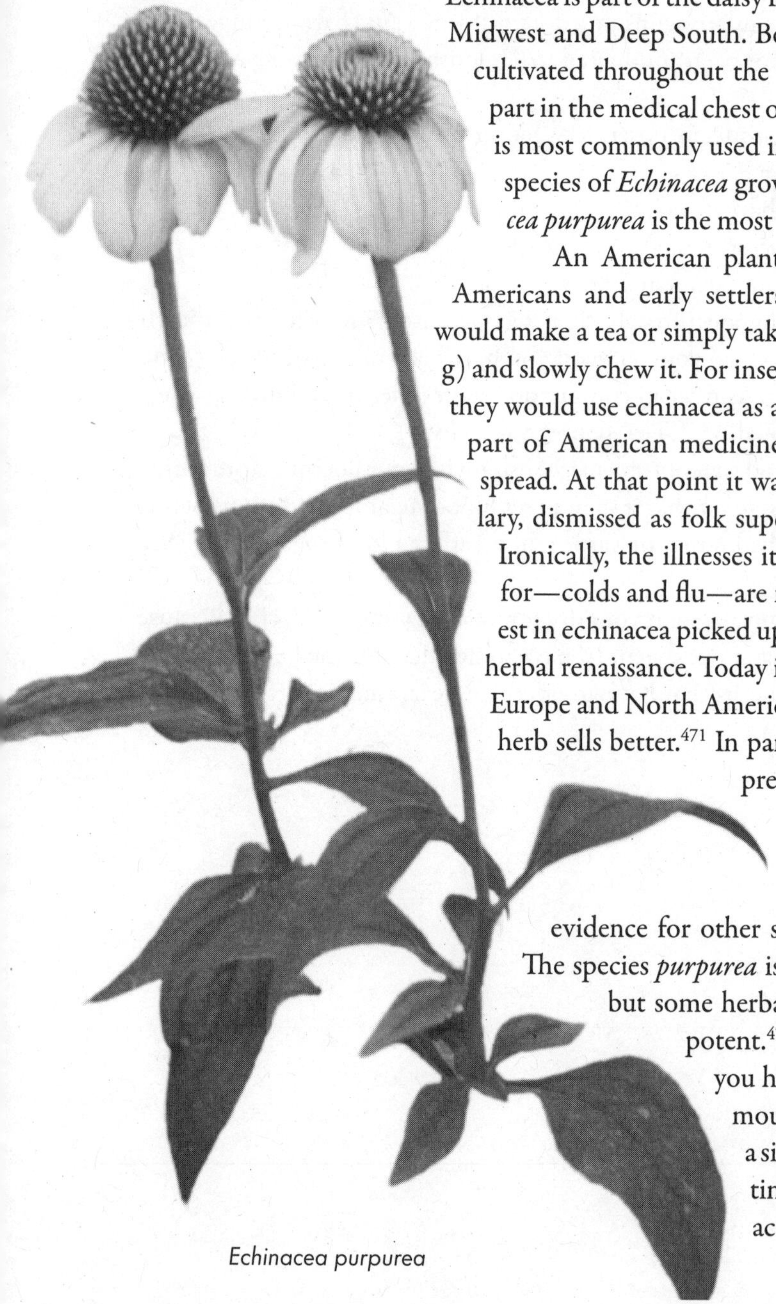

Echinacea purpurea

Echinacea is part of the daisy family. It is native to the American Midwest and Deep South. Because of its popularity, it is now cultivated throughout the world. Though the flower had a part in the medical chest of early American settlers, the root is most commonly used in modern herbal medicine. Nine species of *Echinacea* grow in North America, but *Echinacea purpurea* is the most commonly used medicinally.[469]

An American plant, echinacea was used by native Americans and early settlers alike. For colds and flu, they would make a tea or simply take a small piece of the root (1 or 2 g) and slowly chew it. For insect bites, snake bites, and wounds, they would use echinacea as a poultice. The herb was a crucial part of American medicine until antibiotics became widespread. At that point it was taken off the National Formulary, dismissed as folk superstition, and its use declined.[470] Ironically, the illnesses it had been most commonly used for—colds and flu—are not affected by antibiotics. Interest in echinacea picked up again in the 1970s as part of the herbal renaissance. Today it is one of the most used herbs in Europe and North America. In the United States, no other herb sells better.[471] In parts of Europe it can be medically prescribed.

Commission E recommends only *E. pallida* root and *E. purpurea* herb, citing a lack of evidence for other species and parts of the plant.[472] The species *purpurea* is the most commonly cultivated, but some herbalists believe *angustifolia* is more potent.[473] One way to tell if the echinacea you have is potent is to hold it in your mouth for a little while. Echinacea is a sialogogue: If it makes your tongue tingle or stimulates salivation, its active ingredients are still intact.[474]

What is it good for?

Common cold, upper respiratory infections, other infections. Echinacea is most commonly used to help speed healing from colds and flu. The Cheyenne used it for colds and sore throats, the Kiowa for coughs and sore throats, the Choctaw for coughs, and the Comanche for sore throats.[475] *A Modern Herbal* recommends it for resistance to infection. The Eclectic School recommended it for fevers. The traditional attestation in North America is strong, so much so that echinacea can now be found all over the world.

Test-tube studies show that it kills viruses, including influenza.[476] They also show macrophage activation and activation of polymorphonuclear leukocytes and natural killer cells.[477] A study in mice showed immune stimulation and a quicker recovery from radiation exposure.[478] Another uncontrolled study of upper respiratory infection in dogs showed positive results.[479]

In humans, a study that looked at activation of the immune system showed that tinctures of echinacea stimulated the immune system within 24 hours of when they were taken.[480] A study of a proprietary echinacea extraction (Echinilin®) showed that it enhanced the non-specific immune response and elicited free-radical scavenging properties.[481] Other studies, however, have found no such activation.[482]

What about human clinical studies? Do they show that echinacea works? The jury is still out. Some studies have showed no difference between echinacea and placebo either in the likelihood of getting an induced cold or in decreasing the severity of symptoms.[483] Others, however, have found a decreased severity in those who take echinacea at the first sign of a cold.[484] A study of children with upper respiratory tract infections showed that those who took echinacea had a 28% less chance of developing a second upper respiratory infection within four weeks.[485] But another study of children found no difference in the duration or severity of upper respiratory tract infection in those taking echinacea versus placebo.[486] Still others see little enough improvement that the results may not be statistically significant.[487] The evidence that it improves quality of life in people with upper respiratory tract infections is also inconclusive.[488]

These equivocal findings, however, may say more about the studies themselves than echinacea. The problems with echinacea studies have been fourfold: First, studies show a complete lack of standardization. From study to study, we see different species (*Echinacea purpurea*, *E. pallida*, and *E. angustifolia*), different parts of the plant (leaves, flowers, roots), different modes of administering the herbs (juice, tablets, dried herb in capsule, teas, and tinctures), different quantities of the active ingredient, different doses.[489] Second, some studies simply used over-the-counter echinacea without any check of the contents of the formulation. Recent studies have found that some brands of echinacea supplements contain herbs from species not on the label, and some actually contain little or no actual echinacea.[490] Third, echinacea can lose its potency quickly, especially if not handled well. Most studies did nothing to control for the potency of the echinacea they were using. Fourth, there is more than one kind of cold/flu. We now suspect that echinacea works least well with rhinovirus, the most common kind of cold.[491]

Fortunately, we now have enough echinacea studies that we're able to get meta-analyses. A small Swiss meta-study looked at echinacea and induced colds and found that across three studies, the likelihood of experiencing a clinical cold was 55% higher with placebo than with echinacea.[492] A much larger meta-study sorted through the studies, discarded the problematic ones, and found that in the remaining studies, echinacea decreased the chance of getting a cold by 58% and shortened the duration of a cold by 1.4 days.[493] ◊ ◊ ◆ ◆ ◆

Poorly healing wounds and chronic ulcerations. This use was a common one among settlers on the Great Plains.[494] The Lakota also used echinacea on wounds and sores. The Cheyenne used it for sore gums. The Dakota, Winnebago, Ponca, Pawnee, and Omaha all used it on burns.[495] Commission E also recommends *purpurea* for this purpose.[496] Echinacea contains caffeic acid derivatives and glycoside which help the wound healing process.[497] It also has some antibiotic properties.[498] One study looked at vocal fold wounds in pigs and found that an extract of echinacea helped heal induced injuries.[499] But the clinical trials are still not there to support this use. ◊ ◊ ◊ ◆ ◆

How do you use it?

Commercial *preparations.* Numerous forms of echinacea are available for purchase. It can be found in tablets, capsules, tonics, and as a part of numerous cold remedies. Preparations vary widely. The way it's processed has some effect on its potency.[500] Purchase your echinacea from a reputable source. According to one study, price is one mark of quality.[501] If echinacea preparations are too cheap, be suspicious. Echinaforce® is one brand that has been tested and found effective.[502]

Decoction. If you choose to use the root itself, store it whole,[503] and don't use it after it's lost its smell.[504] One way to tell if the echinacea you have is potent is to hold it in your mouth for a little while. Echinacea is a sialogogue: If it stimulates salivation, it has its active ingredients still intact.[505] Make a decoction of 2 teaspoons of the chopped root material, per cup of water.[506] Bring it to a boil and then simmer for 10–15 minutes. You can take the decoction a cup at a time, three times daily, or you can take it in small doses (2 teaspoons to 2 tablespoons) every 1 or 2 hours during the acute stage of colds and flu. If you want to use it on wounds, you can use the decoction or diluted tincture as a wash. Be aware, however, that echinacea infusions and decoctions tend to lose their potency quickly. Even if you store them in the refrigerator, they change significantly in a few days time.

Infusion. One analysis of research to date suggests that the aerial parts of the plant are more effective than the roots in treating colds.[507] Aerial parts of the plant will need less cooking than roots. Use a standard infusion method to make a tea.

Extracts. The juice pressed from the plant is available commercially.

Tincture. 1:5, 45–50%. If you want to hold a homemade echinacea preparation for a while, an alcohol tincture is a better bet than a preparation made with water.[508] If you make a tincture using at least 50% ethanol (e.g. 100 proof vodka), the tincture should hold for more than a year.[509] Studies show that tinctures effectively carry the active ingredients into the body, with maximum concentration of the main alkamides hitting the bloodstream in less than 30 minutes.[510]

Oils, salves and creams. These can be used to treat wounds. Commercial preparations are available. We have, however, no clear consensus in either the research literature or marketplace about what echinacea cream is good for.

Dosage: How much do you use?

The probable effective dosage is :

Root extract capsules: 250 mg 3 times per day[511]

Tincture: 30–60 drops, 3 times per day[512] (roughly ¼ to ⅔ of a teaspoon)

Expressed juice: 1¼–1¾ teaspoons per day, divided into two or three doses, for five to seven days[513]

Don't take echinacea for more than three weeks. After three weeks of use, discontinue for at least a week to avoid a decrease in effectiveness.[514] Or you can rotate in three-week cycles with astragalus.[515]

What should you be aware of before using it?

A wound wash can do more harm than good if you don't use pure ingredients and careful, sterile procedures. If you have any question about the sterility of your decoction, don't use it on an open wound.

Adverse effects reported generally have been uncommon and minor, including abdominal upset, nausea, and dizziness.[516] High doses increase the chances of dizziness or nausea.

Don't use echinacea internally if you have a progressive systemic disease, such as tuberculosis, leucosis, collagenosis, or multiple sclerosis.[517]

If you have any immune system problems, check with your doctor before taking echinacea.

Avoid, or at least be very cautious about, using echinacea if you are allergic to members of the *Asteraceae* family, for example ragweed, sunflowers, asters, or daisies.

Don't take it if you are taking immunosuppressant, or hepatotoxic drugs such as amiodarone, methotrexate, and ketoconazole.[518]

Some researchers suggest that you not take it at the same time as acetaminophen (such as Tylenol™) because the combination increases the chance of liver damage. This opinion, however, is not universally agreed upon.[519]

Don't take it in conjunction with any other herb or drug known to affect liver function. (See Chapter 5 for a list.)[520]

Elder

Scientific name: *Sambucus nigra* (European Elder), *Sambucus canadensis* (American elder), and *Sambucus ebulus* (European Dwarf Elder).

Also known as elderberry, elder flower, black elderberry, European elder, European alder, ellanwood, ellhorn, red elder, boor tree

Sambucus is the genus of the elder tree. Various species of elder grow as small trees or large bushes throughout the world. The species used medicinally are the European elder, the American elder, and the European Dwarf elder. This article is about the European elder in particular. The fruit, typically referred to as "berries," are rich in vitamins A and C and have nutritional as well as medicinal value when taken internally. For topical uses, the flowers are the main part used medicinally, though historically the leaf and bark were used as well.

What is it good for?

Colds and flu, especially feverish and mucous conditions. The tradition of using elder for colds, flu, and fever spans at least two continents (Europe and North America). Elder has a long history of medicinal use especially among Native Americans. The Cherokee, Iroquois, Yuki, Pima, and Pomo all used it to sweat out a fever.[521] The Quileute, Cahuilla, Kawaiisu, and Costanoan used it as a cold and flu remedy.[522] According to traditional herbalism, elder flower tea is a diaphoretic, meaning that it increases perspiration. It also increases bronchial secretions

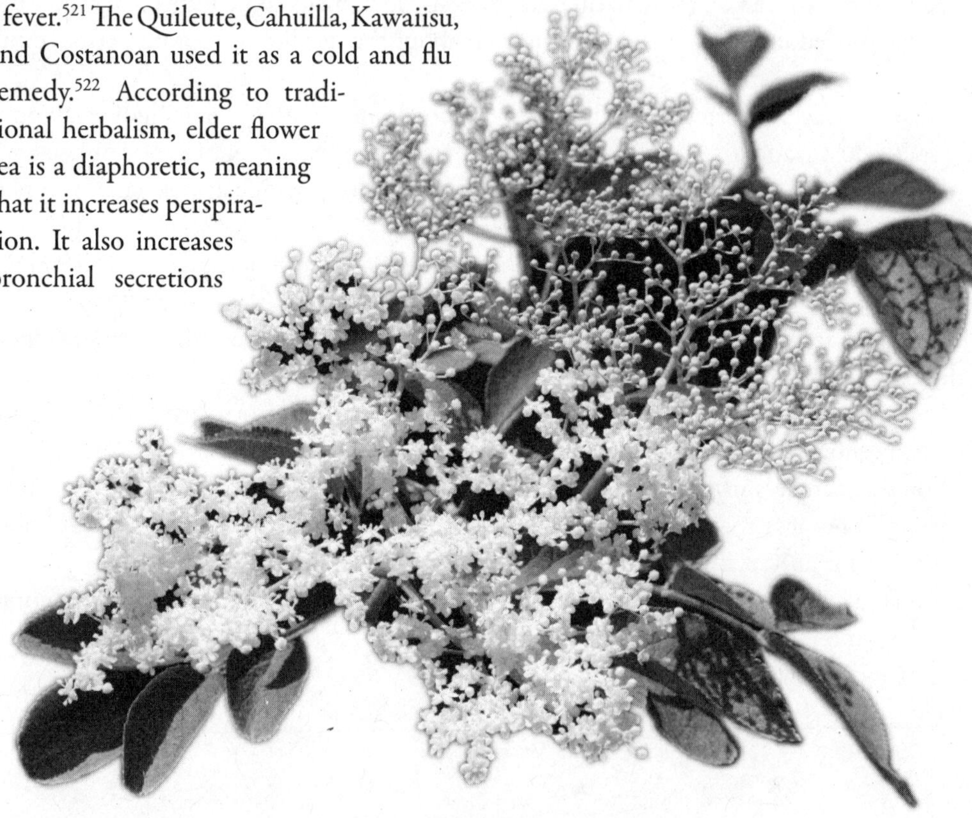

European Elder, *Sambucus nigra*
Courtesy of Renate Eder

and reduces phlegm.[523] The tradition, however, is stronger than the research. In test-tube studies elder shows antiviral activity, albeit fighting viruses that typically infect cats.[524] In a single clinical trial, a placebo-controlled, double-blind study of sixty adults in Norway showed that elderberry syrup relieved flu-like symptoms four days earlier than placebo, with less use of other cold medication.[525] Clinical trials of a proprietary elderberry extract (Sambucol®) showed that it stimulates the immune system.[526] ◊ ◊ ◆ ◆ ◆

Swellings, bruises, and sprains. Topically, elder infusions or decoctions have been used as an anti-inflammatory for bruises, sprains, and other swellings. Again this use has substantial attestation in native American tradition. The Delaware, Houma, Iroquois, Rappahannock, and Choctaw all used elder on swellings.[527] The Cherokee and Hanaksiala used it for rheumatism or arthritis,[528] and the Mendocino on bruises.[529] From animal testing, we know that *Sambucus ebulus* inhibits inflammation in mice.[530] Human research is sparser, but one study shows that it's very useful for inflammation of the gums.[531] ◊ ◊ ◆ ◆ ◆

How do you use it?

Internal use: For internal use (for colds, flu, etc.), the safest way to use elderberry is in commercial formulas. Using the wrong part of the tree in the wrong way can make you very sick. Find a reputable commercial product and follow label directions. One extract that has been tested extensively and found to be effective is Sambucol®.[532]

Infusion: A compress for skin irritations can be made from an infusion of flowers. Use 2 teaspoonfuls of the flowers. Simmer them gently in a half cup of water for five minutes and then strain.[533] Use this infusion externally only unless you first get guidance from a trained herbalist.

Dosage: How much do you use?

The safest way to use elderberry is in commercial formulas. Find a reputable one and follow label directions.

What should you be aware of before using it?

Don't take the bark, stems, or leaves of the plant internally. They contain cyanide and are toxic.[534] Elder flowers, however, are on the FDA's list of substances generally recognized as safe.[535]

Do not eat the seeds of the berries raw. They are quite toxic, especially the seeds of the red berries. Though cooking decreases the toxicity, an even better preparation is to cook and juice the berries and remove the seeds completely. The safest way to use elderberry is to use only commercially prepared extracts. If you want to use anything other than a commercial product, find a trained herbalist teach you specifically how to handle the berries.

Don't take elderberry if you are dehydrated. The herb can increase urination and/or perspiration.

Eleuthero (Siberian Ginseng) Root

Scientific name: *Eleutherococcus senticosus*

Also known as *Acanthopanax senticosus*, eluthera, eleuthera, touch me not, wild pepper, *ci wu jia*, devil's bush, devil's shrub, ussurian thorny pepperbrush. Eleutherococci radix is Eleuthero root

Siberian ginseng is a bristly shrub. As one might expect, it grows in Siberia but also in northern Korea, China, and Japan. A related species, *Eleutherococcus pentaphyllus*, grows wild as an introduced species in North America. The dried roots and/or rhizome are pulverized before use.

Though related to Asian ginseng, Siberian ginseng is not really ginseng because it doesn't contain the ginsenosides that are present in true (*Panax*) ginseng. It is, however, a valuable herb in its own right. Research in China suggests that it might have a more stimulating effect than true ginseng, making it valuable in reducing fatigue. In most people, however, it doesn't increase anxiety the way many stimulants do. Other reports of its ability to regulate blood pressure and insulin have not been sufficiently tested to be credible. Tradition and anecdotal evidence (not to mention herb merchants' hype) would suggest that Siberian ginseng is a very valuable herb. To be frank, however, we still don't have the research yet to be able to zero in on exactly what those benefits might be.

What is it good for?

Adaptogen. Tradition says that eleuthero helps people cope with stress. Such an assertion, however, is hard to test. What tests we do have were conducted in the old Soviet Union. Most showed that the herb increases performance in both mental and physical tests.[536] Increased work capacity was also reported.[537] One study showed modest benefit for patients with moderate chronic fatigue.[538] In China, eleuthero is used as a tonic for times of fatigue, declining concentration, or convalescence. ◊ ◊ ◆ ◆ ◆

Immune-system enhancement. Eleuthero is sometimes hyped as being an immune booster. One study showed that injected eleuthero extract leads to an increase in immune cells like T cells and helper cells.[539] The implications of the study, however, are still unclear. ◊ ◊ ◊ ◆ ◆

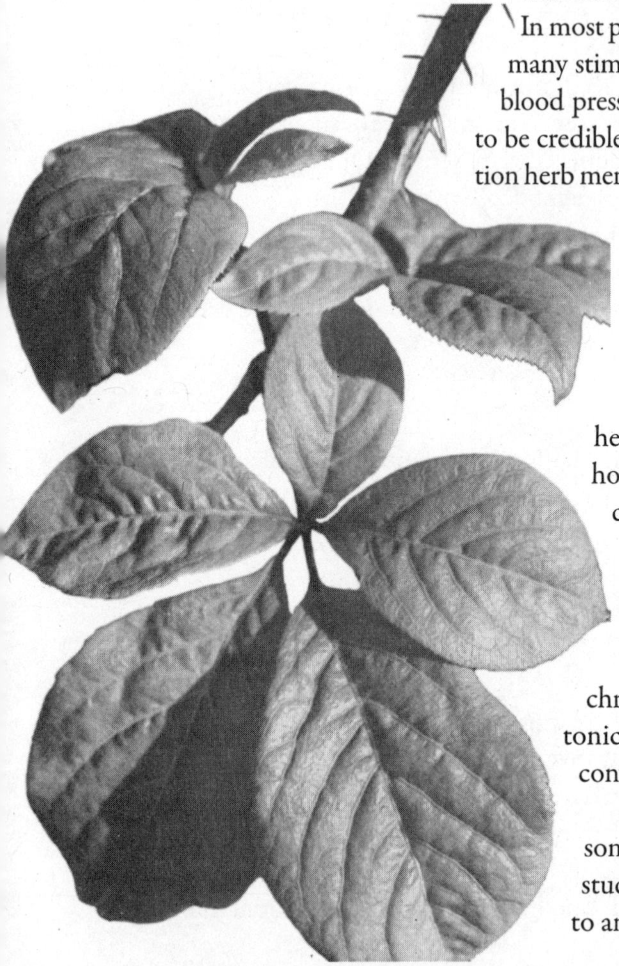

Leaves of the Eleuthero plant, *Eleutherococcus senticosus*
Courtesy of Stanislav Doronenko

How do you use it?

Traditionally decoctions and tinctures were made from the root. However, one of the problems with Siberian ginseng is that it's become a popular enough herb that all kinds of less than reputable companies are producing it. Consequently, the quality of Eleuthero, especially bulk unprocessed eleuthero, varies widely. Your best bet is to find a commercially prepared capsule made by a reputable company and to take the herb that way.

Dosage: How much do you use?

Whole root: A typical daily dosage is 2–3 g of root either made into a tea or in capsule form.[540]

Tincture: 1–2 droppers full of the tincture 2–3 times per day[541]

The Commission E recommends that you don't use Siberian ginseng for more than three months at a time.[542] Other herbalists suggest two months.

What should you be aware of before using it?

The Soviets have been using this herb for some time. Very few adverse reaction have been noted.[543]

Eleuthero is known to be an invigorating herb. This can have a downside as well as benefits. If you have high blood pressure monitor your blood pressure especially closely while using eleuthero.[544] If you have heart disease or tend to have a fast heart rate, keep an eye on your heart rate while taking it. Too much will begin to affect your sleep causing insomnia.

If you get a rash or a flush of the skin, reduce or discontinue use.

If you start getting muscle spasms, discontinue use.

Children should not use this herb.

If you begin to notice heart arrhythmia, discontinue use and seek professional help.[545]

Don't use it if you are using digoxin, insulin, or hormone therapy because it may increase the effects.[546]

Eleuthero could theoretically increase the risk of bleeding, especially when used in conjunction with other herbs with a similar effect. (See Chapter 5 for a list.) If you plan to have surgery, tell your surgeon you have been taking eleuthero and discontinue use.

If you have blood sugar problems, consult a doctor before taking eleuthero. Also exercise caution when using other herbs known to affect blood sugar. (See Chapter 5 for a list.)

Eucalyptus

Scientific name: *Eucalyptus globulus*, *E. polybractea*, *E. smithii*, and *E. australiana*. Of these *E. globulus* is the most common.

Also known as *E. fructicetorum*, blue gum, gum tree, fever tree, cider gum, crown gall, gum tree, *kafur ag*, *malee*, mountain gum, stringy bark tree

The eucalyptus tree is a huge, fast growing, Australian evergreen. Its leaves are full of eucalyptus oil. In fact, on warm days, the oil in eucalyptus forests can vaporize and hang in the air like a blue haze. Leaves are picked from older eucalyptus trees, and the oil is extracted using steam distillation. Eucalyptus trees grow in North America as an introduced species.

The Cook expeditions were the first to bring eucalyptus samples back to Europe. Because eucalyptus trees are known for their ability to dry out swampy areas, they are now planted on every continent of the world. That ability, however, is not what they are best known for. Eucalyptus was used by Aborigines as a fever medicine as well as on sore joints and troubled skin. As one of the most powerful antiseptics in the plant world, the oil quickly gained a reputation as a powerful medicine. Eucalyptus came to the United States in the mid nineteenth century.[547]

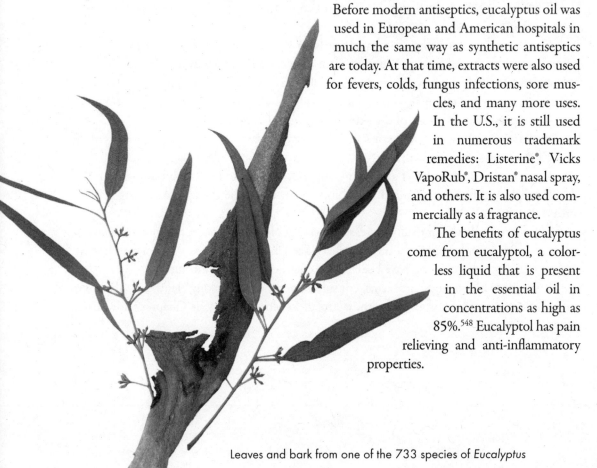

Before modern antiseptics, eucalyptus oil was used in European and American hospitals in much the same way as synthetic antiseptics are today. At that time, extracts were also used for fevers, colds, fungus infections, sore muscles, and many more uses. In the U.S., it is still used in numerous trademark remedies: Listerine®, Vicks VapoRub®, Dristan® nasal spray, and others. It is also used commercially as a fragrance.

The benefits of eucalyptus come from eucalyptol, a colorless liquid that is present in the essential oil in concentrations as high as 85%.[548] Eucalyptol has pain relieving and anti-inflammatory properties.

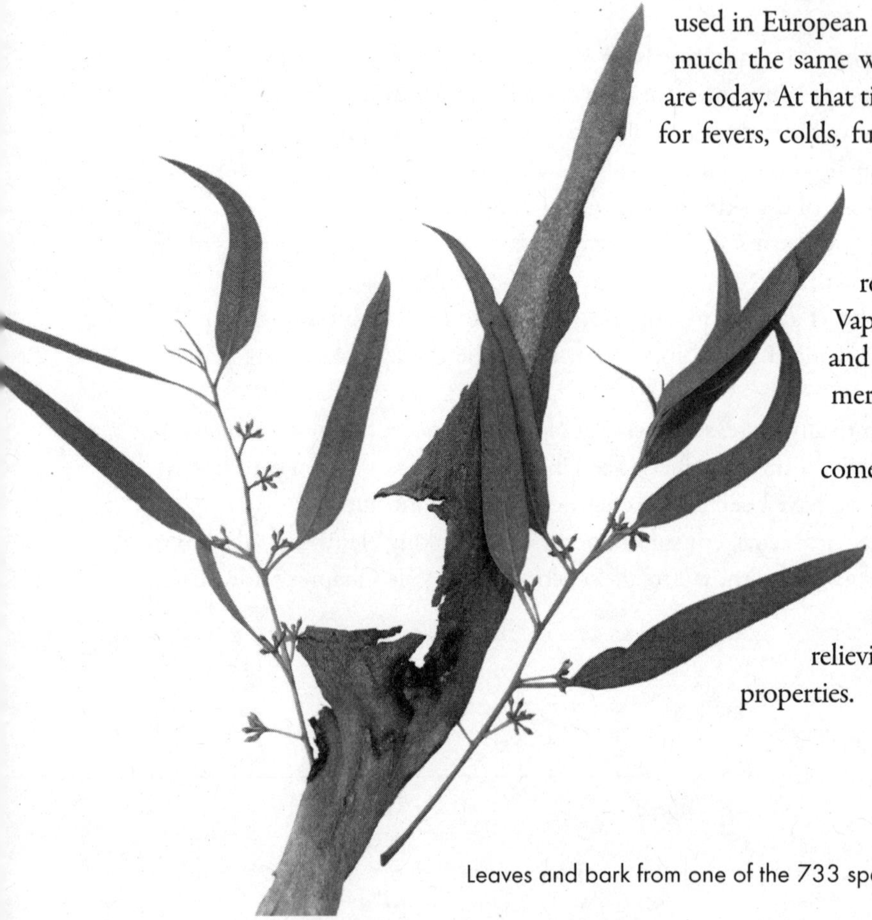

Leaves and bark from one of the 733 species of *Eucalyptus*

What is it good for?

Antiseptic. Eucalyptus' track record as an antiseptic is long and well-known. Australian aborigines have long used it to keep broken skin from becoming infected. Native Hawaiians also used it for sores and cuts.[549] In the early twentieth century, it was used in hospitals to sterilize surgical equipment. The Eclectic School sprayed it on "offensive materials" and to disinfect sickrooms. Modern studies give credence to these uses. They show that eucalyptus is a broad-spectrum antibacterial.[550] In vitro studies have shown that it inhibits the growth of bacteria typically found in the mouth.[551] (That property, however, did not show much benefit in clinical tests of a eucalyptus-based toothpaste.[552]) A Japanese test-tube study found it effective against micro-organisms that cause food poisoning and acne.[553]

Wounds. The antiseptic properties of eucalyptus are well known. Before antibiotics, it was commonly used on minor cuts and scrapes to prevent infection. The Nuholani Indians of Hawaii used it on cuts and sores.[554] The 1918 U.S. Dispensatory notes that an ointment made of eucalyptus oil and paraffin can be used to treat "indolent ulcers" and other skin diseases.[555] A more modern study discovered that it can heal skin ulcers in terminal cancer patients, working better than the standard medical therapies.[556]

Respiratory tract inflammation and congestion. Using eucalyptus for catarrhs is also a time-tested remedy. The most common way of using it is as an inhalant, a couple of drops of the oil being placed in hot water to create eucalyptus vapors. The steam helps open clogged sinuses, while the eucalyptus vapors act as a mild disinfectant. The Cahuilla Indians used it in this way for colds.[557] The 1918 U.S. Dispensatory recommends inhalations of the essential oil as an expectorant and notes that it can also be used to treat asthma.[558] The Eclectic School used eucalyptus vapors as a decongestant. In test-tube studies, eucalyptus has been shown to have some antiviral properties (against viruses other than the cold virus, however).[559] It has an anti-inflammatory effect on bronchitis in lab rats. The rats treated with eucalyptus showed a decrease in mucin (a protein that shows up in overabundance in asthma and bronchitis). Eucalyptus also relaxes the trachea muscles in guinea pigs.[560] One human study showed value in treating asthma.[561]

Fungal infections: athlete's foot, jock itch, ringworm. In vitro, eucalyptus essential oil is effective against most kinds of fungus.[562] A Japanese test-tube study found that eucalyptus extracts were found to be effective against the micro-organisms that cause athlete's foot.[563] One study of athlete's foot, jock itch, and ringworm showed that of the people treated with a eucalyptus ointment, 60% recovered completely and the remaining 40% showed significant improvement.[564] Eucalyptus also shows value in the treatment of toenail fungus.[565]

Muscle spasms and soreness. We have some evidence that eucalyptus might help for muscle soreness and cramps. Commission E notes that eucalyptus is mildly antispasmodic. Animal studies show that eucalyptus oil has both pain analgesic and anti-inflammatory properties in rats.[566] It increases circulation to the area.[567] And we know it does permeate the skin into the layers beneath.[568] But we don't have any human trials showing an effect on the muscles themselves.

Alertness and improved reaction time. Aromatherapy suggests that eucalyptus oil may improve alertness. A study conducted in Munich, Germany, put that claim to the test, testing eucalyptus' influence on reaction time and speed of information processing. Though some people seemed to improve, the results were not statistically significant. Their conclusion: if you *believe* eucalyptus help alertness and reaction time, you might get a bit of a boost from it.[569]

How do you use it?

Infused oil. Infused oil is not as strong as the essential oil, but the infused oil can be made at home, and it is safer. Use the standard method of infusing. Gargle five drops of infused oil in a glass of water for upper respiratory congestion. (Read the "What should you be aware of before using it" section before using eucalyptus as a mouth rinse or gargle.)

Essential oil. Always dilute essential oil before using it. Use a 1:50 ratio of essential oil to water or oil. (See chapter 3 for help choosing an appropriate carrier oil.) That's about two drops eucalyptus oil in a teaspoon of the carrier. (Read the "What should you be aware of before using it" section before using the essential oil of eucalyptus.)

Infusion. An infusion can be made with 1–2 teaspoons of the leaves.[570] This infusion won't have the most important active ingredient, however, because eucalyptol is not soluble in water.[571]

Tincture. 1:5. Eucalyptol can be extracted using alcohol,[572] so if that's what you're looking for, tinctures are a better choice than infusions in water.

Ointment. Use method seven for creams and salves (in Chapter 3), adding 5–10 drops of essential oil to a teaspoon of prepared salve or cream (5–10%). If you're using eucalyptus for muscle aches, rub the preparation into the skin well. That's a better way of getting the oils into the muscles than a patch or compress.[573]

Commercial preparations. Because of eucalyptus' toxicity, the safest way to use it internally (or in mouth rinses) is in commercial preparations where the amount of the active ingredient is carefully controlled. For example, using Listerine® as a mouth rinse is safer and more reliable than making your own with essential oil and a carrier.

Dosage: How much do you use?

Internal use. A traditional dose is 4–6 g of the leaf daily, divided into doses spaced 3–4 hours apart or 3–9 g of the tincture, also in divided doses.[574]

Eucalyptus essential oil should be standardized to 70% to 85% eucalyptol. Approximately, 0.3–0.6 g (0.05 to 0.2 milliliters) eucalyptus oil is the traditional dose for internal use of the essential oil; however, the U.S. National Institute of Health's Medline article questions the safety of this amount, noting that even that small amount could cause toxic side effects.[575] The safest way to use eucalyptus is to stick to commercial preparations and use them only at recommended doses.

External use. 5–20% in oil and semi-solid preparations.[576] and 5–10% in aqueous-alcoholic preparations[577]

What should you be aware of before using it?

Eucalyptus contains a chemical called eucalyptol (also known as cineole), which irritates the skin. The higher the concentration, the more this becomes an issue.[578] Eucalyptus' essential oils should be diluted.[579] Eucalyptus preparations should not be applied to the face, especially the nose, of children and adults with sensitive skin.[580] If you have sensitive skin or allergies, try a small amount of diluted eucalyptus externally before inhaling the steam or gargling with it.

Some people are allergic to eucalyptus (both the pollen and the topical administration). If you have other allergies, be quite cautious the first time you try eucalyptus. Though eucalyptus is a common treatment for asthma and allergies, it causes a worsening of symptoms in some people who are sensitive to eucalyptol. [581]

The essential oil should not be taken internally.[582] It can cause nausea, vomiting, and other gastrointestinal irritations. It can also cause seizures,[583] or even death. (Cough drops and the like contain a small enough amounts that they don't pose a problem.) When making preparations using eucalyptus essential oil, follow safe handling practices: keep it away from foodstuffs, don't get it near your nose or mouth, wear gloves and eye protection, be careful that anything that may have a residue on it (pots, strainers, spoons, etc.) doesn't come in contact with food, and label all preparations as "external use only." The safest policy is to avoid internal or oral use of eucalyptus in anything other than commercially prepared products.

Eucalyptus oil affects the enzyme system of the liver involved in the detoxification process. Therefore, the effects of other drugs can be weakened and/or shortened if you are using eucalyptus.[584]

Don't use eucalyptus internally, even in small amounts, if you have inflammation of the gastrointestinal tract or the bile ducts, or a serious liver disease.[585]

The most conservative advice says that children under the age of 12 shouldn't use eucalyptus.[586] Less conservative advice says it shouldn't be used for those under two.[587] The amount of eucalyptus that a child can tolerate varies widely. Some have an immediate reaction even to a small amount topically; others can tolerate it comparatively well.[588] Ingesting too much can cause problems in breathing and unconsciousness.[589] In fact, even topically, too much can also cause muscle weakness and changes in consciousness.[590] In short, the reported range of toxic doses in children is wide.[591] At the very least, parents should be extremely moderate when using eucalyptus on children, and they should store it out of children's reach.

Traditional wisdom says that eucalyptus worsens the negative effects of borage, coltsfoot, comfrey, hound's tooth, or *Senecio* species. We have no reliable research to that effect, but caution is advised.[592]

Eucalyptol is flammable. Take appropriate precautions when storing eucalyptus essential oil.

We do not know the effect eucalyptus may have on pregnant or nursing women.[593]

Evening Primrose Oil

Scientific name: *Oenothera biennis*

Also known as *flor de Santa Rita*, German rampion, fever plant, night willow-herb, scabish, sun drop, fever-plant, weedy evening-primrose, hog weed, king's cure-all

Evening primrose is a tall wildflower that is native to the United States. It is also found in Europe and parts of Asia. The flowers open in the evening, hence the name. The fleshy, turnip-like root used to be eaten as a table vegetable, much like potatoes are today.[594] Oil extracted from the seeds is the part of the plant most commonly used medicinally. Evening primrose is hardy in any location with enough sun to suit its tastes, so much so that it has become an invasive plant in some parts of the U.S.

Evening primrose is grown commercially in more than fifteen countries because of the oil found in its seeds.[595] The oil in the mature seeds contain 7–10% gamma-linolenic acid (GLA), an omega-6 essential fatty acid with anti-inflammatory properties.[596] Evening primrose oil (EPO) also contains about 50–70% cis-linoleic acid, which can be converted by the body into GLA. EPO has become a common alternative to the borage oil as a source of GLA. Borage oil contains about double the concentration of GLA as EPO, and it's generally cheaper, but it also contains pyrrolizidine alkaloids, which are toxic to the liver. For that reason EPO is becoming the more common GLA supplement.[597]

What is it good for?

Cardiovascular health. This is not a traditional use, but a modern one. Supposedly EPO—more specifically the GLA in EPO—alters the lipid levels in the body in such as way as to benefit cardiovascular health. We have animal studies that suggest a rationale behind this use. In rats, supplementation with EPO lowered the LDL cholesterol levels.[598] EPO lowered both cholesterol and body weight in a second animal study where rats were fed a high cholesterol diet.[599] It reduced platelet aggregation (the formation of blood clots) in rabbits fed an atherogenic diet (one

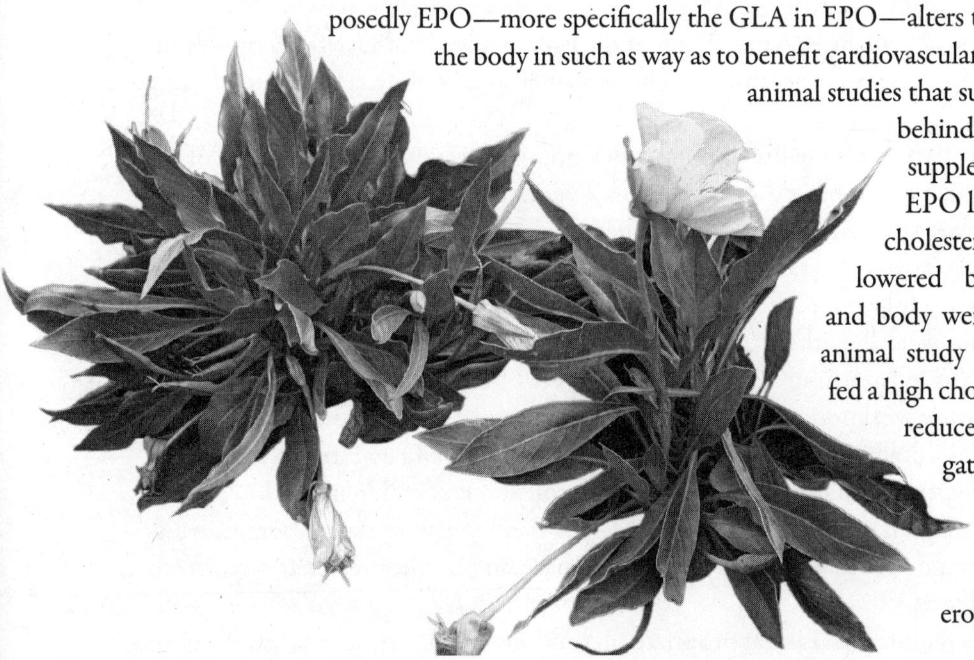

Evening Primrose, *Oenothera biennis*
Courtesy of Karel Jakubec

that would normally cause their arteries to become lined with fatty deposits). As such, it shows potential in reducing the conditions that lead to arteriosclerosis and thrombotic strokes.[600] In two other studies using rabbits, EPO helped undo some of the negative effects of a high fat diet.[601] In short, at this point what we have is a significant number of artificially fat rats and rabbits benefiting from EPO. Human trials are lacking. ◊ ◊ ◆ ◆ ◆

Arthritis. One common use for EPO is to treat the inflammation associated with arthritis. Again, this is a modern use with little traditional backing. We do know that EPO contains lipophilic triterpenoidal esters, compounds that have scavenging and anti-inflammatory properties.[602] What we don't know is the mechanism by which EPO suppresses inflammation in the human body.[603] Clinical studies at this point are small. Several small studies show reduction in symptoms.[604] Others show no benefits.[605] ◊ ◊ ◆ ◆ ◆

Wounds and sores. The Navajo used it on sores.[606] Early American settlers used it for hemorrhoids, sore throat, and bruises.[607] The 1918 U.S. Dispensatory notes that a decoction can be used for eruptive skin diseases.[608] It is also approved for treating eczema and atopic dermatitis in several countries.[609] As we've already noted, EPO has some anti-inflammatory properties.[610] A single in vitro study also shows that compounds in EPO have fungicidal properties[611] though a second study showed no antimicrobial effect at all.[612] Neither study has been repeated. We also have no clinical trials or animal studies. At this point, we don't have enough information to tell whether EPO might be useful in treating bacterial or fungal infections in humans. It may, nevertheless, have some anti-inflammatory properties that could be useful for bruises and swollen wounds. ◊ ◊ ◊ ◆ ◆

Fatigue. One of the uses is treating fatigue—either chronic fatigue or fatigue after recovery from a viral infection. Though we have anecdotal evidence that EPO might be helpful for these conditions, the cross-cultural attestation and scientific evidence are not there.[613] ◊ ◊ ◊ ◊ ◆

How do you use it?

Commercially prepared capsules: Buy capsules from a reliable source. Cheap evening-primrose preparations are sometimes mostly soy or safflower oil.[614] Store it in a cool place.

Dosage: How much do you use?

The concentration of GLA in evening primrose oil varies, depending on how the oil is extracted.[615] Existing studies often did not use standardized oils. Toxicity studies are lacking. Consequently, we're not sure what a good dose of EPO is. In arthritis studies, a typical dose is roughly 540 mg per day.[616] Some herbalists recommend as much as 1,000 mg three times a day.[617] For short term use to treat dermatitis, daily doses as high as 4–8 g (4,000–8,000 mg) have been used.[618] Your best bet is to buy from a reputable company and follow package instructions. Take it with food to help absorption and minimize the chance of gastrointestinal upset.[619]

What should you be aware of before using it?

Reported side effects include occasional headache, abdominal pain, nausea, and loose stools.[620]

Don't take it if you are using phenothiazine drugs. It may pose an increased risk of temporal lobe epilepsy in schizophrenic patients taking epileptogenic drugs such as phenothiazines.[621]

If you have a seizure disorder, check with your doctor before using evening primrose. Several reports of seizures have been filed, some, but not all, of them involving individuals with a preexisting seizure disorder.[622]

Theoretically, evening primrose oil could increase the risk of bleeding. If you plan to have surgery, tell your surgeon you have been taking evening primrose oil and discontinue use at least two weeks or so before the surgery.[623] Use caution when taking it with other herbs that also increase that risk. (See Chapter 5 for a list.)

In animal studies, gamma-linolenic acid (an ingredient of EPO) is reported to decrease blood pressure. Human studies don't show consistent changes in blood pressure, but those studies are still preliminary at this point.[624]

Don't take EPO with drugs or herbs that have monoamine oxidase inhibitor (MAOI) activity or that interact with MAOI drugs. Headache, tremors, mania, and insomnia may occur.[625] (See Chapter 5 for a list.)

Don't take it if you are pregnant.[626]

Fennel

Scientific name: *Foeniculum vulgare*

Also known as finocchio, carosella, *xiao hui xiang* Foeniculi aetheroleum is fennel oil.

The plant is a perennial herb with a long straight stem and an umbrella of seeds. The seeds, which have an anise-like flavor are the part most used medicinally. The essential oil is distilled from the dried, ripe seeds by water steam distillation.

Fennel is indigenous to the Mediterranean region. From there, it spread to Europe, Asia, South and North America, where it now grows wild as an introduced species. Fennel has a long history of use both as a medicine and as a spice. Pliny used it extensively in his remedies. In the Middle Ages, it was used medicinally as a carminative as well as a means of warding off

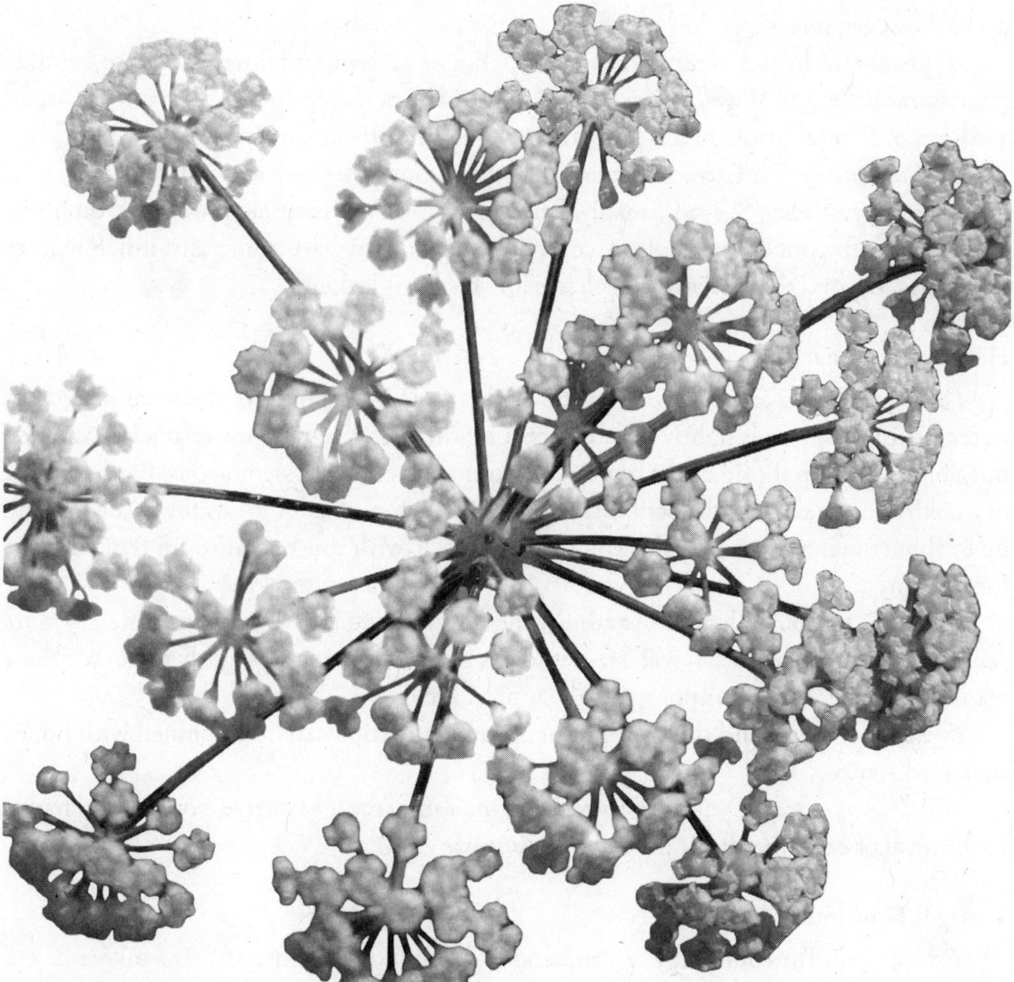

Fennel, *Foeniculum vulgare*

Courtesy of Foodista

evil. Especially during the Midsummer festival, it was hung over the doors of houses to keep away evil influences. It also has a history of use as an insect repellant.

What is it good for?

Throat irritation and colds. We have traditional evidence from at least two continents for this use. The Chinese call fennel *xiao hui xiang* and use it for upper respiratory tract mucous membrane inflammation, cough, and bronchitis.[627] Commission E recommends it for "catarrhs of the upper respiratory tract" and notes that it has mild expectorant properties.[628] In the lab, it relaxes muscle chains in the trachea of pigs it was tested on.[629] We have no clinical evidence for whether it does anything for human beings, however.

Flatulence. The Cherokee used fennel for flatulence.[630] Commission E recommends it for this use, as did the 1918 U.S. Dispensatory and the Eclectic School.[631] Scientific evidence, however, is lacking.

Antibacterial. In vitro, fennel kills several kinds of bacteria and fungi, including candida yeast, salmonella, and *Shigella dysenteriae* (a cause of bacterial dysentery),[632] staphylococcus, and listeria.[633] Implications of this property for human health remain untested.

Anti-inflammatory. Extract of fennel may have some untested anti-inflammatory and/or analgesic properties.[634] Traditionally, fennel decoction or essential oil was used on bruises. Fennel does contain anethole, a compound known to have some anti-inflammatory properties. Beyond that, scientific evidence for this use is lacking.

How do you use it?

Decoction. To make a decoction of the seeds, use 1–2 teaspoons of the seeds per cup of water, bruising the seeds lightly before decocting them.[635] Keep the water at a low simmer, not a boil, and keep the lid of the pot on to minimize the loss of essential oils. For flatulence or a cold, you can use this decoction as a tea. Drink before or after meals for flatulence and up to three times a day for a cold. You can also gargle with this tea (at room temperature) for sore throat.

Tincture. 1:5, 60% alcohol. Anethole, the anti-inflammatory agent in fennel, is more soluble in alcohol than it is in water. Anethole is also an irritant and slightly toxic. For these reasons, tinctures are more appropriate to topical uses.

Syrup. For coughs and throat irritation, fennel decoction can be combined with honey to make a syrup.

Whole or as a spice. If you tend to get gas from eating meat or cheese, you can add fennel to the meal or eat some afterward to help minimize gas.[636]

Dosage: How much do you use?

Essential oil. The commonly recommended dose is no more than 0.1–0.6 ml per day.[637] That's about 2–10 drops per day. The conservative recommendation is to completely avoid taking the essential oil internally. The essential oil can be dangerous (see the "What should you be aware of before using it" section). As little as ¼–1 teaspoon of the essential oil taken orally can have severe adverse effects.[638] Besides, the internal uses are just as well served by decoctions and tinctures.

Whole seed. 5–7 g herb (the crushed seed) daily[639]

Tincture. no more than ½–1 teaspoon, three times (or fewer) per day.[640] Watch to see how you react to tinctures. But anethole in them can be irritating. Too much anethole can be toxic, so stay within the recommended doses.

Infusion. Lightly crush 1–2 teaspoonfuls of seeds. Pour a cup of boiling water over them and leave to infuse for 10 minutes. Drink one cup, up to three times per day.[641]

Don't take fennel for more than a few weeks unless directed by a doctor.[642]

What should you be aware of before using it?

Fennel in food concentrations is on the FDA's list of substances generally recognized as safe. Whole seeds and tinctures, taken short term and in moderation, are generally safe. The problems come to light when it's the essential oil and medicinal quantities that are being used.

The essential oil of fennel can be toxic. Reports of hallucinations and seizures have been reported with its use. Don't use the essential oil without professional supervision.[643]

It's possible to be allergic to fennel. If you are allergic to celery, be especially careful.[644]

The estragole in fennel causes cancer when given to rats in incredibly high doses.[645]

Don't use the herb in medicinal quantities while pregnant.[646]

Children under the age of six shouldn't be given medicinal quantities of this herb.[647]

Be especially careful of your sun exposure while taking this herb medicinally as it can cause photodermatitis.[648]

Don't take it if you are using ciprofloxacin, because fennel may decrease the effect of this drug.[649]

In the wild, fennel looks a lot like hemlock. Don't pick wild fennel for yourself unless you know what you're doing.

Fenugreek

Scientific name: *Trigonella foenum-graecum*

Also known as bird's foot, Greek hay seed, *hu lu ba*, trigonella

Fenugreek is a flowering annual plant with small, hard seeds. These seeds, along with the other above-ground parts, are the parts of the plant used medicinally. It's a native of Asia and southeastern Europe and is not typically grown in North America except for a few isolated areas in California.

This herb has been used for centuries both as a spice and a medicinal herb. It was first cultivated in Assyria in the seventh century B.C.E.[650] The first record of its medicinal use dates back to Hippocrates, the father of modern medicine. From there, use spread through the Mediterranean region to the Far East and South Asia. In China, fenugreek is called *hu lu ba* and is used for impotence and abdominal pain.[651] It also has a place in Ayurvedic

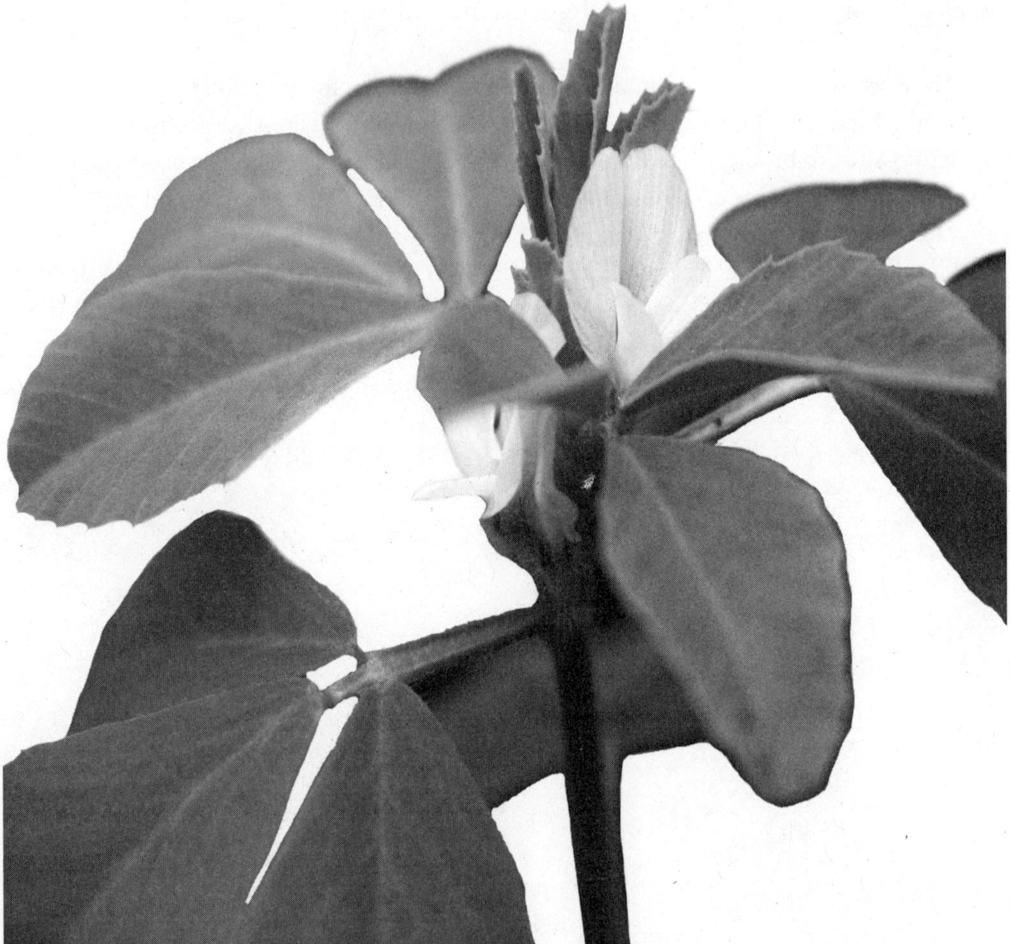

Fenugreek, *Trigonella foenum-graecum*

Courtesy of Anne-Miek Bibbe

medicine. In Western countries, it has much less of a history. In the last thirty years, however, it has begun to gain attention as a help for metabolic syndrome (also called syndrome X). Metabolic syndrome is characterized by blood sugar problems (fasting hyperglycemia, type 2 diabetes, impaired glucose tolerance or insulin resistance), high blood pressure, central obesity (too much fat around the abdomen), increased LDL and decreased HDL cholesterol, elevated triglycerides, and elevated uric acid levels. Fenugreek shows promise for controlling just that complex of symptoms—blood sugar, cholesterol and triglycerides, and possibly weight control.

What is it good for?

Blood sugar control. This use is a modern one and has little traditional attestation. Animal studies abound. Fenugreek lowers the blood glucose level in rats with induced diabetes[652] as well as in dogs and cows. We have fewer clinical studies regarding fenugreek and diabetes in people, but the few we have look promising. One study shows that using fenugreek seeds in conjunction with changes in diet improves blood sugar control and decreases insulin resistance in mild type 2 diabetic patients.[653] Another study of patients with mild non-insulin-dependent diabetes mellitus showed that fenugreek lowered both fasting and postprandial blood sugar. However, people with more serious type 2 diabetes showed less benefit.[654] A small-scale study of patients with type 1 (insulin-dependent) diabetes also showed a decrease in fasting blood sugar and improved glucose tolerance with fenugreek use.[655]

Cholesterol and triglyceride control. In rat experiments, daily fenugreek reduced the accumulation of triglycerides in the liver of obese rats.[656] In one human study, fenugreek lowered blood lipids (both cholesterol and triglycerides) in patients with coronary artery disease but not in healthy subjects.[657] Another human study found that fenugreek seed powder reduced LDL cholesterol.[658] The quality of these studies, however, is not what one might hope.[659]

Sore throat and congestion. Fenugreek contains mucilage, up to 30%, in the seeds. It has been used traditionally for soothing a sore throat, and the presence of mucilage would seem to indicate that that use may have value. We have no studies, however, confirming its effectiveness.

Skin inflammation. Commission E recommends fenugreek as a poultice for local inflammation.[660] Again fenugreek's main value probably comes from the mucilage content, which acts to soothe irritation. Tradition says that it is an emollient, in other words, that it has skin-softening properties. But tradition is all we have for this use.

Exercise recovery. One lone study of bicyclists suggests that fenugreek might help exercise recovery. Following an overnight fast and a ninety-minute ride, a muscle biopsy was taken. The cyclists were then given either dextrose alone or dextrose with an extract of fenugreek. After a period of time, a second biopsy was taken. Those who received the fenugreek had a 63% greater net rate of muscle glycogen resynthesis.[661] In other words, their muscles refueled more quickly. The study has been neither replicated nor challenged.

Weight control. Rats who were fed a high fat diet while simultaneously taking a fenugreek supplement showed decreased plasma triglyceride gain. The researchers postulate that this effect might prevent or slow weight gain caused by a high fat diet.[662] We should note, however, that the rats were not actually weighed. Moreover, fat rats have much more in common with other rats than they do with fat human beings. Combined with the traditional use of fenugreek to stimulate the appetite, this evidence does not suggest that fenugreek is a useful tool for weight loss. ◊ ◊ ◊ ◊ ◆

How do you use it?

Powdered. Commercially prepared capsules are available.

Poultice. A poultice made of the seeds can be used on boils or local skin inflammations. Powder or pulverize the seeds and mix with water to make a paste for the poultice.

Infusion. To make a tea, soak one tablespoon of seeds in a cup of cold water for twenty minutes. Slowly bring the water to simmer. Turn off the heat and steep for 10 to 20 minutes. Strain and drink. To make a cold infusion, which helps preserve the mucilage, soak a tablespoon of the seeds in cold water for three hours. Strain and use.

Whole seeds. The cooked seeds can be eaten as well.[663] Don't boil the seeds because doing so destroys a number of components.[664]

Sprouted. Sprouted seeds were used in one cholesterol-control study.[665] Sprouted seeds also have higher antioxidant properties than cooked seeds.[666] To sprout the seeds, soak the seeds in cool water for twelve hours. Drain, rinse, and drain. Let the seeds sit out of direct sunlight to sprout. Every twelve hours rinse and drain them again. Taste the sprouts at each rinse to see when you like the taste best. They will be ready in 3–6 days.

Gargle. A gargle is made by infusing 1 teaspoon of pulverized seeds in 8 ounces of water. It can be used up to three times per day.[667]

Tincture. Tinctures are not recommended if you want the mucilage of fenugreek to remain intact.

Salve. Use method two for making creams and salves (see Chapter 3). Use a low simmer and avoid boiling the fenugreek.

Dosage: How much do you use?

Internal: Probable effective dosage is .5–2 g, 3–4 times per day made into a tea.[668] One study used 2.5 g twice a day to good effect (on both blood sugar and blood lipids).[669] Don't exceed 6 g per day. It can also be taken as a capsule: typical dose is one 626 mg capsule two to three times per day.[670]

External: 50 g powdered drug with one cup water.

What should you be aware of before using it?

Fenugreek has been used for centuries without significant adverse reactions. The FDA has placed it on its GRAS (generally recognized as safe) list for food use. Studies have also found it to be apparently safe for healthy adults in typical medicinal doses.[671]

It is possible to be allergic to fenugreek.[672] Symptoms reported are runny nose, wheezing, and fainting when it is inhaled; and numbness, rapid facial swelling, and wheezing when it is applied topically.[673] According to Commission E, repeated external applications can result in dermatitis or other undesirable skin reactions. You can become sensitized to fenugreek.

Fenugreek can affect blood sugar levels. If you are diabetic, discuss any herbal supplements you may wish to take (especially ones that affect blood sugar levels like fenugreek) with your doctor before taking them. Be cautious using fenugreek if you are hypoglycemic. Be cautious when using it in conjunction with herbs known or suspected to affect blood sugar levels. (See Chapter 5 for a list.)

Any herb containing mucilage can theoretically interfere with the absorption of other drugs.

If you have any liver problems, check with your doctor before using fenugreek because it does seem to affect the way the liver processes fats.

If you are on heart or hormonal medicine, talk with your doctor before using fenugreek.[674] Don't take it with herbs that have monoamine oxidase inhibitor (MAOI) activity or that interact with MAOI drugs. Headache, tremors, mania, and insomnia may occur [675] (See Chapter 5 for a list.)

Don't take fenugreek if you are pregnant or trying to conceive. Fenugreek has an antifertility effect in laboratory rabbits and rats.[676] One of its traditional uses is to induce labor.

Some people experience more bruising or bleeding than usual when taking fenugreek.[677] It may also change the effects of bloodthinning drugs.[678] Be a bit more careful about training with gear or a partner until you know how you react to it. If you plan to have surgery, tell your surgeon you have been taking fenugreek and discontinue use. Be cautious when using it in conjunction with other herbs known or suspected of increasing the risk of bleeding. (See Chapter 5 for a list.)

Fenugreek has a way of working itself through the body and out your sweat glands, making you smell a bit like curry. The effect is more pronounced for some people than it is for others. It can also do odd things to the smell of your urine.[679]

Feverfew

Scientific name: *Tanacetum parthenium*

Also known as *Leucanthemum parthenium*, *Matricaria capensis*, *Matricaria parthenium* L., *Crysanthemum parthenium*, *Parthenium hysterophorus*, *Pyrenthrum parthenium* L., featherfew, altamisa, featherfoil, midsummer daisy, Santa Maria, wild quinine, bachelor's button, camomille grande, febrifuge plant, federfoy, flirtwort, mother herb, mutterkraut, nosebleed, parthenolide, wild chamomile

Feverfew is a short, bushy perennial that grows wild as an introduced species throughout North America. The above-ground parts—the daisy-like flower and (most commonly) the yellow-green leaves—are used medicinally.

Ancient Greeks and Early Europeans used feverfew for headaches and other aches and pains. They also used it externally for wounds and internally to take down fevers. In fact the name is from the Latin word *febrifuga*, which means to drive a fever away.[680] Ironically, modern research has yet to find evidence for that particular use.[681] In 1978, the first paper was released suggesting that feverfew might be useful for preventing and treating migraines. As more and more evidence has been amassed for that use, feverfew has become better and better known.

What is it good for?

Migraines. According to traditional British herbal thinking, feverfew is best for the "cold" type of migraine, the kind that's made worse by cold such as cold treatments, cold weather, or cold drafts and eased by applying a hot towel to the head.[682] How it works is not entirely known. We do know that it has an anti-inflammatory effect. It contains parthenolide, an anti-inflammatory, which is the chemical constituent believed to affect migraines.[683] Several studies show that when taken on a regular basis, feverfew can reduce the number and severity of migraines.[684] It doesn't however, seem to have an affect on a migraine already in progress.[685]

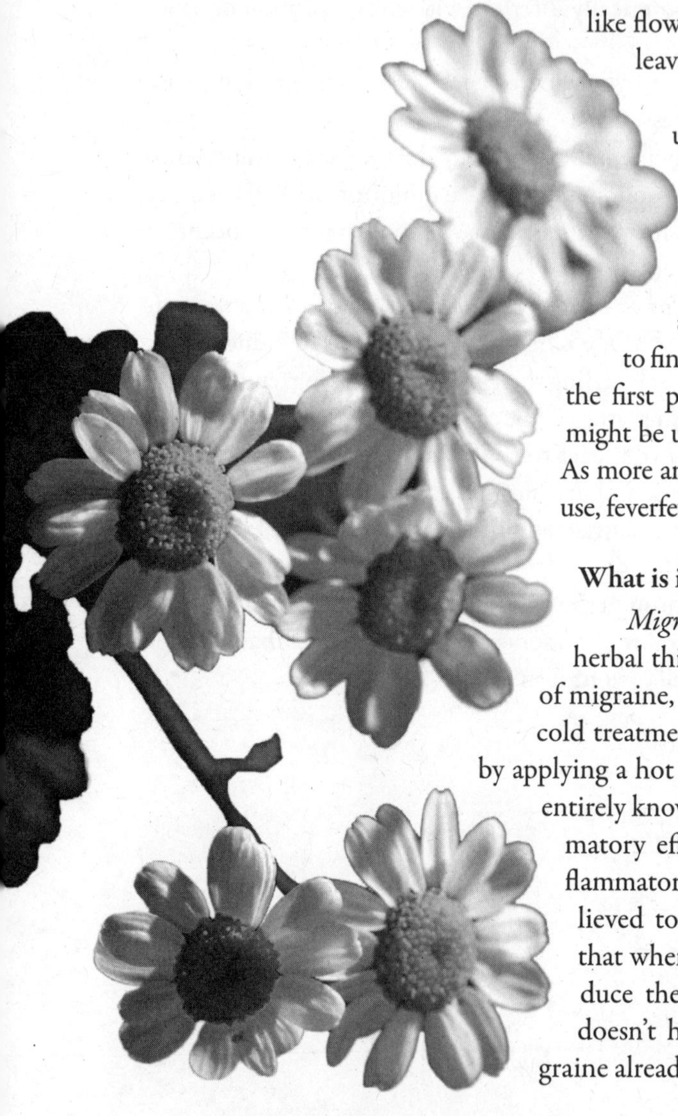

Feverfew, *Tanacetum parthenium*
Courtesy of Renate Eder

Arthritis and joint pain. The Mahuna Indians used feverfew for rheumatism.[686] A 1989 study of forty-one people with rheumatoid arthritis, however, failed to find benefit (at the dose of 70–86 mg per day for six weeks).[687]

Localized swelling or inflammation. The Cherokee used feverfew to bathe swollen feet.[688] In modern times it's used in Aveeno® skin care products to minimize redness and irritation. In vitro studies show that the parthenolide in feverfew has a possible anti-inflammatory action. But the one animal study investigating feverfew for inflammation didn't support this use.[689]

How do you use it?

A commercially prepared freeze-dried extract is available. The potency of this extract, if made by a reliable company, is more consistent than home-grown leaves.

Fresh. If you do grow your own feverfew, eat one fresh leaf daily as a prophylactic against migraines.

Tincture. 5–10 drops every 30 minutes at the onset of a migraine.

Cold infusion brings out the best in feverfew. Wrap the herb in cheesecloth, pre-moisten it, and suspend it in tepid water at room temperature, overnight. Use a 1:32 (herb to water) ratio. Squeeze out the herb into the tea in the morning.[690]

Dosage: How much do you use?

The quality of prepared tablets and capsules varies widely. Some, especially those sold in countries without regulation (like the United States), can contain little or no active ingredients.[691] If you can find a standardized preparation, 250 micrograms of parthenolide is a typical daily dosage for migraines.[692] Alternatively, you can take 25 mg of the freeze-dried extract per day.[693]

Those who grow their own feverfew can take up to two leaves per day.[694]

Don't use feverfew for more than four months at a time. You can form a physical addiction to it if you use it over an extended period of time.[695]

What should you be aware of before using it?

Some people are allergic to feverfew. Being allergic to plants in the daisy (*Asteraceae/Compositae*) family, including chamomile and ragweed, increases the chance of allergy to feverfew.[696]

In the various trials, about 10–18% of people developed adverse reactions of some kind, the most common being ulcers and other problems in the mouth. People with light-colored skin are more likely to experience this reaction.[697] If the leaves give you mouth ulcers, they can be sautéed briefly before you eat them, or you can go with the commercially prepared freeze-dried preparations. Feverfew also blunts some people's sense of taste.

It is possible to form a physical addiction to feverfew if you use it over an extended period of time. Don't use it for more than four months at a time. Withdrawal symptoms include pain in muscle joints and soft tissues.[698]

Women who are pregnant, nursing, or who have menstrual difficulties should talk to a doctor before taking feverfew.[699] One of the traditional uses was for tardy labor. It may stimulate the uterus.[700]

If you are taking blood-thinning drugs, including aspirin, ibuprofen, naproxen, or related drugs, don't take feverfew because it can affect clotting rates.[701] If you plan to have surgery, tell your surgeon you have been taking feverfew and discontinue use. Avoid taking it in conjunction with other herbs suspected of increasing the risk of bleeding. (See Chapter 5 for a list.)

Don't give feverfew to children. Not enough research has been done into the way that it affects them.

Note: Though chamomile is sometimes known as sweet feverfew, it is not the same as or interchangeable with *Tanacetum parthenium*, true feverfew. Neither is it interchangeable with *Tanacetum vulgare*, sometimes called oil of tansy, which is more toxic.

Fish Oil

Also known as omega-3, marine oil, menhaden oil

Not strictly an herbal remedy, fish oil is just that: oil derived from fish. Fish oil contains polyunsaturated fats called omega-3 fatty acids.

The body needs omega-3 to keep the heart, brain, joints, and other physical systems healthy. Unfortunately, the body can't make its own omega-3, so it must get it from outside sources. To give your body what it needs, you need to either make sure your diet contains enough omega-3 fatty acids or you need to supplement. Three types of omega-3 fatty acids are important for human nutrition: docosahexaenoic acid (DHA), eicosapentaenoic acid (EPA), and alpha-linolenic acid (ALA). The body uses DHA and EPA directly. It can convert ALA into DHA and EPA for use, but it can't use ALA directly. Plants such as flax seeds, chia, lingonberries, hemp, walnuts, and canola oil have ALA. Cold-water fish such as salmon, sea bass, anchovies, sardines, mackerel, herring, and others have DHA and EPA omega-3s. (These fish have taken in ALA from plants and converted it already into DHA and EPA, which they store in their bodies.) EPA and DHA, the fish oil omega-3s, are more biologically potent than ALA, the plant omega-3s.[702] That's why I've included fish oil in a book devoted to herbs. Fish oil has the benefits of the omega-3s in flaxseed, only more so.

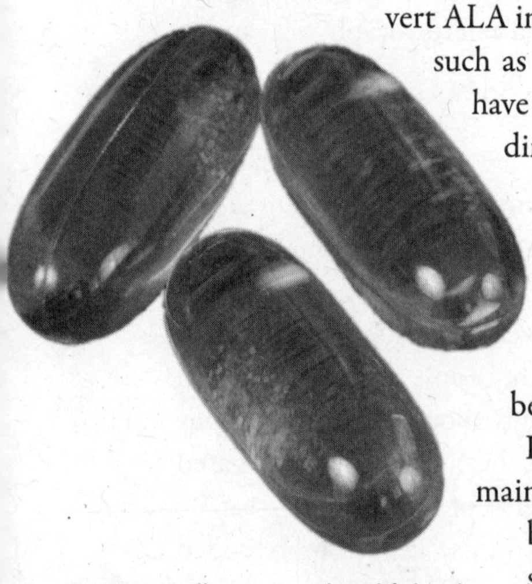
Commercially encapsulated fish oil

It's rare for the Western herbal medical community and the mainstream medical community to agree about much of anything, but they agree on fish oil: in appropriate doses, it's an excellent support for cardiovascular health.

What is it good for?

Supporting cardiovascular health. Fish oil helps with proper blood circulation. A study at the University of California, Davis supplemented the diet of seven healthy subjects with DHA, a kind of omega-3 fatty acid found in fish oil. The subjects then performed a hand-grip exercise while the researchers measured blood flow in the brachial artery, the major blood vessel providing blood to the arm. Those subjects who had taken the DHA had better blood supply to the arm than those who had taken a placebo.[703] ◆◆◆◆

It also helps prevent cardiovascular disease.[704] We now have evidence that fish oil helps lower blood pressure and triglyceride levels in the blood.[705] The American Heart Association recommends fish oil for patients with coronary heart disease. Even the FDA, an agency notoriously difficult to convince about the value of herbs and supplements, has acknowledged the evidence for DHA and EPA's benefits in reducing the risk of coronary heart disease saying that evidence is "supportive but not conclusive."[706] The cardiovascular benefits of fish oil may not extend, however, to people with not just artery disease but also existing heart problems. In one study, people with heart arrhythmias bad enough to warrant implanted defibrillators received no benefit from fish oil supplements.[707]

Exercise capacity and recovery. Horses given fish oil and then put through a training regimen seemed to get more positive physiological changes—lower heart rate, lower packed cell volume, lower serum insulin—than those given a placebo oil.[708] A study looking at the value of fish oil for men with heart disease found that men given DHA and EPA for four months had an improved one-minute heart-rate recovery after exercise.[709] DHA may also help reduce inflammation caused by exercise. Forty men were given a supplement containing mixed tocopherols (vitamin E), flavonoids, and either DHA or a placebo. After ten days of exercise, the DHA group had considerably less exercise-induced inflammation.[710] They didn't, however, have any less delayed onset muscle soreness (also known as DOMS, the inflammatory response of muscle tissue to intense exercise that shows up as soreness and temporary increase in muscle size a day or so after the exercise). A small study done by the University of Kentucky into the effect of fish oil on DOMS also found no help from the oil. According to a second study, fish oil does not help with either the swelling or the pain of DOMS.[711] ◊◊◆◆◆

Exercise-induced bronchoconstriction (EIB). Sixteen asthmatics who typically had attacks during exercise were given fish oil in addition to their normal diet. Though both those who received fish oil and those who received the placebo had continuing problems with EIB, those on fish oil had considerably less severe attacks.[712] A second small study using elite athletes found the same effect.[713] ◊◊◆◆◆

Behavior and developmental disorders. Studies of people with a long history of violent behavior show lower levels of DHA.[714] So do hyperactive children.[715] Studies show that deficiencies in DHA and EPA affect serotonin levels in the brain, which in turn affects development of the neurotransmitters that regulate the limbic system (the fight-or-flight part of the brain).[716] Lower levels of DHA in the blood are also associated with elevated levels of corticotrophin-releasing hormone and increased levels of anxiety, fear, and aggression.[717] Supplementation (DHA taken orally) increases the levels of DHA in the blood and the brain to good effect.[718] For example, young male prisoners given essential fatty acid supplements showed a substantial decrease in violent behavior.[719] Studies with lab animals, school-aged girls, cocaine addicts, and the elderly show similar effects.[720] In normal young adults, fish oil supplements decreased violent behavior during times of stress.[721] Supplementation doesn't, however, seem to affect violence levels in normal adults under nonstressful conditions.[722]

Whether fish oil supplementation affects hyperactivity is a matter of controversy, however.[723] One study found that fish oil doesn't reduce the symptoms of ADHD.[724] Another, one that combined fish oil with vitamin C, found improvements.[725] According to other studies, fish oil can improve behavior and academic progress in children with developmental coordination disorder.[726] It can help with depression.[727] It may even have a positive effect on autism.[728] ◊ ◊ ◆ ◆ ◆

Anti-inflammatory. Omega-3s in general and DHA and EPA in particular have some anti-inflammatory properties.[729] Fish oil may, therefore, be useful in addressing inflammation-related diseases like heart disease, depression, and cancer.[730] Clinical trials show a fish-oil-related improvement in several inflammatory diseases including Crohn's disease, ulcerative colitis, psoriasis, lupus erythematosus, multiple sclerosis, and migraine headaches.[731] Studies investigating the benefit of fish oil for rheumatoid arthritis sufferers show decreased swelling of joints in people taking fish oil.[732] ◊ ◊ ◆ ◆ ◆

Weight loss. One study found that people who took fish oil supplements and combined them with walking lost more weight and body fat than those who just walked or those who walked and took a placebo oil.[733] ◊ ◊ ◊ ◆ ◆

How do you use it?

You can increase the amount of fish oil in your diet by increasing the amount of cold-water fish (herring, salmon, sardines, etc.) you eat. You can also take commercially prepared supplements.

One of the problems, however, with cold water fish and the oils derived from them is the presence of heavy metals. Typically, oils that are refined to extract any heavy metals will say so on the label. Also International Fish Oil Standards, a third-party testing service investigates the quality of fish oil supplements and publishes its finding on the internet (www.nutrasource.ca). One of the contaminants they check for is heavy metals. Alternatively, you can look for fish oil from fish in less polluted area, such as Nordic seas.[734]

Also be aware of the amount of vitamin A in prepared fish oil capsules. Too much is toxic. Fish oil made from the liver (such as cod liver oil) tends to have too much vitamin A.

Finally, be aware that some fish and omega-3 oil capsules contain oils that aren't from fish. Some contain borage, which has dangers that fish oil does not.

Dosage: How much do you use?

The American Heart Association recommends:

Two servings of fish a week for healthy people.[735] Regular intake of oily fish such as salmon, sea bass, anchovies, sardines, mackerel, and herring is the safest way of adding fish oil to your diet.

2 to 4 g per day of EPA and DHA for people with elevated triglycerides[736]

1 g per day dose for patients with existing cardiovascular disease[737]

Some conditions, such as rheumatoid arthritis and Crohn's disease, respond best to higher doses of fish oil.[738] Doses as high as 8 g have been used in some studies without reported problems.[739] As a general rule, however, you shouldn't take more than 3 g of omega-3 fatty acids unless you are supervised by a doctor. In fact, the most conservative advice, that of the FDA, suggests that supplementation be limited to one gram per day or less.[740] Not everyone has a benign response to fish oil; high intake can cause excessive bleeding in some people.[741] High doses can also make you smell a little bit like a bait bucket because the fishy odor comes out through your pores. Also if you eat fish, flaxseed, eggs from free-range chickens or chickens fed omega-3s, walnuts, or any of a myriad of foods containing omega-3s, you may need to adjust your supplementation accordingly. If you have any doubt about the proper dosage for you, consult with your doctor or a naturopath.

If you get fish burps when you take fish oil, break your daily dose into three smaller doses and take them with meals.[742]

What should you be aware of before using it?

Some people experience belching, bloating, flatulence, diarrhea, or nausea when taking fish oil. If you have one of these symptoms, try switching brands first. Some brands are made better than others. If you still have problems, try breaking up the dosage or beginning with a lower dose (as little as 180 mg per day) and increasing it over time. Doing so will gradually build your body's ability to digest the oil.[743]

People who have any seafood allergies should obviously not take fish oil.

Fish oil may affect blood sugar levels. Check with your doctor if you are diabetic or hypoglycemia and want to take fish oil. Be cautious taking it in conjunction with other herbs and drugs that may affect blood sugar. (See Chapter 5 for a list.)

Fish oil increases the risk of bleeding, especially in high doses.[744] If you are taking anticoagulants, including aspirin or NSAIDs, talk with your doctor before taking fish oil. If you plan to have surgery, tell your surgeon you have been taking fish oil and discontinue use. Be cautious when using it in conjunction with herbs known or suspected of increasing bleeding. (See Chapter 5 for a list.)

If you have high LDL cholesterol or triglycerides, talk to your doctor about taking fish oil supplements, whether doing so is advisable and whether you should be taking vitamin E in conjunction.[745]

If you have heart problems, check with your doctor before beginning fish oil.

If you are taking a beta blocker, estrogen, or thiazide, talk to your doctor before taking fish oil.[746]

Flaxseed

Scientific name: *Linum usitatissimum*

Also known as linseed, alpha-linolenic acid (a component oil), lint bells, flax

Flax is a slender-stemmed herb that grows in Europe and North America. The small brown or amber seeds are pressed for oil.

Flax is an immensely useful herb. You can make linen from the fibers. You can use the oil from the seeds medicinally. The oil also has the useful property of drying and hardening when it is exposed to air, making flaxseed oil very useful in paint and varnish. It's no surprise that flax has been cultivated and used for thousands of years.

Oil from flaxseed is called both linseed oil and flaxseed oil. Linseed oil is used in paint, flaxseed oil in herbal remedies. The main difference between the two is the way they are processed, the former using an industrial solvent, the latter by pressing the oil from the seed mechanically. Another difference is in the way the two are handled after processing. When flaxseed oil is exposed to the air or to heat, it goes rancid very quickly.[747] That's the reason flaxseed oil is typically cold pressed and sealed in capsules. Once it has gone rancid, it is no longer fit for consumption and can be used only in paints and varnishes.

Flaxseed oil, like fish oil, contains omega-3 fats, essential oils that the body needs but cannot produce on its own. Three types of omega-3 fatty acids are important for human nutrition: docosahexaenoic acid (DHA), eicosapentaenoic acid (EPA), and alpha-linolenic acid (ALA). Plants such as flaxseed contain ALA. Animals eat the ALA in plants and convert it in their bodies to DHA and EPA. Animals higher up the food chain can get their omega-3s either directly from plants or by consuming the DHA and EPA stored in the tissues of other animals, for example, in cold-water fish.

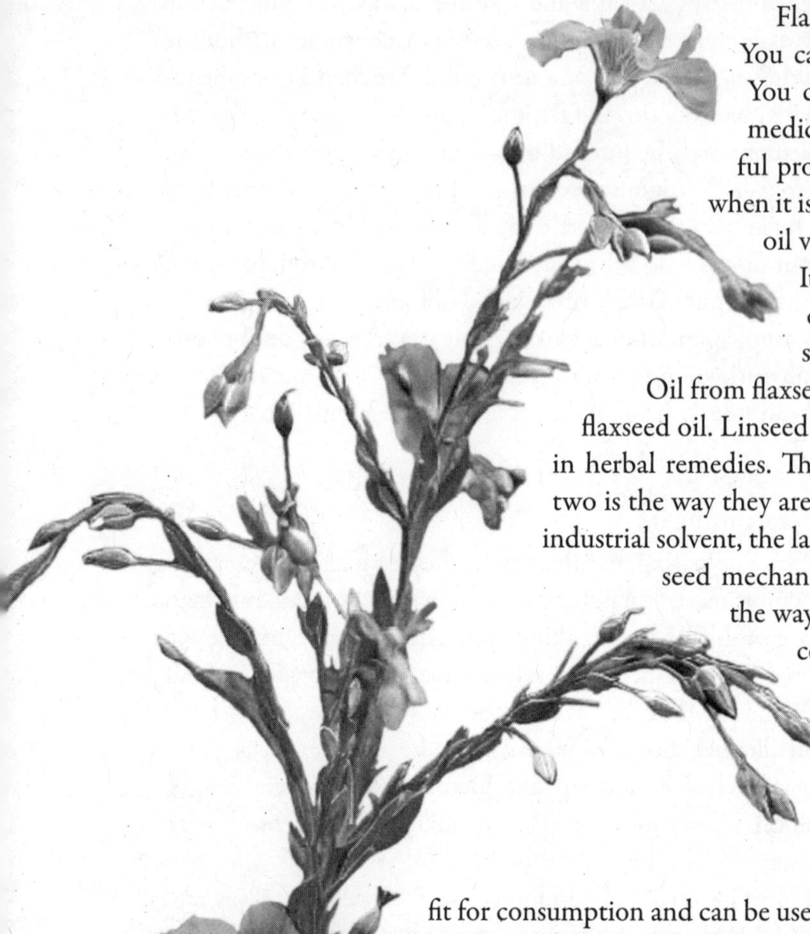

Flax, Linum usitatissimum
Courtesy of Hans-Joachim Fitting

Because they have already been "processed," EPA and DHA fats are more potent than ALA.[748] Studies also show greater effects from EPA and DHA than from ALA. If, however, you are unable or unwilling to take fish oil, flaxseed oil may offer you some of the same benefits. Flaxseeds also contain omega-6 fatty acids in the form of linoleic acid.

What is it good for?

Laxative. The seeds, when eaten whole (with enough water to hydrate them) make a good laxative. This use has been known for at least a hundred years. The 1918 U.S. Dispensatory mentions it.[749] *A Modern Herbal* says that the oil can be used as a laxative, but has a fairly low opinion of the seed, saying, "it affords little actual nourishment and is apparently unwholesome, being difficult of digestion and provoking flatulence."[750] Similarly, the Eclectic School used the oil as a laxative but did not use the whole seed internally. We now know, however, that the value of the seed lies not just in the oil, which may have some mild laxative properties, but mostly in the fiber in the seed itself. Flax seeds have both soluble and insoluble fiber. They also contain mucilage, which swells and softens as it soaks up water. The three properties—oil, fiber, and mucilage—all together make an excellent laxative. Consequently, Commission E recommends it highly for this use.[751]

High cholesterol. Several studies show that flaxseed can lower cholesterol and/or protect the body from the effects of high cholesterol. In an animal study, rabbits with high serum cholesterol were given flaxseeds. The flaxseeds reduced their chance of developing atherosclerosis.[752] In one human study, fifteen obese people with insulin resistance were given 20 g of flaxseed oil per day (in the form of flaxseed oil margarine). All saw improved arterial function.[753] In other human studies, whole flaxseed taken in doses of 15–40 g daily reduced serum cholesterol.[754]

Dermatitis. Flax has demulcent and emollient properties—it softens and soothes irritated skin. These properties come from a thick outer coating of mucilage.[755] Commission E also recommends flaxseed topically for local inflammation.[756] Traditionally, the seed was ground and mixed with hot water to make a poultice to soothe dermatitis.[757] The Eclectic School, for example, used it in this way. Flaxseed, however, may contain more benefit than just mucilage. In a single animal study, it also showed benefit when taken internally. Dogs who took flaxseed oil internally showed an improvement in dermatitis.[758] Several human studies show that fish oil with its related omega-3s has substantial benefit for dermatitis.[759] We don't however, have the studies to make the same claims for flaxseed oil.

Mental performance. The claims of mental and emotional benefit are based on the fact that flaxseed contains omega-3s. Fish oil, which also contains omega-3s has showed significant benefits for the mind and emotions. Studies of flaxseed oil used for this purpose are not nearly as dramatic as the fish oil studies, however. In a study of postmenopausal women with vascular disease, flaxseed lowered blood pressure during a test of induced mental stress.[760] Another study suggests that flaxseed oil had great benefit in treating ADHD.[761] A third study, however, suggests that it doesn't work as well as fish oil for ADHD.[762]

Arthritis. We have some anecdotal evidence that flaxseed may benefit arthritis. The literature, however, has failed to lend support to these claims. A single rat study showed that a flaxseed extract did not reduce inflammation in rats with arthritis.[763] A study of twenty-two people with arthritis who were given a supplement of alpha-linoleic acid showed no improvement in symptoms.[764]

How do you use it?

Whole. Crush or grind the seeds before eating them. If you grind them, do so in a way that doesn't produce heat because heat damages the oils. Always drink extra water (one glass or more per tablespoon of seeds) when taking whole flax seeds. Doing so helps move the seeds through your intestines and decreases the chance of obstruction.[765] Crushed flax seeds have advantages that the extracted oil doesn't have. The seeds are high in fiber. They also have demulcent and emollient properties. Flaxseed contains lignans, an antioxidant, which may be useful in preventing cancer. Flaxseed oil contains no lignans.[766] Studies show that men especially should consume crushed flaxseed rather than taking the extracted oil.[767] (See the "What should you be aware of before using it" section for more information.) Topically, the crushed seeds can be used to make a poultice for boils and abscesses.

Commercially prepared oil. The oil is most commonly sold in capsules. You can, however, buy the oil in bottles, and it is cheaper that way. But flaxseed oil goes bad very quickly, so you should buy it in small quantities and keep it in the refrigerator. Flaxseed oil can be used for any cold use—salad dressings, on bread, etc.—but it should not be used for cooking as heat damages the fatty acids.[768] The oil can also be used externally for dermatitis.[769]

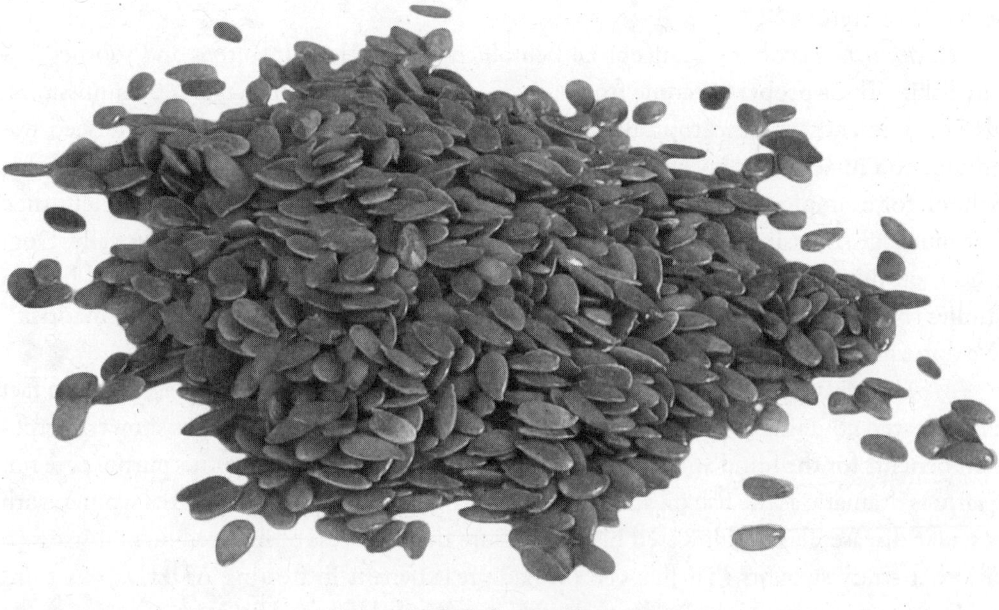

Whole flax seeds

Poultice. Mix 30–50 g of flaxseed flour in warm water and spread the paste on a poultice.[770]

Tinctures aren't recommended if you want the mucilage of an herb to remain intact.[771]

Dosage: How much do you use?

Whole seed. 1–2 tablespoons of the seeds with 1–2 glasses of water per day. If you wish, you can split that into 1–2 teaspoon doses, three times per day.[772]

Oil. The recommended dose of the oil varies widely. The most conservative recommendation is 2 teaspoons per day. Two tablespoons of the oil per day is the highest dose typically recommended. If you are taking the oil in capsules, a typical dose is one 1300 mg softgel capsule of the oil (containing 740 mg of linoleic acid) taken once a day.[773]

For best absorption, take flaxseed and flaxseed oil with food.

What should you be aware of before using it?

For the most part, flaxseeds in reasonable doses are well tolerated. Some people experience flatulence from whole ground flaxseed until they get used to the increased fiber intake. If you take whole flaxseed, you must drink additional water. If you don't drink extra water, it can cause or worsen constipation or even in rare cases cause an intestinal blockage.[774]

It is possible to overdose on flaxseed oil. Symptoms of overdose include shortness of breath, rapid breathing, and weakness. It may also cause seizures or paralysis. Stay within the recommended amounts.[775]

Men should take flaxseed oil only as a part of whole ground flaxseed. They should stay away from flaxseed oil supplements. A meta-analysis of nine studies shows an association between flaxseed oil intake and prostate cancer risk. On the other hand, in other studies, ground flaxseed (the whole seed, not just the oil) may be beneficial for men battling prostate cancer.[776]

If you have macular degeneration or have a family history of the disease, check with a doctor before using any oil containing ALA. One study shows a link between ALA supplementation and progression of the disease.[777]

If you have a hormone imbalance or have a family history of hormone-related tumors, check with a doctor before taking flaxseed, as it does seem to have an effect on hormone production.[778]

Flaxseed is not recommended for pregnant or nursing women.[779]

The seeds contain traces of prussic acid, which is toxic in large quantities. Though prussic acid poisoning is not uncommon in animals that eat green flax, especially after a freeze, human cases of prussic acid poisoning from flaxseed are somewhere between rare and nonexistent. Nonetheless, because the poison is present in the seeds in trace amounts, it is wise to stay within the recommended doses.

Don't take flaxseed if you have a gastrointestinal obstruction or inflammatory bowel disease.[780]

As with any other mucilage, the absorption of other drugs may be negatively affected.[781]

Don't take artist's linseed oil internally. Flaxseed must be processed specifically for human consumption; otherwise it is potentially toxic.

Don't take oil from the related plant *Linum catharticum*, also known as mountain or purging flax. It is a violent purgative.[782]

Note: Flax and New Zealand flax are two completely different plants with completely different medicinal properties.

Garlic

Scientific name: *Allium sativum*

Garlic shares a genus with onions and leeks. Garlic bulbs, which grow at the top of the plants with the flowers, are used medicinally. Originally from Central Asia, garlic is now cultivated throughout the world.

It may not ward off vampires, but it will make your blood healthier for them when the vampires get to you. One of the most common modern uses for garlic is to reduce serum cholesterol. It helps regulate blood sugar. It's also a stimulant for the immune system and an antibiotic. For centuries it has been used on wounds and to treat colds.

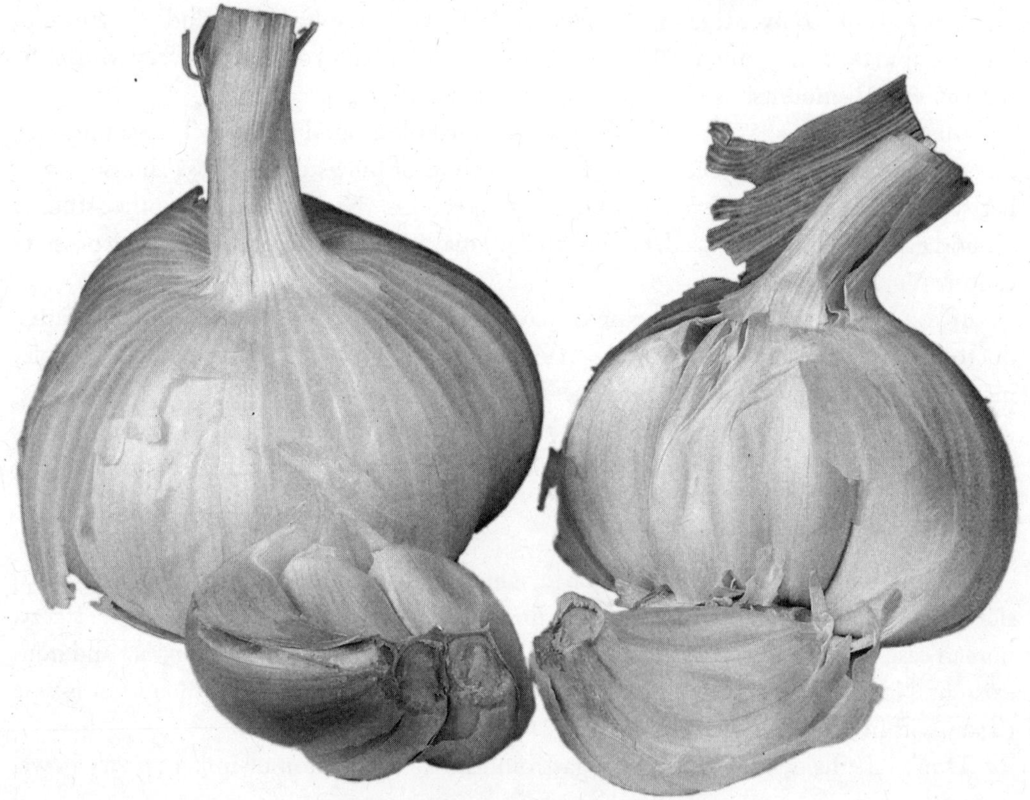

Garlic, *Allium sativum*

Garlic is one of the most thoroughly studied botanical remedies. Louis Pasteur was among the first to study the antibiotic properties of garlic in the 1800s.[783] More recently, its cancer prevention properties are being investigated.[784] Thousands of studies have been done investigating garlic's blood sugar lowering, anti-cancer, anti-oxidant, immune stimulation, and antimicrobial effects.[785]

What is it good for?

Antimicrobial. During World War I, the juice of garlic was expressed, mixed with water, and put on bandages and sterilized mosses, which were then put on wounds.[786] During World War II, it was known as Russian penicillin because its juice was used on wounds in lieu of antibiotics during shortages.[787] Test-tube studies back these uses. Garlic shows the ability to kill bacteria in vitro in concentrations as low as 1:128.[788] In vitro, it also kills the bacteria associated with tooth decay and gingivitis, staph, strep, salmonella, and several other kinds of bacteria.[789] In vitro, it kills the yeast that typically causes yeast infections as well as fungus.[790] It also has antiviral properties.[791] The implications of these properties, however, are not nearly as well studied as the antimicrobial properties themselves.

Hyperlipidemia. Does garlic lower serum cholesterol? Maybe. We have no shortage of studies, but most of those studies are small, poorly designed, or both. Some use dried garlic, some garlic extract. Some studies put the garlic in capsules with various enteric coatings; some don't. Some are long-term, some short-term. Some see cholesterol lowering effects; some don't; some see only short-term effects.

Here is an overview of some of those studies. In one, dried garlic did not lower cholesterol in healthy middle-aged people with normal cholesterol counts.[792] In another study of 23 people with high cholesterol, garlic extract lowered LDL, raised HDL, and lowered blood pressure.[793] Another study gave alliin to people with mild to moderately high cholesterol for 16 weeks. This extract of one of the active ingredients in garlic produced no lowering of serum cholesterol levels.[794] An enteric coated extract of Thai garlic did not lower cholesterol in a study of 136 men with high cholesterol.[795] Garlic lowered cholesterol and triglycerides in subjects who were given a high fat diet.[796] It lowered triglycerides and cholesterol in patients with coronary heart disease.[797] In short, garlic *may* have cholesterol lowering properties, but those properties are not universally observed, and we aren't sure why. Even if garlic does have benefits for high cholesterol, one other factor to consider is how long the benefits lasts. Most of the studies investigating garlic and cholesterol have been short term. At least one study, however, provides evidence that garlic's benefits may not continue past six months.[798]

Colds. The Cherokee used garlic as an expectorant, for croup, and for asthma.[799] It was also used by British herbalists for asthma, hoarseness, coughs, and even whooping cough, both as an infusion made into a syrup and as a salve made from pressed garlic and lard, rubbed on the back and chest.[800] The Eclectic School also recommended either garlic juice or garlic syrup for the common cold. We don't have much clinical evidence for this use, particularly for the topical use, but one study did show that 100+ people who took a garlic supplement every day for twelve weeks had fewer colds during that period.[801]

Cardiovascular health. Beyond the lowering of serum cholesterol, garlic may have other benefits for cardiovascular health. We now have fairly good evidence that it reduces the risk of blood clots (inhibits platelet aggregation).[802] It may also help slow or even reverse the build up of plaque in the arteries and help prevent arteriosclerosis.[803] A study using mice and rats found that aged garlic increases nitric oxide (a compound that helps control the functioning of the cardiovascular system) while protecting against oxidative stress.[804] Garlic lowered blood pressure in both rats and humans.[805]

Exercise performance. In a rat study, rats that were given 2.86 g/kg of aged garlic showed improvements in three markers of fatigue after exercise, suggesting that garlic may help ameliorate the negative physical effects of fatigue.[806] In another mouse study, aged garlic enhanced the production of nitric acid, a sign that it might improve the function of the cardiovascular system.[807] Garlic oil improved exercise tolerance in thirty patients with coronary artery disease.[808] We have no evidence, however, for performance benefit in healthy adults.

How do you use it?

Fresh. For antibiotic purposes, the best way to use garlic is fresh.[809] An odorless amino acid called alliin converts into allicin, the active antibiotic ingredient, when the garlic bulb is ruptured.[810] Get the freshest garlic you can and mash the clove or put it through a garlic press to release the allicin. Use it as soon as possible after pressing it because allicin breaks down quickly. Also be aware that heat causes allicin to break down so that putting garlic in cooking lessens its effects.[811] If you wish to make an infusion, use the cold infusion method and store the infusion in the refrigerator, because allicin tends to break down at temperatures higher than 4 degrees Centigrade.[812]

Garlic can be used topically on fungal infections. Crushed, fresh garlic contains more potent antifungal properties than processed. You can simply smear a little fresh juice on the fungal infection and wait for it to dry, or you can use the crushed garlic as a poultice. If you have sensitive skin or are putting garlic on a sensitive area, consider diluting the juice with a little oil or water or using a plaster instead of a poultice. Garlic can cause rashes and burns. Use caution and test it on a small area of skin before using it more widely.

Capsules. Garlic capsules may work (depending on the quality of the preparation) for cholesterol, but they won't do much for you if you're looking for an antibiotic.[813] Boiled garlic retains its antioxidants and cholesterol lowering ability (in a rat study).[814] And fried garlic helped break down blood clots in patients with heart disease.[815] But another study that used steam-distilled garlic oil showed no cholesterol lowering properties.[816] The problem is with the allicin breakdown. Some supplements are made using methods that preserve allicin, others are not. Even if your brand claims to contain allicin, make sure it has addressed the problem of allicin disintegrating when exposed to stomach acid. Many preparations release 15% or less of their allicin in the digestive tract.[817] Kwai® and Kyolic® are brands that have been clinically tested and found effective.[818] If you are taking garlic to help with cholesterol, check with your doctor to get a beginning cholesterol level. Take the garlic for three months, and then go back and get another test. If your cholesterol hasn't changed, check with your doctor about other options.[819] Even if you do see some cholesterol lowering effects, you need to check in with your doctor periodically for retesting. Some studies seem to suggest that the effect may be temporary.

Infused oils are not recommended. Allicin does not always remain intact in oil.[820]

Essential oils can cause skin irritation, and often don't work as well as fresh garlic again because of the instability of allicin. However, they may have some benefit for fungal infections.

Syrup. Felter of the Eclectic School recommended "covering bruised garlic with sugar" which then could be taken to treat colds. Honey can be used instead of sugar.

Tincture. 1:5, 45% alcohol.[821]

Taking garlic with food can help to minimize the strong taste and aftertaste, but it doesn't do much for garlic breath. The allicin in garlic contains sulfur, and that's what causes garlic breath. After a short while, the garlic smell is no longer coming from your mouth but from your gut. Consequently, mouthwashes no longer are able to help the problem. Deodorized capsules are often depleted of therapeutic effects.[822] However, capsules with enteric coating help with the problem of the sulfur fumes rising from the stomach. They also help keep the allicin from disintegrating in stomach acid.[823] No method, however, can offer a 100% guarantee of eliminating garlic smell.

Dosage: How much do you use?

Fresh garlic. 1 clove or 1000 mg a day in 2–3 doses. Up to five cloves per day is OK.[824]

Dried garlic powder. 400–600 mg per day is a common dose for high cholesterol.[825] And 400–700 mg, three times a day for five days, is a slightly higher dose for treating colds and flu.[826]

Garlic oil. The World Health Organization recommends 2 to 5 mg of the oil daily.[827]

Tincture. The European Scientific Cooperative on Phytotherapy (ESCOP) recommends ½–1 teaspoon of tincture by mouth three times a day for upper respiratory tract infections.[828]

What should you be aware of before using it?

Some people experience unpleasant sensations when taking garlic: burning of the mouth, digestive tract discomfort.[829] Other reported side effects include dizziness, increased sweating, headache, itching, fever, chills, asthma flares, and runny nose. Allergies to garlic are rare but potentially serious. They can also cause swelling of the throat and anaphylaxis when garlic is applied to the skin, inhaled, or taken orally.[830] If you are allergic to members of the *Liliaceae* (lily) family—hyacinth, tulip, onion, leek, or chives—you should avoid taking garlic medicinally.

If you eat garlic, its nature will almost certainly prevent you from taking too much. It's when you take it powdered in capsules or liquid "pearls" that you have to be more careful. It is possible to get a harmful amount of garlic. Garlic in very high doses causes heart arrhythmias in frogs.[831] In people, it can cause stomach ulcers, bronchial asthma, anemia, vertigo, and suppression of testicular functions.

Get professional supervision if you want to take the essential oil internally. Too much can be lethal.

Garlic burns are not unheard of. Keep an eye on garlic poultices especially when they are made with fresh garlic. Don't put them on and then go to sleep. Don't use garlic topically on infants and children.

Be especially careful taking garlic in therapeutic doses if you are pregnant or nursing.[832] It can reduce the infant's feeding.[833] In some cultures, garlic has been used as an abortifacient.[834]

In rare cases, garlic can affect the natural flora in the intestines.[835] If you are prone to intestinal ailments, check with your doctor before using garlic.

Animal studies suggest that garlic may lower blood sugar levels, though human studies don't corroborate this effect.[836] If, however, you are diabetic, hypoglycemic, or taking insulin, glyburide, or a related drug, check with your doctor before taking garlic in therapeutic doses as he/she may want to monitor the effects.[837] Be cautious when using it in conjunction with herbs known or suspected to affect blood sugar levels. (See Chapter 5 for a list.)

In many herbs, the risk of increased bleeding and the interaction with anticoagulant medications is theoretical. In garlic, it has been demonstrated in studies and adverse reaction reports. Don't use garlic without medical supervision if you have any kind of clotting disorder. Also check with your doctor before taking garlic supplements if you are taking any anticoagulant (including warfarin, aspirin, ibuprofen, or any NSAID) or if you are planning surgery or dental work because garlic in therapeutic doses can increase the risk of bleeding.[838] Be cautious when using it in conjunction with other herbs known or suspected of increasing the risk of bleeding. (See Chapter 5 for a list.)

Garlic can interfere with drugs that target the immune system.[839] If you are taking such drugs or if you have an immune disorder, check with your doctor before taking garlic medicinally.

Ginger

Scientific name: *Zingiber officinalis*

Also known as ginger root, garden ginger, *sheng jiang*

Ginger is a perennial plant native to southeast Asia. It produces green-purple flowers, but the rhizomes, the underground stems, are the part that is used medicinally. It's not grown in the continental U.S. but does grow in Puerto Rico and the Virgin Islands.

Despite the near universal use of the term, ginger "root" is not actually a root but rather a rhizome, an underground stem. This tan-to-beige knotted "root" can be used fresh, dried, raw, or cooked. The juice is extracted by pressing, and the essential oils by steam distillation. Originally from tropical Asia, it's now cultivated in the West Indies. It's been used medicinally in the West for 2000 years. It's known in China as *sheng jiang*, where it has been used for twenty-five centuries.[840] It's also a relative of turmeric and has some overlapping properties.

What is it good for?

Motion sickness and nausea. In China, ginger has been used for millennia for nausea of all kinds, including motion sickness.[841] The North American colonists also used ginger for nausea, usually in the form of ginger beer.[842] Ginger has two main active ingredients—gingerols and shogaols—that neutralize stomach acid and tone the muscles of the digestive tract.[843] These actions allow ginger to act directly on the digestive tract, unlike most prescription medicines that act on the nervous system and are consequently likely to cause drowsiness. Ginger also interacts with serotonin in the brain in a way that is not completely understood but that seems to have an effect on nausea.[844] For those whose motion sickness is related to plugged ears, ginger also clears breathing passages and has a mild antihistamine effect which helps with motion sickness.[845]

As for clinical studies, results are mixed. One study showed no benefit of either powdered or fresh ginger for motion sickness.[846] At least two studies showed it to be ineffective against postoperative nausea and vomiting.[847] Yet a study of Danish naval cadets showed that one gram of dried ginger daily quelled the nausea and cold sweats associated with motion sickness.[848]

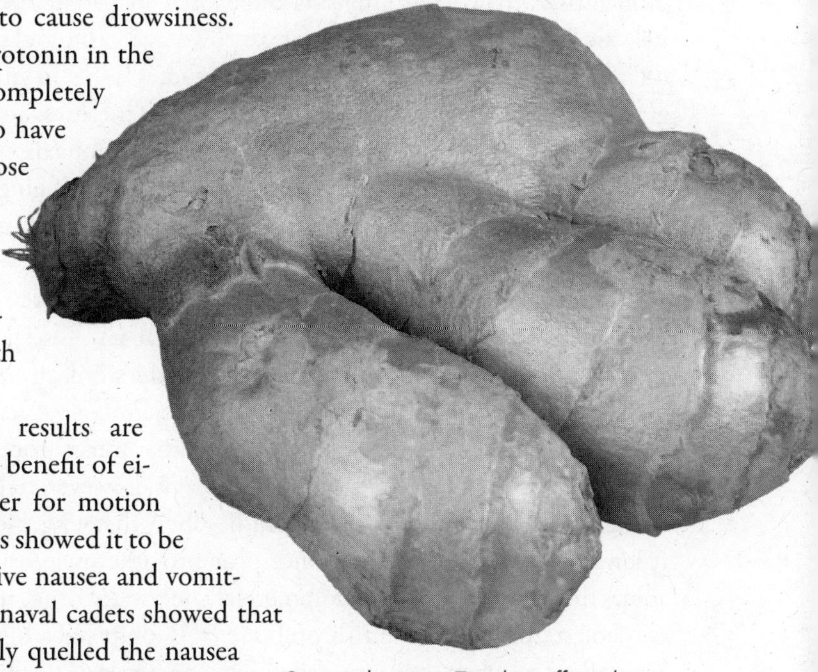

Ginger rhizome, *Zingiber officinalis*

In another study of thirty-six college students, 940 mg of ginger powder worked better than 100 mg of Dramamine® at keeping away the nausea associated with motion sickness.[849] In another randomized, double-blind study of tourists with seasickness, ginger was shown to be as effective as five out of six common motion sickness medicines and superior to transdermal scoplolamine.[850] In another study, ginger was not as effective at treating motion sickness as scopolamine, but it did have fewer side effects.[851] In a study of chemotherapy patients, a 1,000 mg ginger dose was as effective as the prescription drug metoclopramide, but less effective than the prescription drug Ondansetron® in managing nausea and vomiting.[852] Commission E recommends it for this use.

Arthritis. Conventional wisdom has it that ginger helps the pain associated with the inflammation of arthritis. We know that though ginger does not quell inflammation in the same way as NSAIDs, it does indeed seem to do so.[853] In a test-tube study involving bits of cartilage taken from sows, ginger showed an anti-inflammatory effect.[854] In animal studies, rats with arthritis showed less inflammation and joint swelling after taking ginger.[855] As for human clinical studies, results are mixed but hopeful. In a small study of rheumatoid arthritis sufferers, those who took ginger experienced a reduction in symptoms.[856] In three separate studies, it was shown to be more effective than placebo for the pain associated with arthritis in the knee joint.[857] In another double-blind, placebo-controlled human study, however, it showed no benefit for osteoarthritis of the hip and knee.[858]

Colds. Most of the evidence for ginger use in fighting colds is anecdotal. In China, ginger is used as an expectorant, as well as for upper respiratory tract infections, cough, and bronchitis.[859] Powdered ginger is often used in patent decongestant herbal teas.[860] The Eclectic School suggested that one take powdered garlic and cold water before bed to "break up" a cold. What we know from scientific studies is that in vitro, the essential oil inhibits the growth of bacteria and kills influenza virus.[861] (Tinctures, however, are less effective for this purpose.[862]) Clinical studies for this use are all but nonexistent.

Flatulence and colic. In France, a couple of drops of ginger juice or tincture on a sugar cube is used as a remedy for flatulence. The 1918 U.S. Dispensatory recommends tincture of ginger as a carminative and for "debilitated states of the alimentary canal."[863] *A Modern Herbal* recommends ginger for flatulent colic.[864] Felter of the Eclectic School recommended it for digestive problems and hypothesized that it "causes an increased flow of saliva and gastric juice and increases muscular activity of the stomach and intestines." Fyfe of the Eclectic School also recommended it for this use. Preliminary research using mice is beginning to support this use.[865] Animal studies suggest that ginger tones the muscles of the digestive tract.[866] We have no clinical studies on humans, however, to back this use.

Cardiovascular health. Animal studies show that ginger lowers cholesterol. In one study, it lowered LDL cholesterol in mice prone to atherosclerosis.[867] In fact, at least one study shows that it works as well as commercial cholesterol drugs in rabbits.[868] In rats, ginger lowers cholesterol and is an antithrombotic.[869] Rabbits fed a high cholesterol diet showed less artery damage when they were fed ginger concurrently.[870] Human studies, however, are not nearly as promising. In one human study, neither raw nor cooked ginger showed any antithrombotic benefit.[871] In another, 10 g of powdered ginger showed no effect on blood lipids.[872] Still another showed that 4 g per day had no significant effect on platelet aggregation, but a single dose of 10 g did have an effect.[873]

Skin inflammation. In China the fresh juice of ginger applied topically is used for treating thermal burns.[874] The native Hawaiians used it to treat bruises.[875] In animal studies, it reduces skin edema, but burns per se have not been tested,[876] and we have no clinical studies to back this use.

How do you use it?

Fresh ginger root. Take a ¼- to ½-inch (peeled) slice every four hours or up to three times a day.[877] Ginger root also comes candied.

Ginger juice. Grate the ginger root and squeeze out the juice. It can be mixed with honey for colds.[878]

Ginger ale. An eight ounce glass of ginger ale, if it's made of real ginger (some aren't—check the ingredients), contains roughly 1 g of ginger.[879]

Capsules. Like most botanicals, the quality of commercially prepared ginger capsules varies widely.[880] When ginger is standardized, it is standardized for gingerols and shogaols, the two main active ingredients. For motion sickness, take 100 mg a couple of hours before traveling and then 100 mg every four hours thereafter until the motion stops.[881]

Dried and powdered. You do not necessarily have to take dried ginger in capsules. You can take ½ to ¾ teaspoon of dried ginger stirred into in a whole glass of water.[882] Capsules, however, are more convenient and less messy.

Decoction. Place 1–2 slices in a cup or two of water and simmer for 10–20 minutes. A pinch of cinnamon can be added. This is a traditional use for colds with phlegm.

Infusion. Steep ½ teaspoon of grated ginger root in 8 ounces of very hot water for five to ten minutes.[883]

Bath. Put a cup of grated ginger or ½ cup of powdered ginger into a cloth bag. Put the bag under the spout as you draw a bath. Once in the bath, you can use the bag directly on aching joints.

Tincture. According to the 1918 U.S. Dispensatory, alcohol brings out the active ingredients in ginger quite well.[884] Ginger tincture is most commonly used for flatulence and nausea.

Massage oil. Use a couple of drops of the essential oil mixed into a carrier oil (almond works well) as a massage oil for rheumatism.[885] Juice, decoctions, or tincture can also be massaged into sore muscles and joints directly. Use 1 g of powdered ginger or 5 to 50 g of fresh ginger.[886]

Dosage: How much do you use?

Fresh ginger. Recommendations vary widely. On the one hand, one to two inches of the root or three teaspoons of grated fresh ginger are commonly recognized as safe.[887] On the other hand, other sources recommend no more than 4 g of fresh ginger per day, the equivalent of one thin slice.[888]

Dried ginger. ½ to ¾ teaspoon every four hours or up to three times a day.[889] Don't exceed 2–4 g of the dried rhizome per day (including ginger eaten in food).[890] (One teaspoon is roughly five g.) Studies show that doses over 6 g of dried ginger begin to cause problematic changes to gastric surfaces.[891]

Essential oil. Don't take it internally. Get professional help if you want to use it topically. It is extremely strong.

What should you be aware of before using it?

Ginger is on the FDA's list of foods that are generally recognized as safe, and most people tolerate it well.

Ginger, particularly powdered ginger, can cause heartburn. If you have heartburn, ulcers, gall bladder problems, or acid reflux, avoid using ginger medicinally.

Though studies conflict, ginger may increase the risk of bleeding.[892] Check with your doctor if you are taking an anticoagulant (including regular aspirin or an NSAID) and want to take ginger in therapeutic doses.[893] If you plan to have surgery, tell your surgeon you have been taking ginger and discontinue use. Be cautious when using it in conjunction with other herbs known or suspected of increasing the risk of bleeding. (See Chapter 5 for a list.)

Ginger could theoretically lower blood pressure. It did so in one rat study but not another.[894] If you have blood pressure problems, consult with your doctor before taking it.

Ginger may affect insulin sensitivity. If you have blood sugar problems, check with your doctor before using it medicinally. Then watch your sugar carefully as you experiment.[895]

Whether ginger is safe for morning sickness during pregnancy is debatable. One animal study showed a loss of fetus after using ginger.[896] Another showed a reduced birth weight in rats exposed to ginger.[897] Other animal studies show no such effect.[898] The *HerbalGram* of the American Botanical Council sees no problems with using ginger for morning sickness, but the *PDA for Herbal Medicine* and Commission E advise against it.[899] The American Herbal Products Association says that fresh ginger can be used widely, but dried shouldn't be used during pregnancy.[900] If you are pregnant or nursing, check with your doctor and weigh the risks and benefits with him/her before using ginger.

In very large doses, it may cause depression or cardiac arrhythmias.[901]

Don't give ginger in medicinal doses to children under the age of 2.

Don't take the essential oil internally.

Note that not all ginger has the same medicinal properties as *Zingiber officinalis*. A North American species known as wild ginger, Canadian wild ginger, or Indian ginger (*Asarum rubrocinctum* Peattie or *Asarum canadense* L.) contains aristolochic acid and has been associated with nephropathy, a kidney disorder.

Ginkgo Biloba

Scientific name: *Ginkgo biloba*

Also known as gingko, kew tree, maidenhair tree

Ginkgo is an ancient plant, a gymnosperm, that dates back more than 200 million years. It was already well established throughout the northern hemisphere when the dinosaurs arrived on the scene. During the last Ice Age, all of the members of the *Ginkgoaceae* family were wiped out except for *Ginkgo biloba*, which survived in only a small part of its range, in what is now China. Ginkgo is a large shade tree, growing to over eighty feet tall under the right conditions. The leaves of the ginkgo tree are picked, dried, and processed to produce a concentrated, standardized gingko extract known as GBE.[902]

Ginkgo has been prescribed for thousands of years in China. There it is mostly the inner kernel of the seed that is used medicinally. Ginkgo came to the West with Engelbert Kaempfer, who brought it from Japan to Holland in the seventeenth century. Not until the late 1950s did Western medicine begin to study its medicinal uses. The Schwabe Company in Germany produced the first extract from the leaves in 1965.[903] Since then, virtually all studies of ginkgo and use in Western countries has been of this extract. In fact, the American Botanical Council says that it "must be standardized in order to deliver the intended benefits."[904]

Most of ginkgo's value comes in its ability to promote vasodilatation. In other words, ginkgo improves the rate of blood flow in small blood vessels.[905] Thus, it's able to help circulation-related problems such as memory loss, tinnitus and vertigo, age-related decline, varicose veins, and erectile dysfunction.

What is it good for?

Increased memory and learning capacity, especially in cases of dementia. Animal studies show some benefit. In rats, ginkgo reduced post-stress memory dysfunctions.[906] In elderly dogs, ginkgo helped reduce age-related complaints (disorientation, sleep or activity changes, behavioral changes, general behavior, and general physical condition and vitality).[907] In humans, the results are not as unequivocal. Subjects with insufficiency of blood flow, whether due to disease or age, seem to have better success than healthy subjects. In one study, 112 people with a mean age of 70.5 years took 120 mg of ginkgo per day. After a

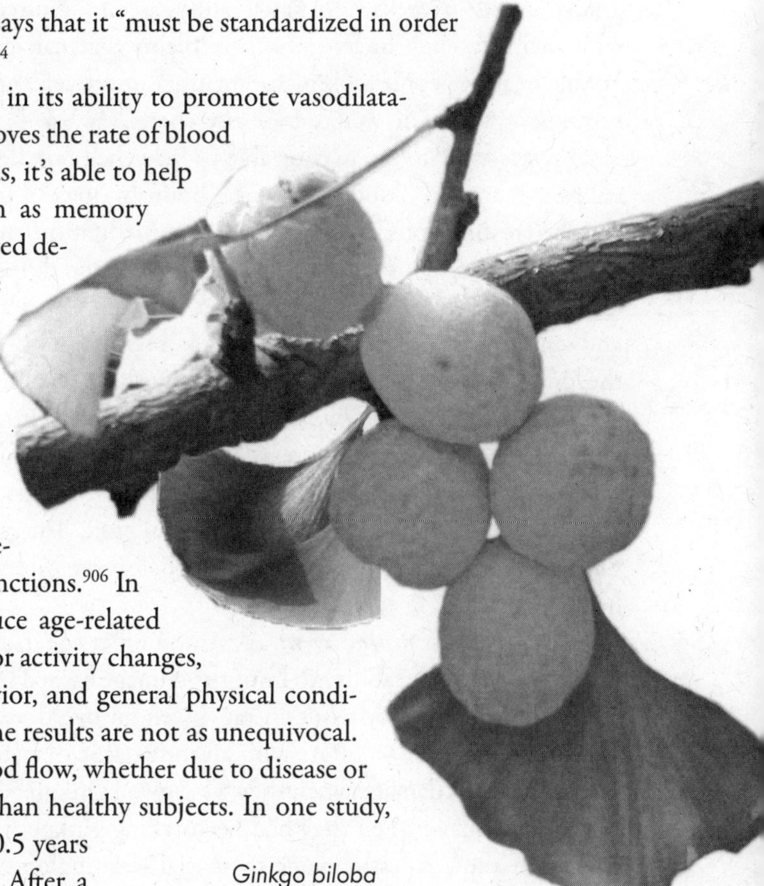

Ginkgo biloba

Courtesy of Love Krittaya

year, most people had significant reduction in short-term memory loss, headache, vertigo, tinnitus, mood disturbances, and loss of vigilance.[908] A study of middle-aged volunteers showed similar improvements.[909] Another showed improvement in the speed of information processing.[910] In fact, a meta study showed a positive outcome in 39 of 40 pre-2000 clinical trials using ginkgo to treat cerebral insufficiency.[911] Not all age-related memory impairment can be helped by ginkgo, however. Some studies show no benefit to memory and cognitive ability.[912] Furthermore, the evidence for using ginkgo to prevent (rather than treat) memory problems is completely lacking.[913] How long benefits last is another issue. In one study, postmenopausal women who took ginkgo for six weeks showed minimal benefits after the longer trial.[914]

The young and healthy may not derive as much benefit. Studies with rats suggest that we can expect more profound effects among the elderly than among the young[915] though one study of young volunteers showed some improvement in a memory task after taking ginkgo.[916] Young volunteers showed no long-lasting memory improvement.[917] In young healthy people, gingko can help improve sustained attention and pattern recognition memory, but the effect doesn't last, suggesting that young, healthy people may develop a tolerance to ginkgo over 4–6 weeks.[918] In short, ginkgo seems to offer the most benefit to elderly people with memory and concentration problems that can be traced to vascular insufficiency. Young, healthy people looking for memory improvement, especially long-term memory improvement, would do well to look elsewhere. ◊ ◊ ◆ ◆ ◆

Adaptogen. Ginkgo may be able to help the brain deal with the effects of stress. In one study, it increased blood flow to the brain in dogs.[919] In another, it increased alpha-wave activity (resting consciousness and light meditation) in the brain while decreasing beta (normal "doing" consciousness), gamma (sleep and deeper focus like meditation), and delta (sleep) waves.[920] This increase in alpha wave activity is typically associated with relaxation and rest. In rats, it proved to be better as a temporary help with acute stress than as a fix for the long-term effects of chronic stress.[921] We have no clinical studies of ginkgo as an adaptogen, but from what little we have, we can guess that it might have some benefit in dealing with occasional short-term stress. ◊ ◊ ◊ ◆ ◆

Allergies and asthma. In one study, allergy patients were given ginkgo and then challenged with the thing to which they were allergic. The ginkgo seemed to have some protective effect.[922] Further studies are needed before we can make any kind of definite assertion, however. ◊ ◊ ◊ ◆ ◆

Tissue injury-limiting agent. A great number of rats have been mangled to teach us that ginkgo may have the ability to limit the damage caused by various insults to the body. Ginkgo helped protect liver tissue in rats given an overdose of acetaminophen, a known liver toxin (in high doses).[923] Rats with an induced stroke (from a temporarily blocked artery) experienced less damage when they were given ginkgo.[924] Rats exposed to radiation suffered less tissue damage when they had been taking ginkgo.[925] Rats with induced aluminum intoxication showed less damage to spatial learning and memory when they protected by ginkgo.[926] Also in rats it minimized the spatial memory loss induced by scopolamine.[927] It also protected the liver of rats against the effects of aging.[928] Does ginkgo help humans recover from the damage of aging or injury? We don't know. So far only rats have "volunteered" for these kinds of studies.

Tinnitus. Commission E recommends ginkgo for tinnitus, a known symptom of early hearing loss. In guinea pigs, ginkgo has no effect on noise-induced hearing loss.[929] Some studies suggest that it might be useful for treating tinnitus if the condition is caught early.[930] Other studies see no benefit.[931] The quality of these studies is in doubt, however, leading some doctors to suggest that potential for unpleasant side effects outweighs benefit for tinnitus sufferers.[932]

Muscle spasms. Ginkgo does not help every case of muscle spasms, but in a study of intermittent claudication, a disease caused by the hardening of the leg arteries, ginkgo helped improve circulation and decrease muscle spasms in the legs.[933] In other words, if the spasms are due to circulation problems, ginkgo might help.

How do you use it?

Take only commercially prepared ginkgo. Do *not* make your own preparations. The pulp and the seed of the tree are toxic. Even handling the fruit incorrectly can result in severe allergic reactions.[934] Ginkgo extract is typically standardized to a potency of 24% flavone glycosides and 6% terpenes. This extract is known as GBE, and it is the only form in which the plant is used medicinally in Western countries.[935] Bio-Biloba® is one brand of GBE with a good track record in clinical tests.[936] Be sure to store ginkgo in a dark, dry place.

Dosage: How much do you use?

Your safest course is to purchase a reputable brand and follow label directions. Typical doses are:

120–240 mg native dry extract in 2 or 3 doses for memory

120–160 mg native dry extract in 2 or 3 doses for dizziness or tinnitus

Check with a doctor if you want to take ginkgo for more than three months. If you are taking it for vertigo or tinnitus, you will see whatever results you can expect in 6–8 weeks. After that, continuing to take the herb is of no therapeutic value.[937]

What should you be aware of before using it?

Ginkgo has a higher rate of nasty side-effects than most herbs. Though many people use it as a "do-it-yourself herb," you might consider getting help from someone who knows this herb before taking it, especially if you have any preexisting health problems.

Don't use unprocessed, unstandardized ginkgo. Some parts of the plant are toxic; others tend to cause severe allergic reactions.[938] Buy your ginkgo prepared from a reputable company.

Most studies show that ginkgo is safe when taken in daily doses of 240 mg or less.[939] Possible side effects include headaches or allergic skin reaction.

Anecdotal reports indicate that ginkgo may cause heart arrhythmia in some people.[940]

Animal studies show that it can affect blood pressure. In rats, it reduced salt-related elevation of blood pressure.[941] It lowered the blood pressure of rats with spontaneously high blood pressure, but not those with normal blood pressure.[942] If you have blood-pressure issues, you might want to check with a doctor before using ginkgo.

Ginkgo can raise blood pressure when combined with a thiazide diuretic.[943] If you are on blood pressure medication, check with your doctor before using ginkgo. Be careful using it in conjunction with other herbs that have an effect on blood pressure.

About 4% of the people who take ginkgo develop minor gastrointestinal problems.[944]

Ginkgo interacts with omeprazole (Prilosec®). Don't take the two at the same time unless directed to do so by a physician.[945]

Ginkgo may affect the blood supply to the brain. If you are prone to migraines, be cautious about taking ginkgo.

With some herbs the risk of bleeding is theoretical. With ginkgo it is supported by numerous adverse reaction reports.[946] Though clinical trials have yet to nail down the reason for this observed risk, the reports are serious enough to warrant caution.[947] Check with your doctor if you are taking an anticoagulant (including aspirin or an NSAID) and want to take ginkgo.[948] If you plan to have surgery, tell your surgeon you have been taking ginkgo and discontinue use. Be cautious when using it in conjunction with other herbs known or suspected of increasing the risk of bleeding. (See Chapter 5 for a list.)

Ginkgo has been associated with adverse ocular (eye) side effects. One survey found reports of retinal hemorrhages and two cases of hemorrhaging in the anterior chamber of the eye.[949] Another study found increased velocity of blood in the ophthalmic artery.[950] The implications of these studies are not yet clear. Caution suggests, however, that if you have any predisposition to eye or vision problems, you should check with your doctor before using ginkgo.

There may be a connection between ginkgo and risk of seizure. One survey of dietary supplements showed a weak connection.[951] If you have a seizure disorder, consult with your doctor before taking ginkgo.[952]

Be especially careful to keep ginkgo seeds away from small children because the seeds can cause seizure and death.[953]

Don't take ginkgo with drugs or herbs that have monoamine oxidase inhibitor (MAOI) activity or that interact with MAOI drugs. (See Chapter 5 for a list.) Headache, tremors, mania, and insomnia may occur [954]

If you are taking any kind of anti-cancer medication, check with your doctor before taking ginkgo.[955]

Ginseng

Scientific name: *Panax ginseng*

Also known as Chinese ginseng, Japanese ginseng, Korean ginseng, *ren shen*, man root, white ginseng, red ginseng. Ginseng radix is ginseng root

Panax ginseng is a low-growing perennial indigenous to China. The *Panax* species grows throughout the northern hemisphere. The roots are the part that's used medicinally. They are often dried and cured before use.[956] Ginseng is very difficult to cultivate. The roots mature slowly, taking sometimes six years or more to be ready for harvest.[957]

The Chinese name, "*ren shen*," means "man root." The name comes from the fork in the ginseng root that makes it look a little like a human body. The "panax" in the Latin name, *Panax ginseng,* is from the Greek, meaning "all healing." *Panax* is a genus containing eleven species. *Panax quinquefolium*, American ginseng, is related to *Panax ginseng*, but studies have shown that the two are certainly not interchangeable in their effects.[958] The difference between red and white ginseng is one of processing, not of species. Both are *Panax ginseng*. Siberian ginseng, *Eleutherococcus senticosus*, is not a true ginseng. It's listed separately in this book under "Eleuthero Root."

Use of ginseng in China can be traced back at least two millennia. Over the years, ginseng has been used for weight control, clearness of mind, and overall well-being. In Chinese medicine, it is used to increase yang energy. Pere Jartoux, a Jesuit missionary stationed in Beijing in the eighteenth century, was the first European to come across it. He noted that the Chinese placed a very high value on the root and suggested that Europeans would do well to try to bring some to Europe and analyze it. Ironically enough, in the early nineteenth century, American ginseng was shipped to China as a substitute for Chinese ginseng, which had grown so costly that the poor could not afford it. Only since the latter part of the twentieth century has ginseng has been embraced by Western herbal medicine. At that time, ginseng started being shipped from China to Europe and the United States. *Panax ginseng* is now cultivated in the U.S.

Part of the problem with ginseng studies is that in the past ginseng was not differentiated by species. American, Asian, and Siberian ginseng were used interchangeably, and the purity and potency of the herb was not taken into account. Consequently, study results vary widely.[959]

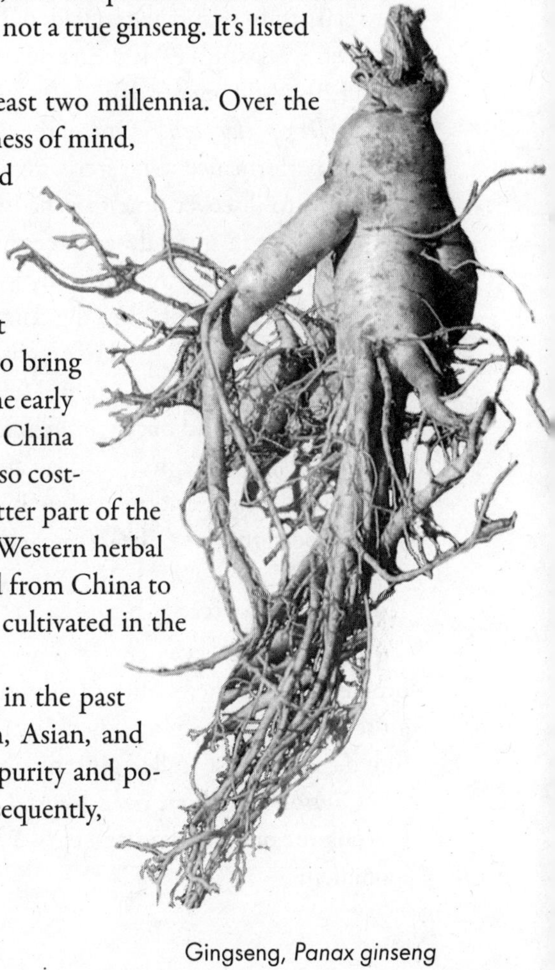

Gingseng, *Panax ginseng*
Courtesy of Katharina Lohrie of FloraFarm, GmbH

What is it good for?

A tonic for fatigue, stress, and problems with concentration. In China, ginseng is used as an adaptogen. The Cherokee, Mohegans, Seminole, and Delaware also used an American species (*Panax quinquefolius* L.) as a tonic.[960] The Iroquois used that species as a stimulant for laziness.[961] The Menominee believed it helped strengthen mental powers.[962] Fyfe of the Eclectic School recommended American ginseng for "nervous debility." Anecdotal studies seem to indicate that ginseng helps chronic fatigue in some patients.[963]

As for scientific study into ginseng's effects, researchers aren't sure exactly how or why it works, but it does have measurable effects in humans. At least thirty ginsenosides have been isolated and studied. Some suppress the central nervous system; some stimulate it. Ginseng also has a measurable effect on the brain. After subjects took a dose of ginseng, EEGs showed changes in brain function.[964] In other studies, *Panax ginseng* helped performance in a mentally demanding arithmetic test and also decreased subjective feelings of fatigue.[965] It helped speed and accuracy in a memory task.[966] It improved quality of memory in another.[967] Middle-aged study participants gained a 7.5% improvement in memory throughout another fourteen week study.[968] It didn't however, seem to have any effect on mood in young adults taking 200–400 mg per day.[969] ◊ ◊ ◆ ◆ ◆

Athletic performance. One of the uses that ginseng has been tested for is ability to improve athletic performance. One study involved a small group of healthy men that were tested on treadmills to discover time to exhaustion. They were tested before and after eight weeks of *Panax ginseng* (2 g per dose, three times a day). Time to exhaustion increased by a minute and a half.[970] Another similar study found an increase in time to exhaustion of roughly seven minutes with a dose of 1350 mg daily for thirty days.[971] A third study suggests that ginseng might help people not used to exercise tolerate beginning exercise better.[972] Yet most studies have been mixed at best. A study of fifteen young athletes showed an improvement in reaction time both at rest and during exercise. It didn't, however, show any improvement in maximal oxygen uptake (VO2 max) and lactate threshold (LAT).[973] Further studies show no increase in aerobic exercise performance, no improvement in aerobic work capacity, and no increase in physical performance or heart rate recovery after exercise.[974] ◊ ◊ ◊ ◆ ◆

How do you use it?

Ginseng is everywhere: in powder, liquid, extracts, tablets, even in chewing gum. The problem is that the quality of ginseng varies widely. Because it takes so long to grow, real ginseng tends to be a bit expensive, and cheap ginseng is often suspect. In fact, one survey found that some so-called ginseng products don't contain any ginseng at all.[975]

Commercially prepared capsules: Gerimax® is a brand with good results in clinical tests.[976] Or look for one standardized to 5–9% ginsenosides, a common concentration of the active ingredient.

Unprocessed root: Alternatively, you can find the actual root at Chinese herb shops and use that. You can make a decoction of the root using ½ teaspoon of the dried pulverized root to every one cup of water. Drink one or two cups per day.[977]

Tinctures: Tinctures bring out the best in ginseng. Use a 1:5 ratio, 70% alcohol.[978]

Wild ginseng of all species is typically more potent than cultivated. However, wild ginseng is becoming endangered due to over-harvesting and the fact that a ginseng root takes years to reach maturity. For the sake of conservation, it is better to go with cultivated ginseng.

Dosage: How much do you use?

Dried root. 1–2 g of root per day is the most you'll want to take.[979] The usual recommendation by Western authorities is 300–500 mg per day. However, studies that used smaller doses, in the range of 300–500 mg, were more likely to fail to show any effects. The amount of a commercial preparation that you take varies with the strength of the preparation. Get a reputable brand and follow label directions.

Tincture. (1:5): 1–2 teaspoons[980]

Topically. We have some historical basis for using ginseng topically. The Chinese used it in lotions and soaps. The Iroquois rubbed a decoction on the legs of lacrosse players.[981] No scientific evidence exists, however, for the effectiveness of topical use.

Though some people do, it's best to avoid taking ginseng long-term. We don't yet know what a toxic dose might be, what a reliably effective dose might be, and what the long-term effects are.[982] Some studies suggest that ginseng may lose its effect after eight to twelve weeks. Some herbalists suggest that use be limited to three weeks.[983] At the very least, if you're beginning to have trouble sleeping, or if you're experiencing unexplained muscle aches, stop taking it.

What should you be aware of before using it?

Ginseng has been used widely for millennia and has gained a reputation for being safe. However, some people do have adverse reactions: nervousness, insomnia, diarrhea, or skin eruptions.[984]

Taking too much or taking it for too long a period can lead to chronic sleeplessness, muscle tension, and swelling.

Some people are allergic to ginseng, some seriously. If you allergic to anything in the *Araliaceae* (Ivy) family, you should exercise extra caution.

If you are taking estrogen or have an estrogen imbalance, talk with your doctor before taking ginseng. Modern research has found it contains steroidal components similar to human sex hormones. Preliminary research indicates an adverse interaction is possible.[985]

If you are diabetic, hypoglycemic, or are taking insulin, glyburide or another related drug, check with your doctor before taking ginseng because it can affect blood sugar levels.[986] Be cautious when using it in conjunction with herbs known or suspected to affect blood sugar levels. (See Chapter 5 for a list.)

Don't use ginseng if you have a bleeding or clotting disorder. It can also interact with warfarin and related anticoagulants, possibly decreasing their effectiveness.[987]

Be cautious about drinking tea, coffee, cola or other caffeine drinks when taking ginseng. The two tend to compound each other's stimulant effects.

Don't take ginseng if you are using an MAOI inhibitor.[988]

Though the effect seems to be temporary, ginseng can increase blood pressure.[989] If you are prone to hypertension, check with your doctor before using ginseng.

Check with your doctor before using ginseng while pregnant. Its safety is not proven.[990]

Get your ginseng from a reputable herb company. Many so-called ginseng remedies have little or no active ingredient.[991]

Notoginseng, a related species has different properties and may be more dangerous than Panax ginseng. Get supervision if you want to use notoginseng.

Siberian ginseng (*Eleuthero*), Prince ginseng, Female ginseng (*dong quai*), Indian ginseng (*ashwagandha*), Brazilian ginseng, Peruvian ginseng (*Maca*), and Southern ginseng (*Jiaogulan*) are not true ginseng and have very different properties.

Goldenrod

Scientific name: *Solidago virgaurea* (European), *Solidago odora* Ait. (American)

Also known as Solidaginis virgaureae herba, woundwort, Aaron's rod (virgaurea), anise-scented goldenrod (odora), sweet goldenrod (odora), common goldenrod, and blue mountain tea

A wild flower—some would say "weed'—with mustard-yellow flowers that bloom in the late summer, goldenrod is a member of the daisy family that grows in North America and Europe. The genus *Solidago* has about 80 different species. *Virgaurea* and *odora* are the two most commonly used by herbalists. The leaves and flowers are used medicinally.

It has a flavor similar to licorice or anise.

Goldenrod is best known as a diuretic. It has been used for centuries to treat urinary tract problems.[992] Chinese herbal medicine

Goldenrod, *Solidago virgaurea*

Courtesy of Renate Eder

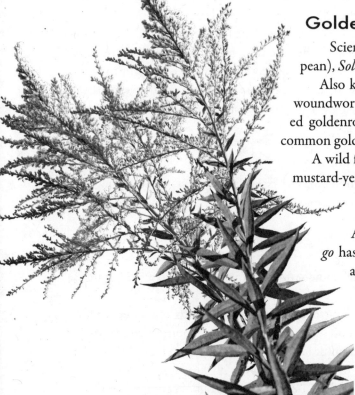

uses a related *Solidago* species, *Solidago virgo-aurea* L, for influenza, headache, sore throat, and other uses.[993]

What is it good for?

Wounds with inflammation and swelling. The use of goldenrod on wounds dates back to the Middle Ages in Europe. The Cherokee chewed the root for a sore mouth.[994] This use has some scientific attestation. At least two tests show that goldenrod reduces induced inflammation and edema in rats.[995] The herb contains astringent tannins that can help constrict tissue and reduce bleeding.[996] It also contains rutin, a bioflavonoid that strengthens capillaries and helps prevent and heal bruises.[997] A related species from Brazil, *Solidago microglossa*, shows powerful antimicrobial properties in vitro.[998] Another study shows it is effective against yeast.[999] ◊◊◆◆◆

Colds. The Cherokee used goldenrod to treat coughs and colds.[1000] It contains benzyl-benzoates, which are known to have immune stimulant properties.[1001] The anti-inflammatory properties might help a sore throat, but we don't have enough research to conclusively support this use. ◊◊◊◆◆

How do you use it?

Commercial preparation. A commercial preparation (for oral use), Urol mono, has been shown to be effective against inflammation in animal studies.[1002] It isn't, however, widely available outside Germany.

Infusion. Infusions have been shown to have similar properties to the commercial preparations.[1003] Use a cold infusion or pour one cup of near boiling water over 2–3 teaspoons of goldenrod.[1004] Let the infusion sit covered for 15 minutes and then strain. Don't boil goldenrod.

Topical use. Commission E doesn't say anything about topical use. In fact, most of the studies have been about internal use. We have, however, some traditional evidence for the topical use of goldenrod. For mouth injuries, swish and spit. You can also use it as a gargle for laryngitis and sore throat. Use it on a compress for wounds with swelling.

Tincture. 1:5, 45% alcohol

When storing goldenrod, protect it from light and moisture.

Combinations: It combines well with echinacea or elder for colds and sore throats.[1005]

Dosage: How much do you use?

Internally. Use 3–5 g of the herb as tea 2–4 times daily.[1006] Don't exceed 12 g per day.

You can take up to 10–20 drops of the tincture 2–3 times per day. Always drink plenty of water when taking goldenrod internally.

Externally. We don't know how much is safe for external use.

What should you be aware of before using it?

Don't use it internally if you have cardiac or renal problems.[1007]

Don't use it internally if you are pregnant.[1008]

It is a mild diuretic and may increase the effects of other diuretics.[1009] (See Chapter 5 for a list.)

If you are taking lithium, don't use goldenrod without the supervision of a physician.

Note that using diuretics to lose weight in order to fit into a lower weight class to fight is foolish and counterproductive. Being dehydrated causes your muscles and your brain to function less efficiently. It also makes you more prone to injuries.

Be cautious about applying goldenrod to broken skin. It is possible to contaminate a wound with an herbal preparation. If you aren't sure about how sterile your preparation is, don't use it on broken skin.

Goldenrod can cause dermatitis when applied topically.[1010] Goldenrod is a member of the *Compositae* family. If you are allergic to any of the members of the *Compositae* family (ragweed, daisies, aster, etc.), you have a greater chance of being allergic to goldenrod.

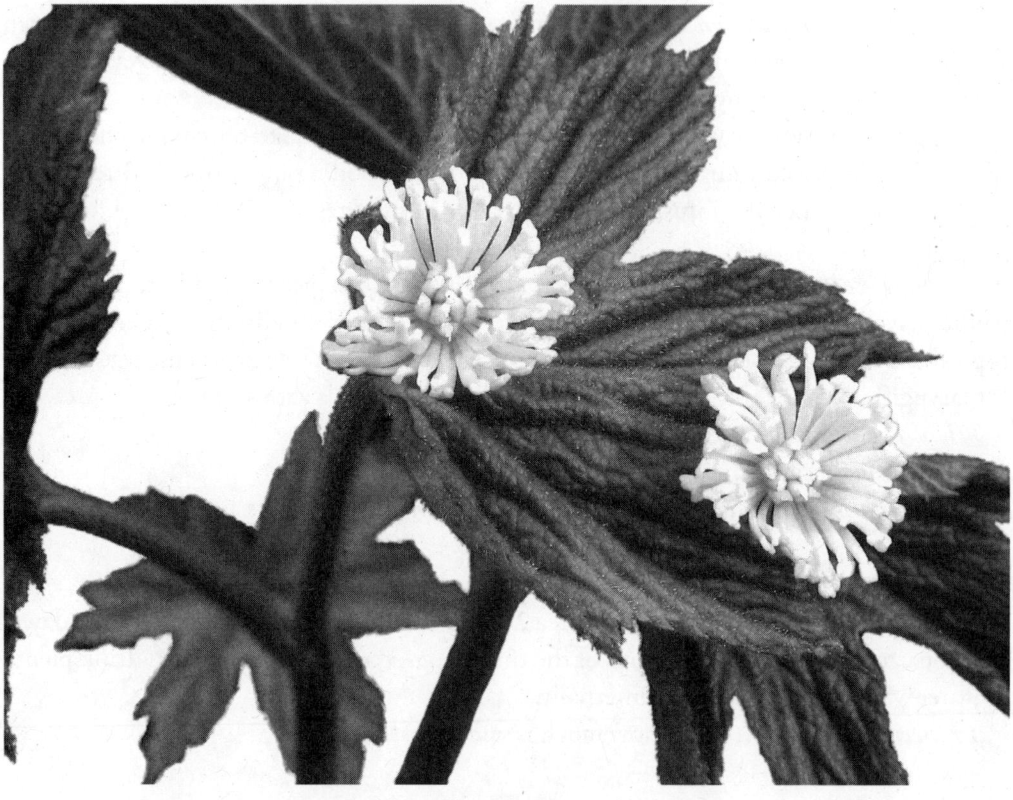

Goldenseal, *Hydrastis candensis*

Courtesy of Alan Cressler

Goldenseal

Scientific name: *Hydrastis canadensis*

Also known as eye balm, Indian paint, orange root, jaundice root, orange root, yellow root, yellow puccoon, ground raspberry, wild curcuma, turmeric root, Indian dye, eye root, eye balm, jaundice root, hydrastis

Goldenseal is a small perennial that grows in the woods in the East, Midwest, and Deep South regions of North America. The dried rhizome is used. Goldenseal is a member of the buttercup family (*Ranunculaceae*).

The taste is bitter, and the smell is strong and nasty. Despite it's nastiness, goldenseal used to be one of the most commonly used medicinal plants in North America. The Cherokee and Iroquois used the herb for a variety of ailments, but without much consensus about what it was good for. It was part of several patent medicines, including "Dr. Pierce's Golden Medical Discovery." In the early part of the twentieth century, 200,000 to 300,000 pounds of goldenseal were used annually as medicine.[1011] Even today in the U.S., goldenseal sells about as well as echinacea and better than the better-known valerian and St. John's wort.[1012] Because of heavy use, wild goldenseal has been seriously depleted, so much so that it is classified as an endangered plant in many states. Sticking with cultivated goldenseal will help wild goldenseal recover.

What is it good for?

Scrapes and burns. The Cherokee used goldenseal for inflammations.[1013] Micmac Indians used it for chapped and cut lips.[1014] In traditional British herbalism, it was used for general ulceration and hemorrhoids.[1015] Traditional uses in the U.S. include using the root tea as a rinse for sores in the mouth—canker sores, cracked lips, etc.[1016] Felter of the Eclectic School said, "Hydrastis is one of our most efficient topical medicines." Goldenseal was even used for cancers before the advent of modern cancer treatments. Fyfe of the Eclectic School suggests that it may have antiseptic properties. Does the research back the hype? Maybe. We know that goldenseal contains the alkaloids hydrastine and berberine. Both are astringent and have mild antiseptic properties.[1017] Beyond that, however, we can't say much. We don't have any clinical evidence either for or against goldenseal's use on skin injuries.

Immune support for colds and flu. Goldenseal has been used as a remedy for just about any viral or bacterial infection accompanied by mucus, most especially colds and upper respiratory tract infections. The Iroquois used it for whooping cough.[1018] The 1918 U.S. Dispensatory notes its use in cases of rhinitis.[1019] Traditional Chinese healers use it for immune support for patients whose immune system has been weakened by chemotherapy and other conventional treatments. In vitro experiments suggest that it might have some immune system enhancing properties.[1020] We have, however, no clinical evidence for this use. Given this lack of evidence and the dangers of taking goldenseal internally, it is probably wise to look for immune support elsewhere.

Exercise recovery. Goldenseal is known as the poor man's ginseng. In the West, goldenseal has been used like a tonic. Proponents claim adaptogenic and exercise recovery properties. The research evidence for this use, however, is lacking. Given the dangers of taking tannins internally and on a regular basis, it is probably best to avoid taking it for this use.

Plantar warts. We have some very limited traditional evidence for this use. Goldenseal can irritate the skin, a characteristic that's common to most do-it-yourself wart remedies. Irritation alone, however, does not make a wart remedy.

How do you use it?

Tinctures. For tincture of the dry root use 1:5, 70% alcohol. Goldenseal is typically used as a tincture for topical use. Two of its active ingredients, berberine and hydrastine, are poorly soluble in water but soluble in alcohol. Add ½ teaspoon of the tincture to a glass of water for a gargle or mouth wash. The tincture can be applied to wounds full strength (on those who tolerate it well), or it can be diluted.[1021] To make a wash or compress, add 1 teaspoon of the tincture to a half cup of water for skin inflammations. For plantar warts, apply the undiluted tincture three times a day. In the evening, apply a piece of gauze soaked in the tincture and leave it on overnight.

Infusions. An infusion is made by steeping ½–1 teaspoon of goldenseal powder or 2 teaspoons of the dried herb in a cup of water.[1022] It can be used as a mouthwash or gargle. The safer course of action when using goldenseal is to spit and not swallow.

Capsules. If you are taking goldenseal internally, take only preparations specifically marked as safe for internal use, and follow recommended dosage carefully. Some herbalists recommend that goldenseal not be taken internally at all.[1023] A common standardization for commercial extracts is 8 to 10% alkaloids or 5% hydrastine.

Dosage: How much do you use?

Internal. Limit yourself to only those preparations labeled for internal use and get professional supervision while taking it. Back off if you notice any laxative effects. Do not use goldenseal long-term. Limit to three weeks of use with two weeks between use.

External. Topical goldenseal can cause irritation or ulcers especially in people with sensitive skin. Start with a low dose well diluted to see how you tolerate it.

What should you be aware of before using it?

Large doses can be toxic.[1024] Taking too much (or too large a dose or a moderate dose for too long) can lead to digestive disorders, vomiting, hallucinations, difficulty in breathing, heart problems, and even central paralysis. If you are taking goldenseal internally, take only preparations specifically marked as safe for internal use, and follow recommended dosage carefully. Some herbalists recommend that goldenseal not be taken internally at all.[1025]

Avoid all internal use if you are pregnant. Animal studies show that it can induce contractions of the uterus.[1026]

Avoid internal use if you tend to have high blood pressure.

If you're using it as a mouthwash or rinse, don't use it long-term. It can cause drying of mucous membranes.[1027]

Don't take it if you are using heparin.[1028]

Topical goldenseal can cause skin irritation or ulcers especially in people with sensitive skin. Start with a low dose well diluted to see how you tolerate it.

Though traditionally goldenseal was used as an eye wash, that use is not recommended because of concerns about both the sterility of the solution and possible irritation.

Goldenseal could theoretically affect blood pressure, blood sugar, and clotting time. Use caution especially if you have issues in any of these areas.

Be careful about your source of goldenseal. Tainted preparations and preparations containing other less safe herbs have been reported.[1029]

Goldenseal is sometimes called "Indian turmeric" or "curcuma." It is not, however, true turmeric (*Curcuma longa* Linn.), and it has very different properties and uses.

Gotu Kola

Scientific name: *Centella asiatica*

Also known as Indian pennywort, marsh penny, Asiatic pennywort, white rot, *antanan*, and *pegaga*

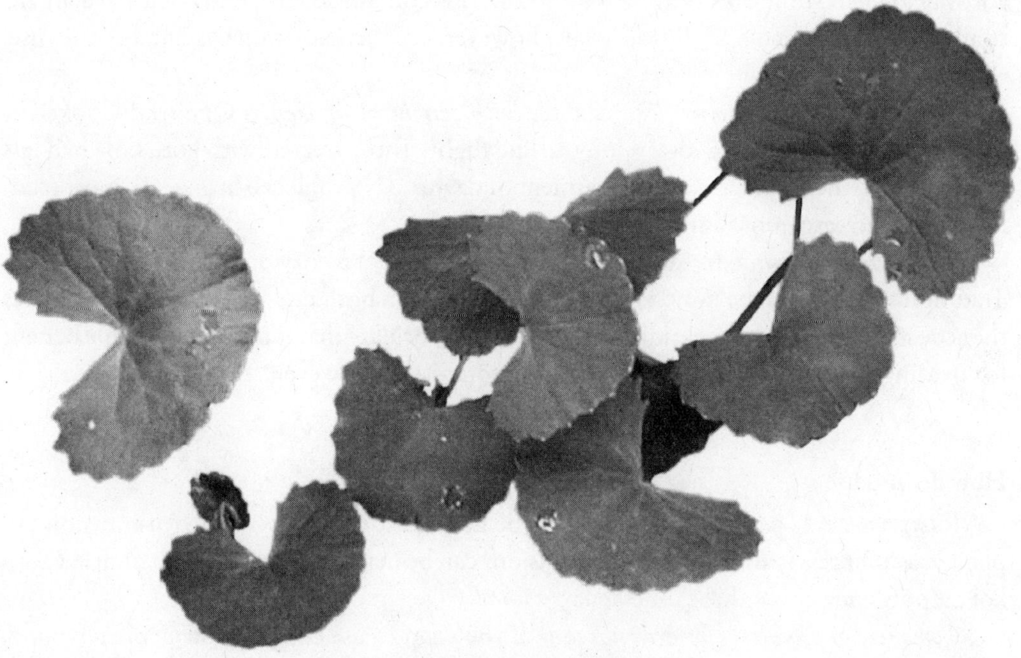

Gotu Kola, *Centella asiatica*

Courtesy of Forest and Kim Starr

Gotu kola is a creeping annual with pink or red flowers. It prefers swampy tropical environments. A native of India, Sri Lanka, South Africa, and Madagascar, it now grows as an introduced species in Oregon and Hawaii. The leaves are used medicinally.

Sri Lankans observed that elephants are fond of gotu kola and that they have a long life span. The plant became known as a life-giving herb.[1030] Both Ayurvedic medicine and traditional Chinese medicine make use of gotu kola. One of its most common uses is for skin problems.

What is it good for?

Helps minimize scarring. Gotu kola has been used for centuries both internally and externally to facilitate wound repair.[1031] One of the common uses in India has been to treat the wounds caused by leprosy.[1032] Animal studies show promise. In a study of rats with induced wounds, various gotu kola extracts fostered wound healing. The most effective extract was asiaticoside, one of the active ingredients in gotu kola, which induces collagen formulation.[1033] Putting asiaticoside topically on rats' wounds led to an increased presence of antioxidant in the newly formed tissue.[1034] Again in rats, both delayed-healing wounds (such as those found in diabetics) and normal wounds benefited from topical application of gotu kola.[1035] Studies in humans are a bit more scarce. In one, extracts simulated scar-free wound healing for a number of different types of scarring.[1036] As part of a combination cream, gotu kola has been shown to help reduce the incidence of stretch marks in pregnancy.[1037]

Healing of hyperextended joints, stretched or injured ligaments. Gotu kola contains asiaticoside, which stimulates healing. Gotu kola also contains compounds that have an anti-inflammatory effect.[1038] Clinical trials, however, are virtually nonexistent for this use.

Improves circulation to the legs for those with venous insufficiency. One study looked at swelling in the feet and legs after a long airline flight. Those treated with gotu kola had less swelling.[1039] Others have looked at treatment of day-to-day problems. In general, most studies show a decrease in swelling and circulation.[1040]

Strengthens the mind. In India, gotu kola is sometimes taken as an aid to meditation.[1041] Tradition says it clears the mind and helps memory.[1042] In both rats and people, it attenuates the acoustic startle response, leading researchers to speculate that it might have some benefit for treating anxiety disorders.[1043] Beyond that one study, however, all we have is tradition.

How do you use it?

Compresses and poultices. Poultices can be applied to closed wounds. An infusion applied to a compress is also effective.[1044] Infusions can be made from either fresh or dried gotu kola. Apply compresses three times a day.

Commercial products (for external use). If you want to use gotu kola on an open wound, use a reputable commercial product that has been made for that particular use. Ointments are available. Madecassol® and Centelase® are two common European brands.

Commercial products (for internal use). Gotu kola tablets and capsules are commercially available.

Infusions (for internal use). You can also make the leaves into a tea using the standard infusion method.

Dosage: How much do you use?

Internally: A probable effective dose for internal use is .6 g of the herb infused into a tea, taken 3 times per day[1045] If you wish to take capsules, the American Botanical Council recommends splitting the daily dose into three doses. They recommend 0.5–1.0 g per day. They also note that it should be taken only for short-term occasional use.

Externally: If you get commercial preparations for external use, use it according to label directions.

What should you be aware of before using it?

Tests of sensitivity in guinea pigs show that you are not likely to develop an increased sensitivity to gotu kola with use over time.[1046] However, some people do get contact dermatitis from it[1047] and it may increase sensitivity to the sun.

A 1972 paper reported that mice that were subject to repeated applications of concentrated gotu kola (twice a week for eighteen months) developed cancerous skin tumors.[1048] Though the study has not been reproduced nor the effect seen in humans, it is probably wise to use gotu kola judiciously, avoiding long-term use.

Too much taken internally can cause headaches and loss of consciousness.[1049]

Don't use gotu kola if you are pregnant, nursing, or trying to conceive.[1050]

Check with your doctor before taking gotu kola if you are taking diabetic drugs. Be cautious when using it in conjunction with herbs known or suspected to affect blood sugar levels. (See Chapter 5 for a list.)

Check with your doctor before taking gotu kola if you are taking cholesterol drugs or sedative drugs.[1051]

Gotu kola causes sedation in animals in large doses.[1052]

Large doses and prolonged use may adversely affect cholesterol levels.[1053]

Note that gotu kola is *not Cola* spp.

It is sometime incorrectly called Brahmi. Gotu kola is related to brahmi (*Bacopa monniera*) and has similar effects, but they are different plants.

Hops

Scientific name: *Humulus lupulus*

Also known as lupulin, lupulus, hummulus, humulus, common hops, European hops, hop, hop strobile

Hops is a fast-growing perennial bine native to North America and Europe. (Bines are like vines, but instead of tendrils or other appendages, bines wrap and use stiff, downward facing hairs to help attach themselves to whatever they're climbing on. However, though not technically accurate, "hops vine" is much more commonly used than "hops bine.") It's generally the flower that's used medicinally, though the strobilae is sometimes used as well.

Hops is in the same family as cannabis (*Cannabaceae*). The expression "hopped up" comes from experiments with smoking hops that had less than desirable results.[1054] Hops is also related to stinging nettles. The word "hops" comes from the Anglo–Saxon word "to climb." Given the right framework, hops vines can climb to more than thirty feet.

What is it good for?

Insomnia. The Cherokee used hops for alleviating pain and producing deep sleep. The Meskwaki used it as a treatment for insomnia.[1055] *A Modern Herbal* says that both infusions and tinctures are commonly used for nervousness and insomnia.[1056] The Eclectic School also recommended hops for this purpose. Commission E recommends it for sleep problems but suggests that it might work best when combined with other herbs that have a sedative effect.[1057] ◊ ◊ ◆ ◆ ◆

The precise nature of hops' sedative effect is tricky to pin down. The herb does contain very small amounts of methylbutanol, a compound with sedative effects.[1058] Whether or not it has enough of this compound to cause sleep in humans is another matter. A 1992 German study showed that 150 g in a single dose (*a lot* of hops) are necessary to make an adult human drowsy.[1059] Another study done in Germany in 1967 showed that hops did *not* work by depressing the central nervous system as does most sedatives.[1060] Most of the clinical sleep studies we have combine hops with valerian. We know that a valerian-hops mixture inhibits the stimulant effect of caffeine.[1061] We also have a few studies that suggest that the mixture improves sleep efficiency.[1062] These studies, however, have been neither large nor well-

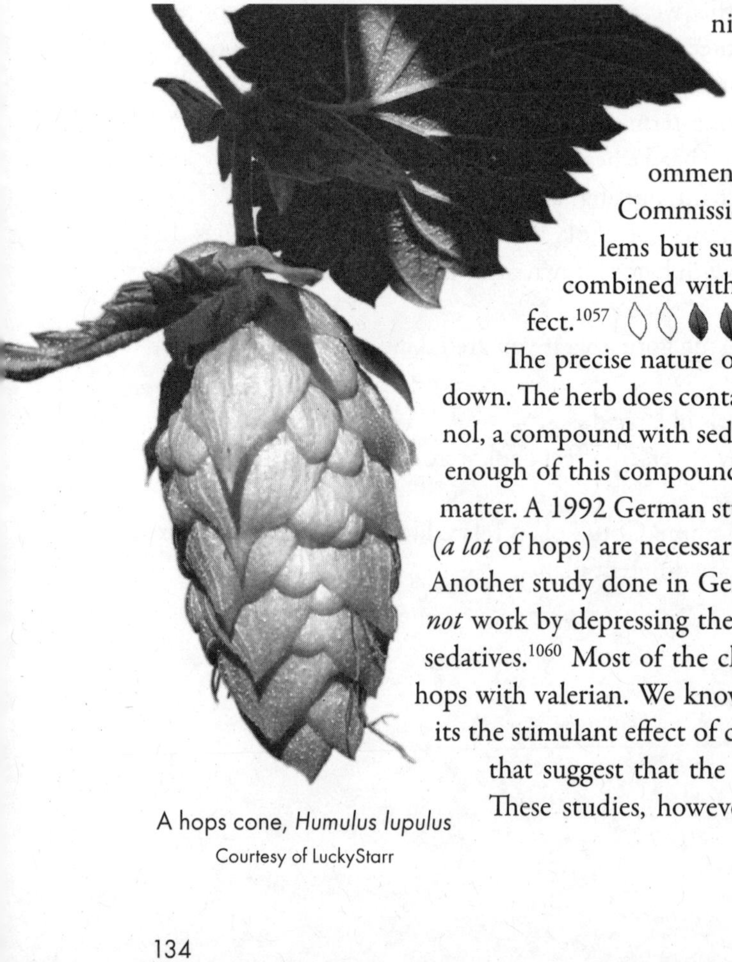

A hops cone, *Humulus lupulus*
Courtesy of LuckyStarr

controlled. Moreover, we don't have much evidence about what hops can do on its own because it is often combined with valerian.

Anxiety. The Delaware Indians used the blossoms for nervousness.[1063] The Mohegan used hops as a "nerve medicine."[1064] Commission E recommends it for sleep anxiety.[1065] Fyfe suggests it for "deranged conditions of the brain and nervous system." Clinical studies for this use, however, are absent. ◊ ◊ ◊ ◆ ◆

Wounds. The Round Valley, Dakota, and Omaha Indians used hops for wounds.[1066] Traditional British herbalism says that it allays pain and inflammation and is often combined with chamomile as an external remedy for bruises and swellings.[1067] Fyfe of the Eclectic School recommends it for "inflammatory and painful local affections." Another traditional European use is for facial neuralgia. The Eclectic School recommended a "hops bag," made by sewing hops into a pillow then using the pillow for face ache. We now know, however, that hops dust is prone to carrying harmful bacteria that should not be inhaled, throwing the wisdom of the dry "hops bag" into question. A better alternative is to use it as a plaster, moistening the bag with water or vinegar to control the dust before applying. One in vitro test shows that hops does have some antimicrobial actions, but the test was very limited.[1068] It also contains tannins. In other words, tradition suggests that it might have some benefit for wounds, but we have very little scientific corroboration for this use. ◊ ◊ ◊ ◆ ◆

How do you use it?

Infusion. Infusion works well for hops.[1069] Use an infusion of fresh flowers if you can get them, or dried or freeze-dried flowers if you can't. Use 0.5 g (or roughly 1 teaspoonful) per cup of tea and let infuse for 10–15 minutes using the standard infusion method.

Tincture. (1:1 in 45% alcohol) For anxiety, take up to ½ teaspoon three times a day of the tincture.

In combination. Hops is often combined with other sedatives.[1070] For insomnia especially, combining it with other sedating herbs often works better than using it alone. Hops strobilae, with valerian rhizome, and passionflower and chamomile flowers, is a common combination. You can drink hops as a tea, but its not the most palatable beverage. Another more drinkable option is tincture in water. (Check the respective entries for appropriate doses.)

Dosage: How much do you use?

A traditional dose is 1–2 g of the herb daily.[1071]

Tincture. For the tincture, a traditional dose is ⅛–¼ teaspoon per dose up to three times daily.

We have no studies regarding safe levels of hops. The above doses are *common* doses, not necessarily universally safe doses.

What should you be aware of before using it?

The FDA lists hops as one of its GRAS (Generally Recognized as Safe) foods.

In animal studies, overdosing on hops caused seizure, hyperthermia, restlessness, vomiting, stomach pain, and increased stomach acid.[1072]

If you are exposed to hops pollen regularly—if you live in an area where hops is grown—it's possible to develop an allergy. If you suspect you have an allergy to hops pollen, be judicious in your internal use of the herb.[1073] Allergies to hops have also been reported in people allergic to peanuts, nuts, and bananas.[1074]

Don't use hops if you are prone to depression.

Be careful not to inhale the dust from ground hops when making preparations. It can contain harmful bacteria.[1075]

Hops is *supposed to* make you drowsy. Be cautious about driving or engaging in activities for which you must be alert. Be careful about mixing hops with alcohol because each can accentuate the effects of the other.[1076] It may also compound the effect of other sedative herbs. (See Chapter 5 for a list.)

Don't use if you are taking a phenothiazine drug as hops may increase its effects.[1077]

Don't use it without talking with a physician if you have any kind of estrogen imbalance or if estrogen-dependent breast cancer runs in your family. Some traditional wisdom says that hops has a kind of hormonal effect on the body. Research is still unclear what that effect is, but it would be wise to have your hops use monitored by someone trained if you are concerned with its effects on the endocrine system.[1078]

Don't take it with drugs or herbs that have monoamine oxidase inhibitor (MAOI) activity or that interact with MAOI drugs. Headache, tremors, mania, and insomnia may occur[1079] (See Chapter 5 for a list.)

Animal studies suggest that it may alter blood sugar levels.[1080] Use caution if you have blood sugar issues.

It may lower triglycerides and free fatty acid blood levels.[1081] If you have cholesterol or other blood lipid issues, you may want to keep an eye on your levels while taking hops.[1082]

It is possible to become sensitized to the external application of hops.

Horse Chestnut Seed

Scientific name: *Aesculus hippocastanum*

Also known as buckeye (applied most commonly to related American species)

The horse chestnut is a large tree, 40 feet or more tall. It flowers in June, then sets a round, prickly fruit containing a large, shining, brown nut. This nut, and occasionally the bark, is used medicinally. The horse chestnut is native to a small area in the mountains of the Balkans in southeast Europe, as well as in northern Greece and Macedonia. It has been cultivated throughout the temperate world, however, including North America.

The horse chestnut is *not* the same as the same chestnuts of the genus *Castanea*. The Castanea chestnuts—sweet chestnut, American chestnut, Japanese chestnut, Chinese chestnut—are the ones that grow edible nuts, which are roasted and eaten, especially around Christmas (as in *The Christmas Song*: "Chestnuts roasting on an open fire/ Jack Frost nipping at your nose/") If, however, you were to roast and eat the horse chestnut, you would most likely become quite sick because horse chestnuts contain a toxin related to a common rat poison.

The leaves and nut of a horse chestnut, *Aesculus hippocastanum*

Courtesy of Renate Eder

What is it good for?

Problems caused by inflammation or poor tone of veins. The Kawaiisu and the Costanoan used the smashed fruit (of *Aesculus californica* [Spach] Nutt., a related species) as a salve for hemorrhoids.[1083] A modern study shows that the latter use may have scientific merit. Horse chestnut contains aescin which has a vascular tightening effect. Aescin, when tested alone, has been shown to reduce swelling and inflammation.[1084] The best-researched use of horse chestnut is for chronic venous insufficiency, a pathological condition in which the veins are unable to get enough blood to the legs, causing (among other symptoms) leg cramps. Several high-quality studies have shown that horse chestnut can reduce pain, edema, and cramps.[1085] Researchers are not entirely certain how horse chestnut works, but they think that the aescin it contains may help strengthen capillaries

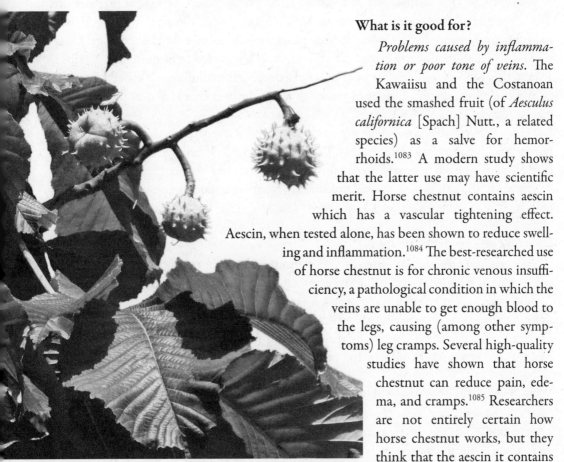

and improve the tone and strength of veins.[1086] That effect is probably not permanent, however. Horse chestnut is typically considered to be a treatment for the symptoms of venous insufficiency, not a cure for the condition itself.[1087] We also have no indication that horse chestnut seed would help with leg cramps brought on by exercise or electrolyte imbalance.

◊ ◆ ◆ ◆ ◆

Bruising. The Cherokee used the nuts of a related species (*Aesculus pavia* L.) as a poultice on inflammations and sores.[1088] Another related species (Japanese horse chestnut—*Aesculus turbinata*) has been shown to have anti-inflammatory properties in vitro and in vivo.[1089] Aescin, one of the active ingredients in horse chestnut, has been show in vitro to have anti-inflammatory properties.[1090] We have one study showing that horse chestnut may be useful for treating bruises when applied topically. Ten grams of 2% aescin gel applied in a single dose within five minutes of bruising reduced the tenderness of the bruise.[1091] ◊ ◊ ◆ ◆ ◆

How do you use it?

Commercial formulations (for internal use). Take only those commercial preparations that have had the toxic component, aesculin (esculin) removed. Venastat® is one such over-the-counter preparation.[1092] Controlled-release capsules minimize the chance of gastric irritation.[1093] Though properly prepared horse chestnut is reported to be quite safe,[1094] this is an herb that is best used with the supervision of a doctor. The conditions it's used for should be monitored by a doctor, and the potential effect on the liver should also be monitored by regular testing.

Commercial formulations (for external use). Topical preparations are available from European companies. One preparation, Reparil-Gel N®, developed by Madaus AG in Germany, has been tested to good effect against blunt injuries and bruises.[1095]

Poultice. You can make a topical preparation from ½ teaspoon of powder in 16 ounces of water.[1096]

Dosage: How much do you use?

Commercial formulation (internal use). Because you will be taking a commercially prepared capsule, your best bet is to choose a reputable brand and follow label directions.

Commercial formulation (external use). Gels or creams, which are more common in Europe than in North America, are typically standardized to contain 1–2% aescin. These preparations can be applied topically three or four times per day for hemorrhoids, skin ulcers, varicose veins, sports injuries, and other trauma.[1097]

What should you be aware of before using it?

Whole horse chestnut is classed as an unsafe herb by the FDA.[1098] It contains aesculin, a compound similar to the rat poison warfarin, which breaks down blood proteins.[1099] The buds, flowers, nuts, leaves, bark, seedlings, and honey of the horse chestnut are all toxic. The effects of taking them internally include gastrointestinal irritation, vomiting, abdominal pain, diarrhea, staggering, trembling, breathing difficulty, and, if enough is consumed, collapse and paralysis, which can in rare instances proceed to coma and death.[1100] Horse chestnut is also is toxic to the liver and kidneys and can cause long-term damage.[1101]

Take only commercial preparations that have had the toxic components removed. Don't use injected horse chestnut preparations.[1102]

Don't take it if you are taking an antithrombotic, including aspirin.[1103] If you plan to have surgery, tell your surgeon you have been taking horse chestnut and discontinue use. Be cautious when using it in conjunction with other herbs known or suspected of increasing the risk of bleeding. (See Chapter 5 for a list.)

Don't take it if you have liver or kidney problems.[1104] If you see any yellowing of skin or eyes, discontinue taking horse chestnut and see a doctor immediately. If you take horse chestnut regularly, or if you have concerns about how it affects liver function, you should have a doctor monitor your liver functions while you are taking it.[1105] Don't take it in conjunction with any other herb or drug known to affect liver function. [1106] (See Chapter 5 for a list.)

Report any unusual bleeding, fatigue, or fever to a doctor.[1107]

Don't take it if you are pregnant or nursing.[1108]

Taking horse chestnut orally can make your urine turn red.[1109]

Topical horse chestnut creams and gels don't have the same hazards as horse chestnut taken internally.[1110] If you are allergic to tropical fruits, you may have a reaction to topical horse chestnut.[1111]

Horseradish

Scientific name: *Armoracia rusticana*

Also known as pepperrot, *Cochlearia armoracia*, mountain radish, great raifort, red cole. Armoraciae Radix is horseradish root

Though native to eastern Europe and western Asia, horseradish is now grown as an introduced species throughout the northern parts of the United States. The plant is a flowering perennial. The large, fleshy root is used medicinally.

Horseradish has been cultivated for about two thousand years. It was brought to North America by the early colonists who used it not only as medicine but as a condiment.[1112] Horseradish's active ingredients are released when the root is cut or crushed. Allylisothiocyanate, butylthiocyanate, mustard oil, and mustard oil glycosides are all present.[1113] Grate a bit of horseradish using an open grater and all the potent chemicals inside will immediately announce their presence. In fact, unless a fast release of secretions from eyes and nose is your intent, you will find a food processor with a tight lid a big help when preparing fresh horseradish.

What is it good for?

Colds. One of the most common uses of horseradish is for colds and catarrhs of the respiratory tract. The Cherokee used it for colds, sore throats, and asthma.[1114] *A Modern Herbal* says it can be mixed in glycerin and used for hoarseness and coughs.[1115] We don't have much research into the medicinal effects of horseradish. It doesn't take an M.D., however, to proclaim that the stuff makes your nose run. If you're clogged up and want to get everything in your nose and sinuses moving, horseradish is a remedy people have been using for centuries. Put some on your tongue and you'll immediately notice the effects on your nose and sinuses. It also has some antimicrobial properties that have been examined only in vitro.[1116]

Muscle aches and joint pain. Horseradish has been a traditional part of liniments and poultices for minor aches and pains. The Delaware used a poultice for neuralgia.[1117] The

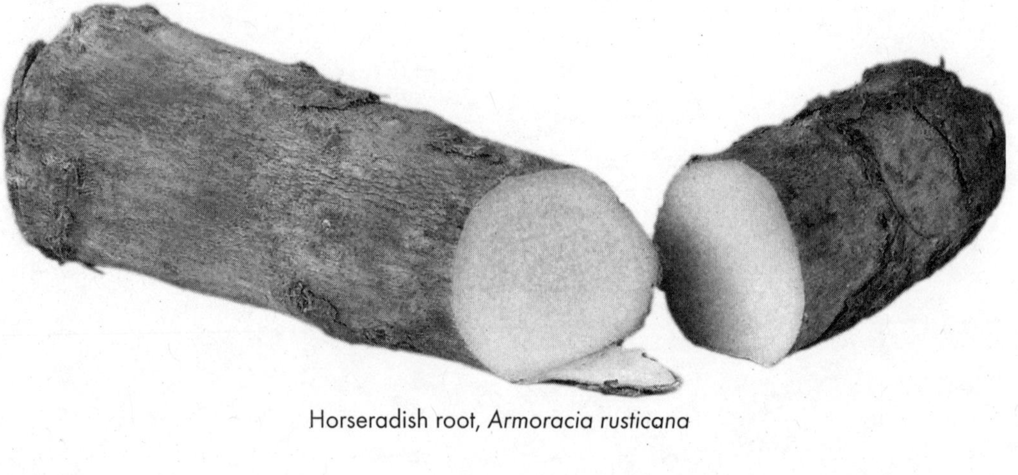

Horseradish root, *Armoracia rusticana*

Cherokee used it for rheumatism.[1118] *A Modern Herbal* says that a poultice can be used for all kinds of aches.[1119] But does it work? We do know that horseradish applied to the skin stimulates blood flow to the area.[1120] It may also be useful as a counterirritant, a substance that depletes neurotransmitters and so decreases pain. That's conjecture, however. We don't have the research to back any of it.

Rheumatism. Horseradish has been used not just topically but also internally for joint aches. *A Modern Herbal* gives this recipe for "chronic rheumatism": fresh horseradish root, orange peel, nutmeg, and spirit of wine—1 or 2 teaspoonfuls in half a wineglass full of water, two or three times daily after meals.[1121] As long as you listen to your nose and mouth and don't force huge amounts of horseradish, this remedy is probably not going to hurt you. Whether or not it will help is another issue entirely.

How do you use it?

Horseradish can be used fresh or dried. The root can be cut or ground, and the juice can be pressed out.

Infusion (for internal use). Mix freshly grated root into hot liquid for colds. Freshly pressed juice can be used instead of grated root.[1122]

Poultice. For a poultice, mix freshly grated horseradish with cornstarch.[1123]

Tinctures. Tinctures don't dissolve any of the essential oils and are not recommended.

Essential oil. Don't use the essential oil at all, either internally or externally. It's just too strong.[1124]

Dosage: How much do you use?

2–4 g of the fresh root before meals is probably an effective dosage.[1125] 20 g of fresh root per day is the maximum dose.

What should you be aware of before using it?

The FDA includes horseradish on its list of food generally recognized as safe. That recommendation applies to use as a condiment, not use in medicinal quantities.[1126]

If you're going to take it internally, listen to your mouth. Your body has a reason to warn you about overuse. Too much horseradish can cause stomach and intestinal problems.[1127] Don't subvert your body's natural warning system by putting it in capsules.

Be a bit cautious the first time you use horseradish topically. In some people large concentrations can cause blistering.[1128]

Don't give it to children under the age of 4.[1129]

Don't use it if you have ulcers or kidney problems.[1130]

Large doses can cause diarrhea, vomiting, and irritation of mucous membranes.[1131]

Don't take it if you are using cholinergic drugs because it may increase their effects.[1132]

If you are taking thyroxine or suffer from hypothyroidism, check with your doctor before using medicinal concentrations of horseradish. The rational for this warning is neither clear nor universally recognized, but prudence suggests you discuss it with your doctor.[1133]

Horsetail

Scientific name: *Equisetum arvense*

Also known as common horsetail, scouring rush, shave grass, bottle brush, toad pipe, Dutch rush, flied horsetail, horse willow, pewterwort, *cola de caballo*, corncob plant, corn horsetail, paddock pipes, running clubmoss, *shen jin cao*, *wen jing*

Horsetail is an ancient plant. It's a perennial, has hollow stems that look a little like bamboo and no flowers. It grows wild throughout most of the North America (except in parts of the Deep South of the U.S.). It also grows in temperate regions of Europe, sometimes so well that it's considered an invasive weed. Approximately 25 species of *Equisetum* exist, each with its own medicinal properties. *Arvense* is the one most commonly used medicinally. Unless otherwise noted, it is the one described in this section. The aerial (above-ground) parts, especially the stems, are used medicinally.

Close relatives of modern horsetail grew 270 million years ago. The dinosaurs probably tromped on a bit of it when they roamed the earth. It also has a long history of medicinal use. The Chinese use the species *Equisetum hyemale*, which they call *mu zei* for wounds and burns.[1134]

Traditionally, horsetail was used as a mild diuretic. That use is fairly well attested to, even in the modern scientific literature.[1135] But for martial artists, its potential as a healer of wounds is more interesting. Since the time of the Greeks, horsetail has been used for the treatment of wounds. Like agrimony, it is rich in silica and has astringent and anti-inflammatory properties. In fact it gets the name "scouring rush" from that silica, which made it good for scouring pots.

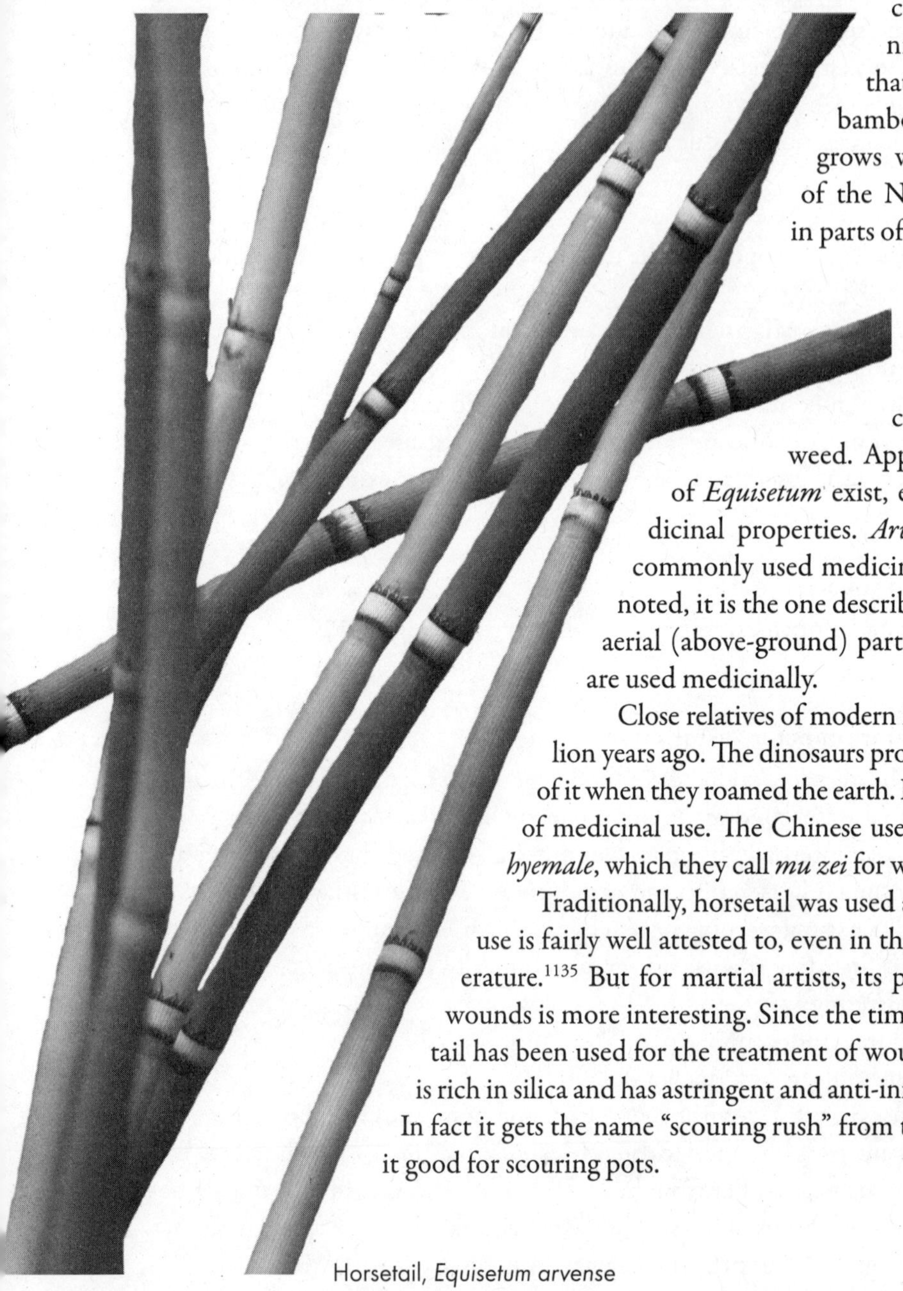

Horsetail, *Equisetum arvense*
Courtesy of Laura Westbrooks

What is it good for?

Wounds. Horsetail is very astringent and functions well as a clotting agent. The Kwakiutl Indians used a poultice of rough leaves and stems on cuts and sores.[1136] The Pomo used a decoction of it as a wash for itching or open sores.[1137] In Chinese medicine horsetail is called *mu zei*, and it is used topically for wounds and burns.[1138] Since the sixteenth century, horsetail has had a place in British herbalism as a way to stop bleeding and heal wounds quickly.[1139] Though we don't have clinical trials to back this use, it makes sense in terms of some of horsetail's properties. In vitro studies show antioxidant properties.[1140] The essential oils are a broad-spectrum antimicrobial.[1141] Animal studies show that an extract of horsetail reduces irritation and inflammation from wounds.[1142] Also of benefit may be the silica. In the 1990s, pharmaceutical companies began experimenting with silica in burn dressings. They found that the presence of silica helped stabilize burns and helped wounds heal more quickly.[1143] Horsetail is very high in silica. ◌◌◆◆◆

Joint injuries. Repair of joint injuries is one of the traditional uses of horsetail. Again, we have no clinical evidence. We do know that the body needs silica to form cartilage and connective tissue, and the silica in horsetail seems to be quite easily absorbed.[1144] The herb also contains calcium and other minerals. ◌◌◌◆◆

Fractures. Tradition says that hand and foot baths containing horsetail decoction may help speed fractures in those areas.[1145] The silica, calcium, and other herbs may also help in bone building. One (rather poorly constructed) study suggests that horsetail taken internally can raise bone density as effectively as calcium supplements.[1146] The scientific recognition of that use, however, is lacking. ◌◌◌◌◆

How do you use it?

Read the warning section before using horsetail internally. The recommendations for how much horsetail to use in any given preparation varies widely. These are some typical recommendations, but they are *not* backed by safety studies.

Infusion. Pour ½–1 cup of boiling water over 2 g (about 2 teaspoons) and continue boiling for 5 minutes. Then allow this infusion to steep for another 10 to 15 minutes before straining. Take it internally three times daily.[1147] To make a larger batch for use as a compress, use 10 g of herb to 1 quart of water.[1148] Boil for five minutes, and then steep for 10–15 minutes.

Cold infusion. Use the cold infusion for external use only. Mix 10 teaspoons of horsetail in cold water and soak for 10 to 12 hours.[1149]

Tincture. (1:1 in 25% alcohol) Take about 2 teaspoons (10 ml), three times daily.[1150]

Capsules. You can also find commercially prepared capsules or commercially packaged teas. If you plan to take the preparation without boiling it, make sure that the thiaminase present in fresh horsetail has been neutralized. If you take it internally, be sure to drink plenty of water because it acts as a diuretic.

Poultice. Make the powder into a paste and use that as a poultice on joint injuries and minor fractures.[1151]

Soak. For a soak use 2 g of the herb per one quart of hot water. Allow it to steep for an hour before soaking.[1152]

Dosage: How much do you use?

Frankly, we don't know how much is safe. Horsetail has been used for centuries without obvious deleterious effects. We now know, however, that it contains equisetic acid, which is toxic and potentially deadly when taken internally in high doses.[1153] 6 g of the cut herb per day is a typical maximum daily dose for internal use.[1154] A safer course of action is to use horsetail externally only.

What should you be aware of before using it?

We don't know as much about the safety of horsetail as we might like. The stem seems safer than the rest of the plant.[1155] In fact, pharmaceutical grade horsetail herb consists solely of the dried, green, sterile stems of *Equisetum arvense* L. in whole, cut, or powdered forms. Don't use horsetail for extended periods of time.

Most of the problems with horsetail occur when people take it internally. It has a toxicity similar to that of nicotine.[1156] Don't take it internally without the supervision of a qualified herbalist or naturopath.

Horsetail contains thiaminase, an enzyme that splits thiamine, a B vitamin, making it inactive and resulting in thiamine deficiency.[1157] The body's energy metabolism depends on thiamine. Alcohol, high temperature, and alkalinity neutralize thiaminase, which means tinctures, or decoctions that are subjected to 100 degrees Centigrade temperatures (boiled) are safer for internal use than dried or fresh horsetail.[1158] The Health Protection Branch of Health in Great Britain and Welfare Canada have banned the sale of horsetail unless it has the thiaminase removed.[1159]

Horsetail also contains equisetic acid, which is toxic and potentially deadly when taken internally in high doses.[1160] The amount of equisetic acid a person can tolerate depends on several factors, including the size of the person. Poisonings have been reported in children using horsetail stems as whistles.[1161]

Horsetail contains small amounts of nicotine.[1162] People who have recovered from a nicotine addiction may wish to avoid taking it internally. People who smoke or use nicotine patches should factor the amount of nicotine in horsetail into their daily intake.

If you take horsetail internally, you should also increase your intake of fluids because it acts as a diuretic and can cause dehydration.

It is an irritant and can cause dermatitis in some people.[1163] Try a little on unbroken skin to see how you react before using it on wounds.

If you cannot guarantee the sterility of your horsetail preparation, don't use it on broken skin.

The herb is not recommended for children.[1164]

One of the traditional uses (e.g., Fyfe) is to promote contractions of the uterus. Though the modern evidence does not exist for this use, it probably should not be used by women who are pregnant.

Note that this horsetail is not the kelp of the genus *Laminaria*, which is also called "horsetail."

Lavender

Scientific name: *Lavandula augustifolia*, *Lavandula vera*, or *Lavandula spica*

Also known as *Lavandula officinalis* L., English lavender, French lavender, common lavender, garden lavender, true lavender (augustifolia), spike lavender (spica), pink lavender, white lavender

So-called "English Lavender" is actually native to the Mediterranean region. It has become, however, a common nonnative garden herb in both Europe and North America. The small evergreen plant produces white, blue, or purple flowers. The flower is used to produce an essential oil. Both the flower and the oil are used medicinally. Some mixtures also contain stem and leaf, but these have less medicinal value. It grows wild in New York and Vermont as an introduced species.

Lavender is best known as an ornamental plant and a culinary herb, part of the *herbes de Provence* blend in French cooking. It also has a long history of medicinal use. The word lavender comes from the Latin word for "to wash," and may refer to its use in washing wounds. For many people, lavender reminds them of their grandmother's perfume. Lavender contains 0.5–1.5% of an aromatic volatile oil, which is where most of the therapeutic effects come from.[1165] Spike lavender yields more essential oil, but true lavender has more of the active ingredients than spike lavender.

What is it good for?

Restlessness and anxiety. This use has both traditional and scientific attestation. A seventeenth century Persian medical text calls lavender "the broom of the brain," because of its reputation to sweep away cares. Fyfe of the Eclectic School suggests its use for "nervous depression and hysteria." Animal studies show benefits, as do human studies,

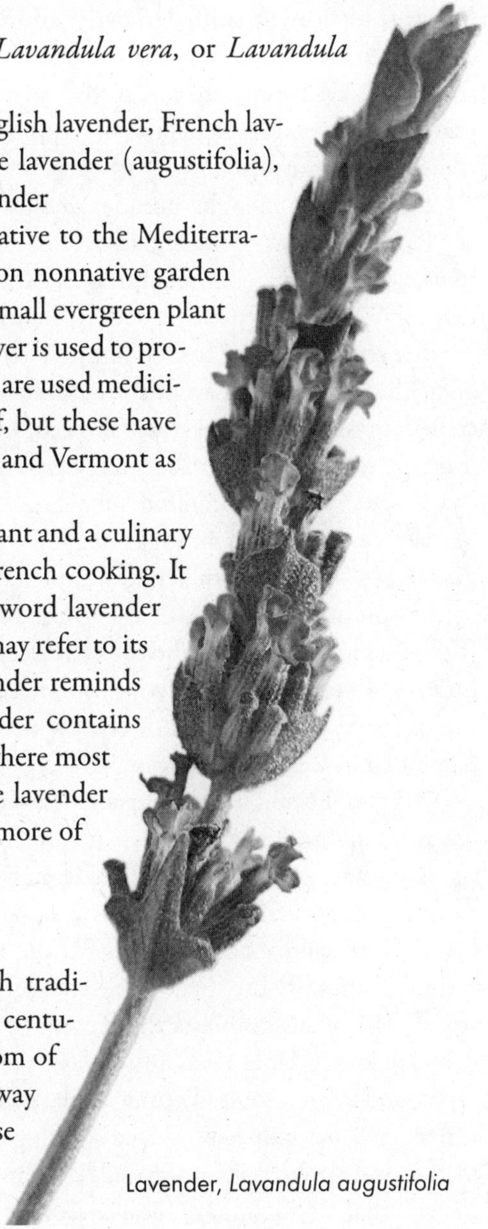

Lavender, *Lavandula augustifolia*

suggesting the benefits are physical and not merely due to a positive association with the smell. In rats, it has been shown to reduce anxiety.[1166] In mice, smelling the aroma of lavender counteracts the effects of a shot of caffeine.[1167] The smell of lavender settles down dogs prone to travel anxiety.[1168]

Human clinical studies also show benefit. In a Japanese study, thirty-six male workers were analyzed during the "afternoon slump" at work. Some were given lavender to sniff during a half-hour break. Others were just given the break. Those that sniffed the lavender were more alert and worked better after going back to work after the break.[1169] A study of male college students who sniffed lavender aroma found a similar benefit in reducing drowsiness in the afternoon.[1170] One study associates lavender aroma with reduced stress and increased arousal.[1171] Unfortunately, in a study of 145 volunteers who took an assessment test in the presence of lavender smell, lavender also decreased working memory and reaction times as compared to controls.[1172]

Interestingly enough, lavender doesn't just increase alertness, it also helps quell anxiety. Lavender scent decreased anxiety in a dentist's waiting room as compared to controls (music, and no smell and no music).[1173] It helps reduce restlessness in elderly dementia patients.[1174] A study of patients with dementia suggests that it can decrease aggression.[1175] In another study, lavender helped improve relaxation and mood, and improved the ability to do math problems.[1176] Lavender tincture taken internally might help improve mild to moderate depression.[1177] One study showed, however, that suggestion enhanced or detracted from the relaxing effects of sedating herbs including lavender.[1178]

Insomnia. In European folk medicine, lavender was sewn into pillows to promote sleep. Modern research is beginning to suggest that the smell of lavender helps with mild insomnia.[1179] In a small study of geriatric patients, lavender used as aromatherapy helped as much with insomnia as hypnotic drugs. Those patients who used lavender were also less restless while sleeping than those who took the sleeping pills.[1180] A Korean study also found benefits for using lavender scent to treat insomnia and mild depression.[1181] The German Standard License (GSL) for lavender flower tea approves its internal use for insomnia and restlessness. Commission E endorses this use.[1182]

Wounds. Lotion or cream made of lavender essential oil has been used traditionally for eczema, sunburns or scalds. Ancient Romans used lavender in their baths to soothe and heal the skin. During World War II, the French Academy of Medicine looked into lavender for antiseptic purposes. At the time essence of lavender was a common remedy in France for bruises, bites, and aches and pains.[1183] We do know that the oil has tannins and antimicrobial properties.[1184] The linalool in lavender essential oil kills various kinds of fungus in vitro.[1185] The oil also inhibits the growth of some bacteria, specifically bacteria involved in dental plaque.[1186] It also has anti-parasitic effects.[1187] In animal studies, we see some benefits for wounds. A mouse study using a related species (*Lavandula multifida*) showed that tincture of lavender reduced induced swelling.[1188] In another mouse study it inhibited inflammation and outward signs of pain.[1189] Animal studies also suggest that topical application of the essential oil might have local anesthetic activity.[1190] However, not all animal studies are unequivocal. One used lavender essential oil on induced wounds in rats and found no beneficial effect from the essential oil. That study did, however, find benefit from lavender honey (honey made by bees from lavender flowers). Human studies are sparse. One found lavender effective in the healing of the perineum after childbirth.[1191]

Nervous stomach. The 1918 U.S. Dispensatory notes that tincture of lavender can be used for "gastric uneasiness," nausea, and flatulence.[1192] The Eclectic School recommended lavender as a carminative and nausea treatment. Modern studies show that spike lavender has antispasmodic actions in smooth muscles, such as those found in the gastrointestinal tract.[1193] It also improves circulation. Commission E approves it for this use.

Tension headache. A Modern Herbal describes how lavender water used to be rubbed into the temples for headache.[1194] We have some modern evidence that it might help modulate pain. Sixteen people were tested to see how the smell of lavender affected their perceptions of pain. Though the lavender did not change perceptions of the level of pain, it did decrease the subjective appraisal of the unpleasantness of that pain.[1195]

Muscle spasms. Lavender has occasionally been used as a rubefacient. One study found good effect when using oil of bergamot (an Italian citrus fruit) and lavender as an ointment for low back pain.[1196] But other than that, we have neither wide traditional use nor scientific backing.

How do you use it?

Infusion. Infusion brings out the best in lavender.[1197] The tea is good for nervous exhaustion and anxiety. To make tea, use 1–2 teaspoons of lavender flowers per cup of water.[1198] Bring just the water to a boil. Remove from heat and add the lavender. Cover and steep for 15 minutes.

Essential oil. For internal use, take 1–4 drops (ca. 20–80 mg), e.g., on a sugar cube. Essential oil can be used undiluted (it's one of the few essential oils that can be used undiluted). For external use, it can be added 1–4 drops per tablespoon to a carrier oil to make it easier to apply.

Tincture. (1:5 in 50% alcohol) The tincture can be massaged into the temples for insomnia and tension headache. It can also be taken internally. Tincture might be more effective than infusion when used topically on inflammation.[1199]

Lotion. A lotion or cream can be made of essential oil for use on eczema, sunburns or scalds. Mix the essential oil with pure vegetable butter (shea butter, sal butter, mango butter, etc.).

Bath. To use lavender as a bath, sew a cup or two of lavender flowers into a muslin bag. Put it under the spout of the tub and run the bath, or put a few drops (1–5) of the essential oil in the water.[1200] Lavender baths are good for tension or insomnia.

Massage. A mixture of 20% lavender oil in combination with 80% grape-seed oil can increase overall well-being, and decrease anger and frustration.[1201]

Aromatherapy. 2–4 drops of the essential oil in 2–3 cups of boiling water. Or put a few drops on a handkerchief. Or you can stitch a cup or two of the flowers into a pillow to keep near your head as you are falling asleep.

Dosage: How much do you use?

Infusions. Don't exceed 3–5 g of lavender daily when taking internally.

Essential oil. A common dose of the essential oil (for internal use) is up to 4 drops per day. However, more conservative herbalists say that lavender oil should not be taken internally.[1202]

Tincture. 2/3 to 1 teaspoon per day is a typical maximum dose.

What should you be aware of before using it?

The FDA has lavender on both its list of spices that are generally recognized as safe and essential oils that are generally recognized as safe.

Lavender essential oil is commonly considered to be one of the mildest of the essential oils. Historically, it has been used on wounds, even open wounds. One study, however, shows some damage to human skin cells in vitro.[1203] Lavender is generally safe in reasonable doses. Too much, however, can cause respiratory depression.[1204] We don't know what the effects are of long-term lavender use.

Lavender smell has a mild sedative effect on some people. Be aware of this fact if you plan to drive or do something else that requires alertness.

Allergy to lavender is not unheard of.[1205] It is also possible to become sensitized to lavender. In some people, lavender taken internally may increase sensitivity to the sun.[1206]

Avoid lavender oil during pregnancy.

Lavender essential oil may have a mild estrogenic effect. In one report, five boys (ages 4–7) experienced abnormal breast development after using products containing lavender oil. Subsequent research found that when tested in vitro on human breast cancer cells, the essential oil mimicked estrogen while reducing the activity of androgens.[1207]

If you have sensitive skin, dilute the essential oil before using it topically.

Don't take it if you are taking a commercial or prescription sedative.[1208] It may compound the effect of other sedative herbs. (See Chapter 5 for a list.)

Licorice

Scientific name: *Glycyrrhiza glabra* (Mediterranean/Middle Eastern), *Glycyrrhiza uralensis* (Chinese), *Glycyrrhiza lepidota* Pursh (American)

Also known as *Liquiritia officinalis*, liquorice, Chinese/Persian/Russian/Spanish licorice, sweet root, sweet wood, DGL (deglycyrrhizinated licorice), *gan cao*, glabridin, glabrene, glucoliquiritin, glycyrrhetenic acid, glycyrrhiza, glycyrrhizin

Licorice is an herbaceous perennial. The genus *Glycyrrhiza* includes about 20 species. *Glycyrrhiza glabra* is native to the Middle East, *G. uralensis* to China, and *G. lepidota* to North American. *Glabra* is the species most often used medicinally. The root or stolon is the part of the plant that's used. The roots are first dried. Then they are boiled, and the resulting syrup is evaporated. The result is licorice extract. Licorice contains a chemical that is extremely sweet, so much so that in some countries the dried root is chewed like a candy. This chemical encourages the production of hydrocortisone, an anti-inflammatory agent.

What is it good for?

Colds and catarrhs *of the upper respiratory tract*. Wherever licorice is found—in eastern and western Asia, Europe, and North America—it's used as a decoction for coughs and a sore throat. The use dates back to ancient Egypt, where *G. glabra* tea was used to soothe the throat. When Americans first went to the People's Republic of China and were allowed to observe Chinese medical practices, they found doctors using *G. uralensis* licorice as a decoction for coughs.[1209] In traditional Chinese medicine, licorice is called *gan cao*. It is one of the fifty fundamental herbs[1210] and is used for sore throat and bronchitis among other many things.[1211] The Cherokee, Keres, Bannock, Blackfoot, Great Basin Indians, Montana, Bella Coola, Haisla, Hesquiat, Kitasoo, Nitinaht, Oweekeno, and Thompson Indians all used

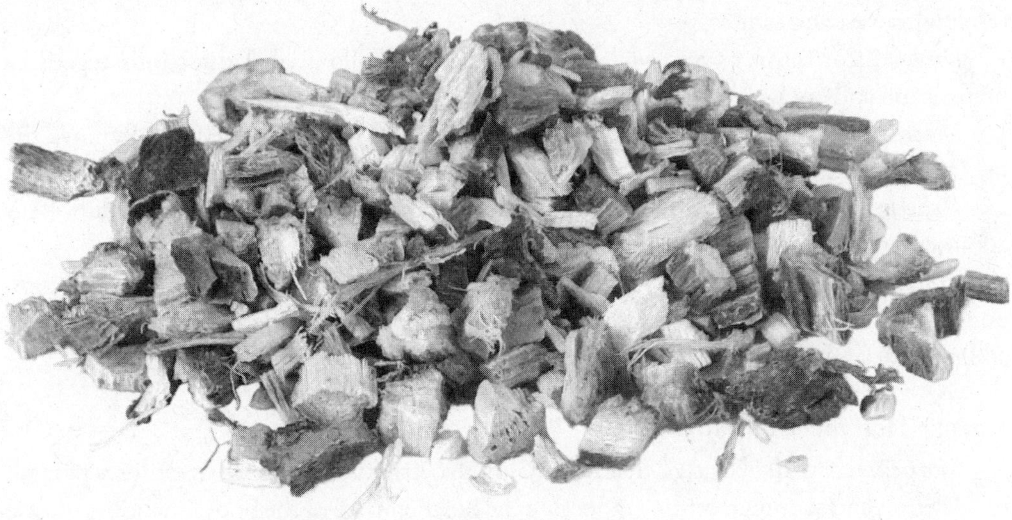

Dried licorice root, *Glycyrrhiza glabra*

licorice for throat problems, making it one of the most widely recognized medicinal herbs in North American Indian lore.[1212] In Ayurvedic medicine, it is used as an expectorant.[1213] The Eclectic School recommended it as an expectorant as well. Some modern over-the-counter cough medicines still use licorice.[1214]

Tradition says that licorice helps loosen sticky phlegm so it's easier to cough up.[1215] It's a demulcent and soothes irritated throats. It is also an antispasmodic. In other words, to say that the tradition is strong is an understatement. We have clear attestation from across continents and centuries for using licorice for upper respiratory problems, but what is the scientific research like? Quite a bit weaker. We know that in test tubes, licorice kills staph and strep bacteria.[1216] It also shows weak antiviral activity[1217] and may have anti-allergic properties.[1218] Though the FDA allows its use in over-the-counter cough medicine, Western medicine has few or no clinical or animal studies to support this use.

Anti-inflammatory. The glycyrrhizin and liquiritin in licorice have steroid-like effects that have an anti-inflammatory and antiarthritic effect.[1219] In Chinese medicine, licorice is thought to diminish excess heat. In Ayurveda, it is used to treat inflamed joints. That's the good news. The bad news is that in order to get this benefit you need to take it orally. That's a problem because licorice's glycyrrhizic acid is the compound with anti-inflammatory properties, and it is the very ingredient that you don't want to ingest too much of.[1220]

How do you use it?

Candy. "Licorice" whips sold in groceries stores as candy generally contain little or no true licorice. Most are made with anise. Be sure to check the label so you know what you're eating.

Sticks. The real thing is sold in juice sticks, a solid version of the extract, or as dried root. Let about a teaspoon of "juice stick" dissolve in an equal amount of water and then mix the result with water or wine.

Drops. Licorice drops are available commercially. Follow label directions regarding preparation and dosage.

Decoction. A strong decoction brings out the best in dried licorice root. Remove the bark and chop the root. Combine the root with cold water at a 1:32 ratio (root to water). Bring the mixture to a boil slowly, boil for ten minutes, cool until warm, and strain. Pour additional water through the root to return the volume to 32.[1221]

Tincture. Do *not* make tinctures of licorice. It tends to bring out the undesirable components as well as the desirable ones. A strong decoction can be made and then preserved by adding 22% (by volume) grain alcohol.[1222]

Dosage: How much do you use?

The problem with licorice is that it contains glycyrrhizin. Long-term use causes potassium deletion and sodium retention, affecting the biochemistry of the body, including muscle function.[1223] Symptoms reported after too much licorice use include swelling, headache, stiffness, and shortness of breath.[1224] One case, in which a man consumed 200 g per day for ten weeks reported extreme sleepiness, high blood pressure, and paralysis.[1225] Another case of chronic use reported kidney failure.[1226] Most herbalists agree that you should not exceed 5–15 g of root, equivalent to 200–600 mg of glycyrrhizin per day. Commission E recommendations are somewhat more conservative, suggesting that you limit intake to no more than 100 mg of glycyrrhizin daily.[1227] The probable effective dosage is probably somewhere between .75 and 4 g, three times a day.[1228] Don't use licorice for more than 4–6 weeks.

Deglycyrrhizinated licorice extract (sometimes called DGL) is also available. Licorice has two classes of bioactive components with known pharmacological effects: glycyrrhizic acid and licorice flavonoids. The glycyrrhizic acid can be removed.[1229] At least one study shows that some therapeutic effects remain.[1230] For DGL extract, use 380 to 1140 mg, three times daily taken by mouth, or follow label directions.[1231]

What should you be aware of before using it?

Licorice is not usually harmful at the levels found in food and candy, though one otherwise healthy individual was hospitalized after eating a pound and a half of licorice in nine days.[1232] If you do choose to take licorice, limit both the amount you use each day and the length of time you take it. Most cases of adverse effects from licorice involve overdoing it. If you get a headache or start feeling lethargic, discontinue use. Too much can lead to severe hypertension (high blood pressure), hypokalemia (low blood potassium levels), fluid retention, and vision problems.

Don't take licorice if you have any of the following: cholestatic liver disorders, liver cirrhosis, hypertonia, hypokalemia, and severe kidney insufficiency[1233]

Don't use it if you are diabetic.[1234] Be cautious when using it in conjunction with herbs known or suspected to affect blood sugar levels. (See Chapter 5 for a list.)

Don't use it if you have high blood pressure, are prone to fluid retention, have rapid heart beats, or any other heart problem.

Theoretically, licorice use may increase the risk of bleeding. If you plan to have surgery, tell your surgeon you have been taking licorice and discontinue use. Be cautious when using it in conjunction with other herbs known or suspected of increasing the risk of bleeding. (See Chapter 5 for a list.)

Don't take it if you are taking a diuretic.[1235]

Don't use it if you are taking digoxin-based drugs,[1236] a corticosteroid such as prednisone,[1237] spironolactone, or a related drug.[1238]

If you are taking birth control pills, talk to your doctor first before taking licorice. Combining the two can increase blood pressure and cause edema.[1239]

Don't take it with warfarin.[1240]

One study showed that licorice lowered serum testosterone levels in healthy men.[1241]

Don't take licorice if you are pregnant. It has been associated with premature birth.[1242]

Marshmallow

Scientific name: *Althaea officinalis*

Also known as althea, kitmi, mallards. *Althaeae folium* is the leaf.

Not surprisingly, marshmallow grows in marshes, bogs, and other low, wet areas. Native to Europe, it now grows both in Europe and in the northeastern parts of the United States. Flowers, leaves, and roots are all used: the flowers for coughs, the leaves for throat irritation and bronchitis, and the roots for wounds and burns.

No, we're obviously not talking about the puffy white things you toast over campfires. Those marshmallows were once made from *Althaea officinalis* but today are made mostly from sugar. True marshmallow may be the oldest herbal medicine we know of. Archeologists excavating a Neanderthal grave site found marshmallow flowers they believe may have been used medicinally.[1243] Hippocrates used it. So did herbalists in medieval Europe and early America.[1244] Pliny said, "Whosoever shall take a spoonful of the Mallows shall that day be free from all diseases that may come to him."[1245] Modern assessments of the plant's usefulness are somewhat less grand.

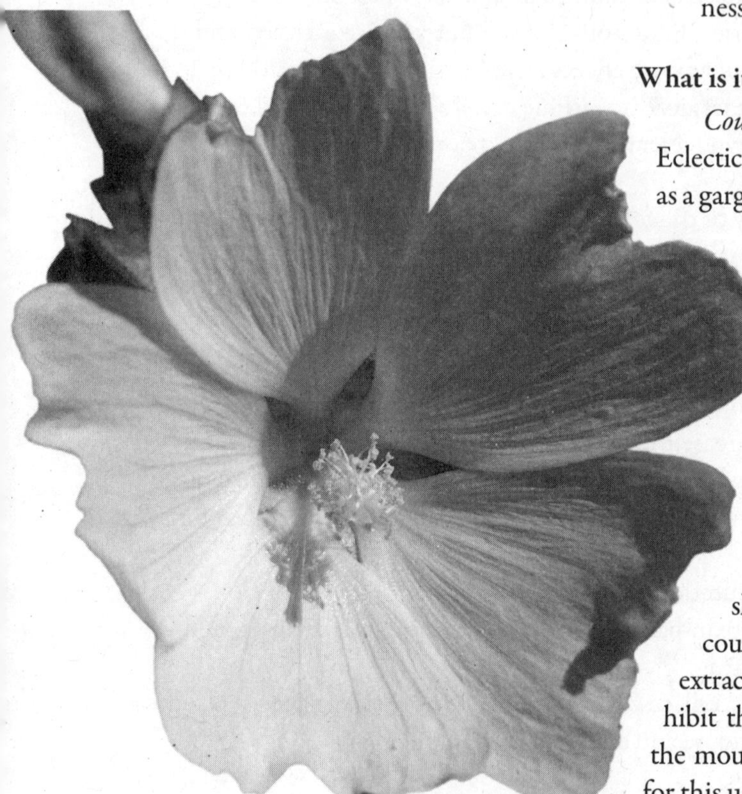

Marshmallow, *Althaea officinalis*
Courtesy of Renata Eder

What is it good for?

Cough, or sore or inflamed throat. The Eclectic School recommended marshmallow as a gargle for a sore throat. Traditionally it was used to soften, soothe, and protect irritated mucous membranes and to break the irritation-cough-irritation-cough cycle. The main benefit of marshmallow comes from the mucilage content. The root contains up to 5–10% mucilage.[1246] The benefit of mucilage to irritated throats is well proven. Beyond that, experiments on cats showed that cats with an induced cough coughed less when fed marshmallow root extract.[1247] In vitro, it has been shown to inhibit the kind of bacteria typically found in the mouth.[1248] Commission E recommends it for this use.[1249] ◊ ◊ ◆ ◆ ◆

Skin irritations. We have traditional attestation for this use. Hippocrates used marshmallow for treating wounds. The Eclectic School also recommended it for skin irritation. It fights some kinds of bacteria in vitro.[1250] It also has antioxidant properties in vitro.[1251] It may even help enhance the ability of white blood cells to fight certain germs.[1252] In a single animal study, tincture of marshmallow helped relieve burns and acid-induced irritation in laboratory mice. These studies, though preliminary, suggest that marshmallow is more than just mucilage.[1253] ◊ ◊ ◊ ◆ ◆

How do you use it?

Decoction. Use 25 g of root to one quart of water. Boil the mixture down until it's reduced to three cups.[1254]

Infusion. Cold infusion brings out the best in marshmallow leaves. Wrap the herb in cheesecloth, pre-moisten it, and suspend it in room-temperature water overnight. Use a 1:32 ratio. Squeeze out the herb in the cheesecloth into the infusion in the morning.[1255] To make a cold infusion of the root, add 2–4 g finely chopped root to a cup of cold water and leave it to infuse overnight. If you want to drink these infusions warm, heat them gently until warm but not hot. Cold infusion helps protect the mucilage in marshmallow, something that's especially desirable if you are using it for an irritated throat. Make sure to make infusions or decoctions of marshmallow as needed because they tend to ferment when stored.[1256]

Poultice. Use a paste of powdered root mixed with water.[1257] For irritated skin, you can use either the poultice or the infusion or decoction on a compress.

Syrup. A syrup for irritated throats can be made using the decoction and honey. (See Chapter 3 for more information.)

Tinctures. Tinctures aren't recommended if you want the mucilage of marshmallow to remain intact.[1258]

Dosage: How much do you use?

Infusions. Make the tea with 1 teaspoon of leaves per cup of water.[1259] Five grams of the leaf can be taken in this way per day.

Decoctions. Six g of root per day.[1260]

Syrup. Ten g (2 teaspoons) of the syrup is a typical dose.[1261]

What should you be aware of before using it?

Marshmallow is generally recognized as being quite safe. We don't have the studies, however, to confirm either safety or danger.

Absorption of other drugs taken simultaneously may be delayed by the mucilage in marshmallow.[1262] Check with your doctor if you are on a prescription drug before taking marshmallow.

Diabetics should look into the sugar concentration of marshmallow before taking it internally. They should also monitor their blood sugar carefully when taking it as it has been known to lower blood sugar levels in animal studies.[1263]

We don't know if marshmallow is safe for children.

Myrrh

Scientific name: *Commiphora molmol*

Also known as *mo yao*, guggal gum, myrrha

Myrrh is the resin from a particular kind of shrub that grows in Arabia and Somalia. It's a pale yellow liquid that oozes from wounds in the bark of the shrub and hardens into globules.

Myrrh is perhaps best known as an incense and embalming ointment. It is burned as part of religious rituals of a number of different religions. Called *mo yao* in Chinese, it has been used for centuries as part of formulas that stop bleeding, heal wounds, and strengthen and heal tendon and ligament injuries. Myrrh contains volatile oil, resins, and gum. The resins are the most likely component to have medicinal value. Myrrh has also been used as a treatment for internal parasites.

What is it good for?

Mouth sores or gingivitis. The 1918 U.S. Dispensatory notes its use for "spongy gums" and mouth sores.[1264] The Eclectic School recommended the diluted tincture as a treatment for bleeding gums and as a gargle after a tonsillectomy. *A Modern Herbal* lists several mouth and throat conditions for which myrrh can be used: canker sores, spongy gums, and ulcerated throat.[1265] It also used to be a common ingredient in tooth powders.[1266] In China, it's still used for mild inflammation of the oral and pharyngeal mucosa, gingivitis, and chapped lips.[1267] As for the research, we know from test-tube studies that it's an anti-inflammatory.[1268] It stimulates white corpuscles, which fight off pathogens. It also has antithrombotic effects (in other words, it keeps blood from clotting).[1269] Animal studies show anti-inflammatory and analgesic properties.[1270] Studies in humans, however, are lacking.

Scars. Anecdote says that myrrh mixed in olive oil helps reduce the appearance of scars when the mixture is rubbed into a wound that has completely healed over. We have no re-

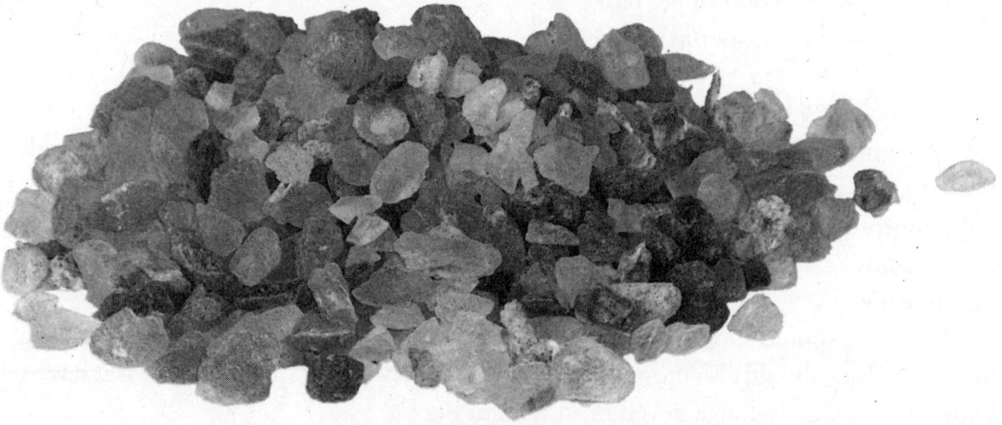

Myrrh, *Commiphora molmol*

search, however, either corroborating this use or shedding light on the safety of using myrrh on recently healed wounds.

How do you use it?

Commercial preparations. A number of commercial preparations using myrrh as an ingredient is available.

Tinctures. If you want to make your own preparations, myrrh can be purchased either as globules of resin or in powdered form. Resins don't dissolve well in water, so infusions and decoctions don't work for myrrh. It can, however, be dissolved in alcohol for a tincture or in oils (1:5). The tincture is used topically.

Wash. A wash for external use can be made by adding a few drops of myrrh tincture to witch hazel.

If you are storing myrrh, make sure you do so in a very dry place, away from light. The powdered form tends to absorb moisture.

Dosage: How much do you use?

Tincture. Dab the affected area 2–3 times daily with undiluted tincture. As a rinse or gargle, you can use 5–10 drops of the tincture in a glass of water.[1271] Rinse and spit.

What should you be aware of before using it?

One study showed that myrrh kills skin cells, while another showed that it protected cells.[1272] The long-term implications (in fact, even the short-term implications) of these studies is unclear. We don't have much in the way of safety studies regarding myrrh. Topical use of myrrh has been going on for centuries with little ill effect. Internal use is another matter, however. We don't know much about the effects of taking myrrh internally either from studies or from the tradition.[1273]

Don't use myrrh if you are pregnant.[1274]

It can cause dermatitis in some people. It's best to see if you tolerate it well before using it on irritated skin.[1275]

Nettles

Scientific name: *Urtica dioica*

Also known as stinging nettle, common nettle, greater nettle

Nettle is a flowering perennial, some would say "weed," that grows in the United States, Canada, and Europe. Anyone with the misfortune to wander through a nettle patch would remember the plant. The bristles on the leaves inject a substance that causes stinging and burning. The leaves and stems are the part of the plant most commonly used, though the roots also have a history of medicinal use.[1276]

One of nettle's most common uses is as a food. The young leaves are rich in vitamin C and are eaten as greens as well as made into wine. Medicinally, the plant has a long use of reducing congestion, controlling coughs, and relieving asthma symptoms.[1277]

What is it good for?

Rheumatic ailments. Considerable anecdotal evidence is available for this use. The Hesquiat used a poultice of steamed nettle leaves on arthritic joints.[1278] The Nitinaht, the Okanagan-Colville, Paiute, Thompson, Chehalis, and Pomo would whip the arthritic parts of the body with raw nettles to relieve symptoms.[1279] Commission E recommends both internal and external nettle use for arthritis and other joint pain. Test-tube studies show some analgesic effect[1280] and anti-inflammatory effect.[1281] A randomized controlled double-blind crossover study of 27 patients with osteoarthritic pain at the base of the thumb or index finger showed stinging nettle leaf had significantly greater benefits than placebo.[1282] How does it work? One hypothesis is that it stimulates circulation while (possibly) cleansing the system of uric acid. Nettle may also function as a counterirritant.

◊ ◊ ◗ ◆ ◆

Improves resistance to allergens (allergic rhinitis). This tradition comes mostly from Europe and North America. *A Modern Herbal* notes that the nettle juice can be used for bronchial and asthmatic

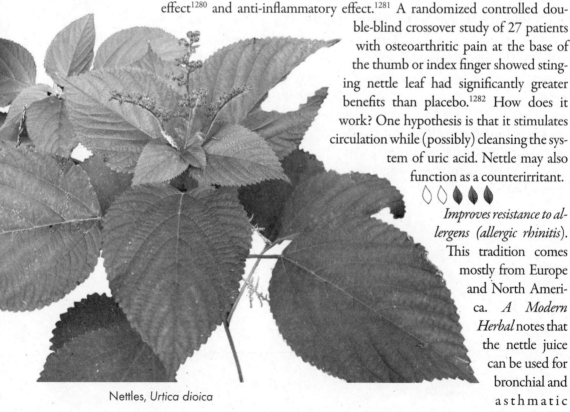

Nettles, *Urtica dioica*

troubles.[1283] The Eclectic School recommended it for excessive mucus discharge. It also has a traditional reputation as a spring tonic. We have a couple of clinical studies to back this use. A randomized, double-blind study looked at the effectiveness of nettles in treating runny nose caused by allergies. The study used 300 mg freeze-dried *Urtica dioica* and found that 58% rated it effective in relieving their symptoms and 48% found it to be equal to or more effective than their previous medicine.[1284] Other studies support this finding.[1285]

Wounds. We have some anecdotal evidence for this use. The Hesquiat rubbed nettles on the body as an analgesic.[1286] The Klallam rubbed an infusion on the body for soreness or stiffness.[1287] The Cahuilla used it for headaches and sore backs.[1288] The Eclectic School used it in rose water for eczema. Topical lotions, poultices, and other preparations have also been used to stop bleeding and heal wounds.[1289] The 1918 U.S. Dispensatory notes one such preparation, sold under the brand name Brandol® for the treatment of burns and wounds.[1290] We have some evidence that an infusion of nettles has antioxidant, antimicrobial, and analgesic properties[1291] But we have no clinical studies to back this use.

How do you use it?

Infusion. Cold infusion brings out the best in nettles. Wrap the herb in cheesecloth, pre-moisten it, and suspend it in tepid water at room temperature, overnight. Use a 1:32 ratio (for example, one ounce of the fresh leaves or a half an ounce of the dried to 32 ounces of water). Squeeze out the herb into the tea in the morning.[1292] If you don't have time for a cold infusion, steep 3–4 teaspoons (4–6 g) of the leaves in a half cup of boiling water.[1293] You can drink the infusion to stimulate circulation and help with arthritis. A compress soaked in the infusion can help with sore arthritic joints.

Capsules. Capsules containing dried leaves are commercially available.

Tincture. A tincture (1:10) can be used as a liniment.

Dosage: How much do you use?

Infusion. 1–2 g as tea, drunk 2–3 times a day[1294]

Capsules. One study found a dose of 300 mg per day of freeze-dried *Urtica dioica* effective for the treatment of allergic rhinitis.[1295] You can, however, take up to two 480 mg capsules two to three times a day.[1296] Don't exceed 8–12 g per day.[1297]

Tincture. ¼–¾ teaspoon of the tincture three times a day[1298]

What should you be aware of before using it?

The FDA has placed nettles on its "herbs of undefined safety" list.[1299]

Some people are allergic to nettles.[1300]

Though historically nettles have been used externally for arthritis pain, using a whip of nettles stalks is not without its risks. At the very least, the whipped site will be highly uncomfortable for a while. At worst, it can cause a severe rash and possible allergic effects.

Nettles taken internally tend to be a diuretic.[1301] If you're taking them internally, drink plenty of water to avoid dehydration.

Too much nettles can result in urticaria, itchy eruptions on the skin. If you start itching while taking nettles orally, discontinue, drink plenty of water, and contact your doctor.[1302]

Too much can cause stomach upset and urine suppression.[1303]

Nettles has been shown to cause uterine contractions in rabbits. Though no reports of miscarriage exist in the literature, pregnant women should avoid taking nettles orally until we know more about their effects.[1304]

Don't use nettles if you have cardiac or renal problems.[1305]

Don't take it if you are taking diclofenac.[1306]

Passionflower

Scientific name: *Passiflora incarnata*

Also known as apricot vine, may pea, maypop, water lemon, wild passionflower, corona de Cristo, granadilla, grenadille, maypops, passiflora, passion vine

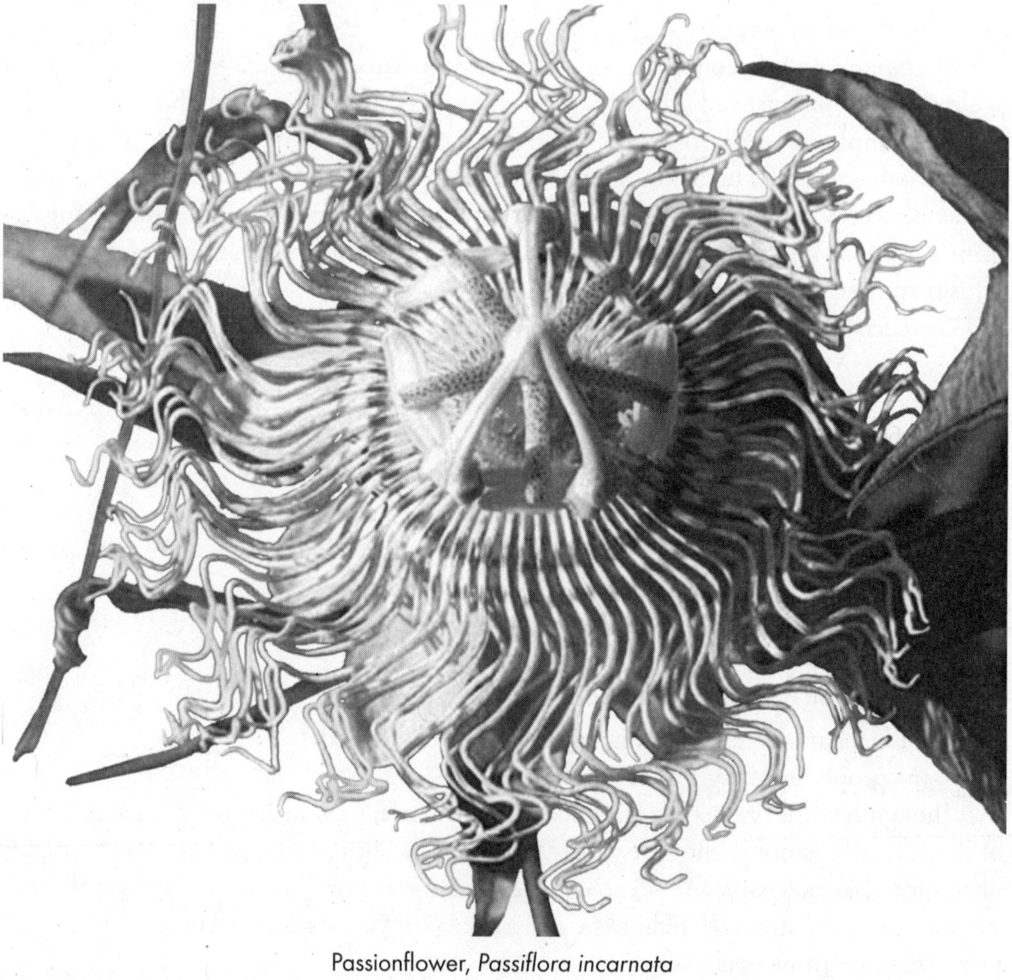

Passionflower, *Passiflora incarnata*

Passionflower is a viny plant with purple flowers. It is native to the southeast part of the United States. The vines, leaves, and flower buds are used medicinally.

Passionflower has a long history as a sedative. You'd think that with a name like "passionflower," it would engender all kinds of emotion and desire. Oddly enough, passionflower is more of a sedative than a stimulant. Unless you're a mouse. Passionflower has aphrodisiac effects in mice. If you're human, however, don't count on it.[1307] The rumors about passionflower's values as an aphrodisiac probably come from the flower's name. The name, though, does not refer to sexual passion but to the passion, or suffering, of Christ. The name was given to the flower by Spanish explorers, who discovered a species of it in Peru and concluded the flowers were symbolic of the Passion, and therefore a sign that God was blessing their enterprise.[1308] It was, perhaps, a use of the flower even more dubious than its use as an aphrodisiac.

What is it good for?

Nervousness, restlessness, and anxiety. We have some traditional evidence that passionflower might benefit nervousness. Tincture has worked in mice as an anti-anxiety medicine.[1309] One human study compared passionflower to oxazepam, a prescription anti-anxiety medicine, and found that it was as effective as the prescription drug for treating anxiety. Though the effect of passionflower was not as rapid, the side effects were less severe.[1310] Commission E recommends it for this use.

Insomnia. *A Modern Herbal* recommends passionflower for insomnia.[1311] The Eclectic School recommended it especially when the insomnia was due to fevers. Fyfe of the Eclectic School suggests it is particularly beneficial for teething children who can't sleep and adults who can't sleep because they've drunk too much "alcoholic stimulants." Passionflower was traditionally thought to slow the pulse, sedate, and deepen sleep. We aren't sure, however, why this is true, or even that it's true. In the nineteenth century, scientists believed that passionflower had narcotic properties.[1312] Modern research has revealed that it's not quite that simple. Passionflower does have low concentrations of chemicals that can slow the nervous system, but it also has some chemicals that are commonly recognized as stimulants.[1313] One theory is that the sedatives overwhelm the stimulants and the net effect is an herb that promotes sleep.[1314] Yet not all studies are unanimous in the opinion that it improves sleep. One animal study saw no benefit to sleep latency or total time of wakefulness (in rats).[1315] Human studies are sparse. In 1978, the FDA banned passionflower from over-the-counter sleep aids because of questions about its safety and effectiveness.[1316] Yet the Herbal PDA notes "no health hazards or side effects. . . with the proper administration of designated therapeutic dosages."

Wounds. The Cherokee used passionflower for boils and to draw out inflammation from brier wounds.[1317] Modern research suggests that it has some antibiotic properties, killing several different kinds of bacteria, yeast, and fungi in the test tube.[1318] In one animal study, it helped with cough due to throat irritation in mice.[1319] A related species, *P. edulis*, has anti-inflammatory properties and speeds wound healing time.[1320] Another, however, showed no benefit in wound healing.[1321]

Nightmares. Fyfe suggests its use for "distressing insomnia," especially when caused by cardiac disturbances. Some herbal sleep aids, valerian in particular, have a reputation for causing nightmares or restless sleep. Combining passionflower with the valerian may help with these problems.[1322] This use is in no way based on scientific research, but it does have some anecdotal evidence behind it.

How do you use it?

Infusion. Make the infusion from dried flowers.[1323] Pour one cup of hot water over a teaspoon of passionflower. Infuse for ten minutes and then strain. A cup, taken like tea in the evening before bed, can help promote sleep. Don't take it more than two or three times per day.

Tincture. Tinctures (1:5 to 1:8, 45% alcohol) are also a possible use for passionflower. If you are taking passionflower to help with anxiety, taking it in tincture form may prove more convenient than the tea. One study suggests that tincture may be more effective than an infusion for the treatment of anxiety.[1324] If you are taking passionflower for anxiety, you may need to take it for several weeks before you begin to feel the effects.[1325]

Capsules. Commercial extracts are also available. Follow the directions on the label.

Dosage: How much do you use?

Infusion. 1–2 g (or 1 teaspoonful) of the dried herb per cup of tea, no more than 2–3 times per day.[1326]

Tincture. If you are using passionflower tincture, use ½–1 teaspoon (or 10–60 drops) up to three time per day.[1327]

Don't exceed 4–8 g of herb per day.[1328]

What should you be aware of before using it?

Passionflower has been used safely for many years. In 1978, the FDA banned passionflower from over-the-counter sleep aids because of questions about its safety and effectiveness.[1329] This decision is not, however, universally accepted. We have very few studies to tell us about the safety of passionflower. Mice injected with extracts suffered no serious harm.[1330] Commission E describes it as a benign herb with no known side effects and no known interactions.[1331] It is not a narcotic and does not have the same addictive potential of many sleep aids.[1332]

Some rare adverse effects—nausea, vomiting, drowsiness, and rapid heartbeat—have been reported.[1333]

Because the herb does contain chemicals that are known to slow down the central nervous system, large doses should be avoided. It may compound the effect of other sedative herbs. (See Chapter 5 for a list.)

Don't use it if you are pregnant or nursing.[1334] Passionflower contains harman and harmaline, which are known to affect the uterus.[1335] Though the medical literature contains no reports of miscarriage, caution is still warranted.[1336]

Don't use it if you are taking antidepressant medication. Be cautious about using passionflower if you are prone to depression.[1337]

Theoretically, passionflower use may increase the risk of bleeding. If you plan to have surgery, tell your surgeon you have been taking passionflower and discontinue use. Be cautious when using it in conjunction with other herbs known or suspected of increasing the risk of bleeding. (See Chapter 5 for a list.)

We don't know for sure if passionflower is safe for children, though it does have some traditional use in treating children.

Note that some species of passionflower (such as *Passiflora caerulea*) contain cyanide and are toxic.[1338] Others like *Passiflora actinia* have been known to cause catalepsy in lab animals.[1339] Check to make sure it is *Passiflora incarnata* that you are getting.

Peppermint Oil

Scientific name: *Mentha piperita*

Also known as brandy mint, lamb mint, black mint, white mint, white peppermint, balm mint, curled mint, Our Lady's mint, pfefferminz, *bo he*. *Oleum Menthæ piperita* is peppermint oil.

Peppermint is a natural hybrid, a cross between spearmint and water mint. Though the leaves and flowers have been used medicinally for centuries, today the more commonly used preparation is essential peppermint oil. Peppermint oil is obtained by steam distillation from freshly harvested, flowering sprigs. Peppermint is native to central and southern Europe. Though it is an introduced species, it grows wild throughout North America.

Mentha, the mint genus, contains at least fifteen species, most of which have been used medicinally. Because of

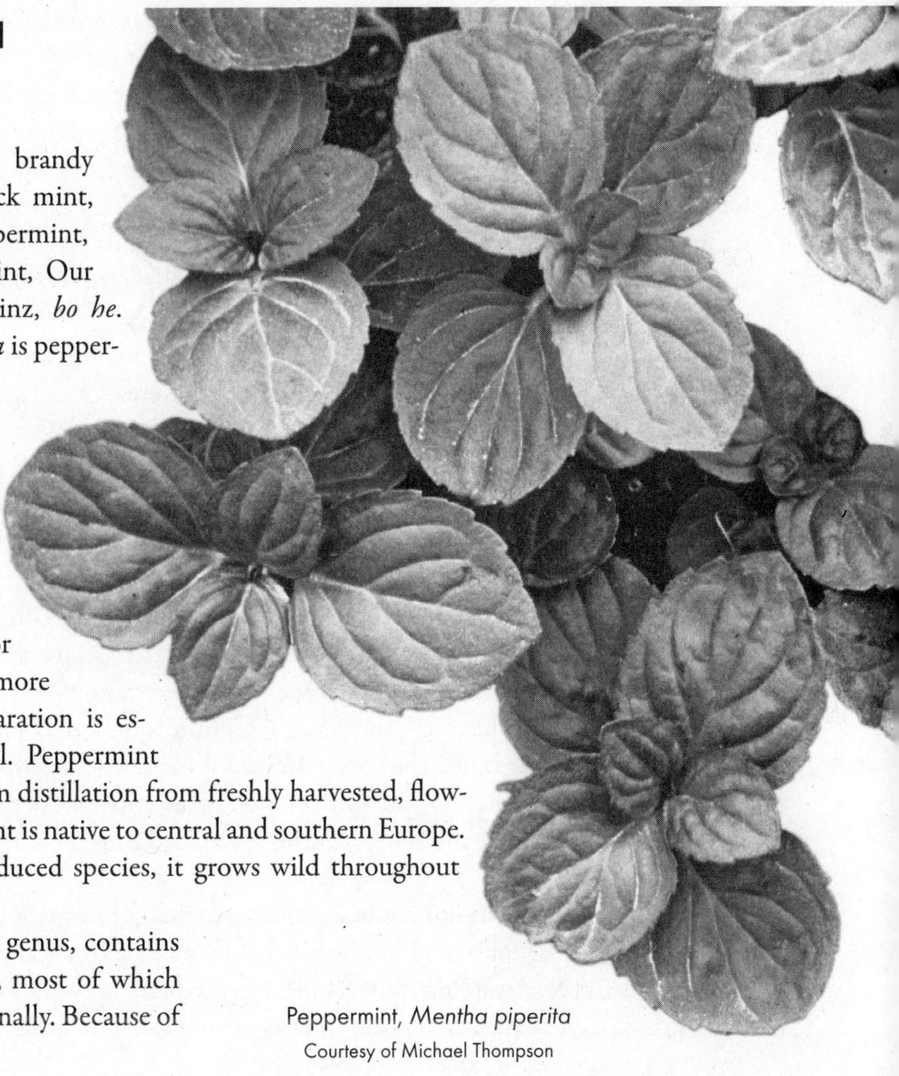

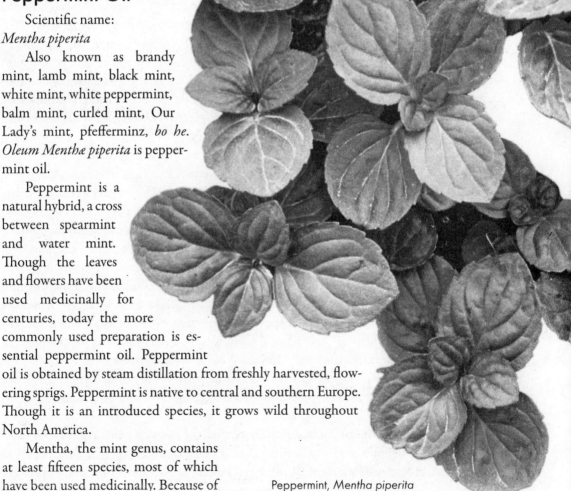

Peppermint, *Mentha piperita*
Courtesy of Michael Thompson

cross-breeding between species, the mint family has hundreds of varieties. We know that peppermint has been used medicinally since the seventeenth century, when it was used in England for "stomach weakness."[1340] Menthol, one of the active ingredients of Tiger Balm®, was first distilled from peppermint oil in the late 1800s. Fifty percent or more of peppermint oil is menthol.[1341] Peppermint has been cultivated commercially since the mid-1700s.[1342] Archeological evidence hints at its use long before that.

What is it good for?

Colds, bronchitis, and cough. In North America, the Cherokee, Iroquois, Flathead, Kutenai, Navajo, Okanagan, Thompson, Carrier, Cree, Gosiute, Paiute, Sanpoil, Shoshoni, Washo, Chehalis, and Cowlitz all used mint as a cold remedy. In Europe it's also used for colds. Even the FDA approves of this use. Peppermint oil and menthol can be found in many over-the-counter cough drops, topical rubs, and nasal decongestants.[1343] In short, this use is very widespread. But does it have any scientific basis? Some. One animal study showed that peppermint inhibits histamine release and runny nose.[1344] Another showed antiviral and other antimicrobial effects.[1345] Clinical trials are, however, lacking.

Neuralgia. Peppermint has been used traditionally for inflammation and itching.[1346] Commission E recommends it for this use. How does it work? The menthol in peppermint oil acts as a counterirritant. Menthol also has mild local anesthetic and antipruritic (anti-itching) properties.[1347] It makes the skin feel as though it has been "cooled." Studies are sparse, but in a single case study of postherpetic neuralgia (nerve pain left over after a case of shingles) peppermint oil was effective.[1348]

Headache. We have traditional evidence from three continents for this use. The Chinese use mint (*bo he*) for headaches.[1349] The Gros Ventre, Keres, Cree, Gosiute, Paiute, Cherokee, and Iroquois all did as well. So did Fyfe of the Eclectic School. We also have a couple clinical studies that show possibilities. One looked at the effect of rubbing peppermint oil in ethanol on the forehead and temples. The results were a significant decrease in headache pain.[1350] Another study found that a mixture of peppermint and eucalyptus decreased the tension of tension headaches but not the pain.[1351]

Myalgia (muscle pain). The efficacy of menthol (one of the components of peppermint oil) as a rubefacient for muscle pain is widely recognized.[1352] The Hoh, Quileute, Kawaiisu, Okanagan-Colville, Cherokee, and Iroquois all used various mints as an analgesic. The Eclectic School used them as rubefacients. Commission E recommends peppermint for muscle pain. We now know that peppermint oil has a mild antispasmodic effect.[1353] The menthol increases circulation and functions as a counterirritant to decrease pain. One study showed that a sport gel containing menthol decreased time away from training in patients with athletic injuries.[1354]

Digestive aid. Peppermint has traditionally be used for stomach pains, nausea, and flatulence. The Eclectic School used it as a treatment for nausea and colic. Fyfe of the Eclectic School notes this use, recommending it for flatulence and diarrhea. We know that it stimulates the liver's production of bile, which helps breaks down fats.[1355] A small-scale study suggests that combined with caraway, peppermint might be useful for reducing heartburn symptoms.[1356] The FDA is not convinced. They no longer allow it to be used for this purpose in nonprescription remedies.[1357] Commission E says it is also helpful in reducing symptoms of irritable bowel.[1358] One preliminary study showed that it reduces bowel spasms.[1359]

Wounds. In vitro peppermint displays antimicrobial properties, killing various bacteria and viruses, including the virus responsible for cold sores.[1360] It has strong free radical scavenging capacity in vitro.[1361] It contains benzoic acid, a vulnerary.[1362] (Vulneraries are substances that promote wound healing.) It also has some antifungal properties[1363] and some analgesic properties were found in animal studies.[1364] It has an anti-inflammatory effect in mice.[1365] The clinical evidence for peppermint promoting healing of wounds in humans, however, is lacking.[1366]

Reaction time and coordination. One study showed that the smell of peppermint improved physical response time.[1367] However, the test used synthetic peppermint odor. Another studied typing with and without the smell of peppermint. This study found that speed, accuracy, and alertness improved in the presence of the peppermint smell.[1368] A study of the effect of peppermint smell on long-distance driving found that the smell increases alertness, reduces fatigue, and lowers drivers' anxiety and frustration.[1369] Yet another suggests that these benefits are not due to some physical change but to psychological factors.[1370]

How do you use it?

Infusion. Pour a half-cup of hot water over a large spoonful of peppermint leaves. Let them infuse for ten minutes, and then strain and drink. Menthol is only lightly soluble in water, so if it's peppermint's counterirritant properties you're looking for, a tincture or the essential oil is a better bet. If you intend to drink the peppermint, however, an infusion is safer than a tincture.

Essential oil. Though tea is one of the most common ways of using peppermint, infusion is unlikely to provide medicinal concentrations of the active ingredients.[1371] The most reliable use of peppermint is commercially prepared peppermint oil, which is produced by steam distillation.

Enteric-coated peppermint oil is available. The coating allows you to minimize the risk of stomach irritation. However, most of the uses for this enteric-coated peppermint—gallstones, irritable bowel, etc.—are serious enough, the effective doses are high enough, and menthol is dangerous enough that you'll want to consult a doctor or naturopath before taking it.

Tincture. Tincture is a good possibility for topical uses as menthol is soluble in alcohol. Alcohol also helps the menthol in peppermint penetrate the skin.[1372] However, the strength of tinctures tends to vary quite a bit.[1373]

Massage. For a liniment, you can use the tincture or you can dissolve the essential oil in grain alcohol. For massage oil, you can dissolve the essential oil in an appropriate carrier oil.

Dosage: How much do you use?

Infusion (for internal use). A typical daily dose of the leaves is 3–6 g, brewed as tea (infused), split between two to three doses.[1374]

Essential oil (for internal use) can be taken in doses of 1–4 drops (.05–.2 milliliters) at a time.[1375] A typical daily dosage of the essential oil is 6–12 drops.

Tincture (for internal use). ¼–½ teaspoon three times a day is a typical dose.

Inhalation. Use 3–4 drops of the essential oil in hot water.

Preparations for external use. In semi-solid and oily preparations (like ointments and massage oils), a 5 to 20% solution (essential oil in a carrier) is a typical concentration [1376] In aqueous-ethanol preparations (like liniments), a 5 to 10% solution is a typical concentration.[1377] In nasal ointments, use no more than 1 to 5% essential oil.[1378] Some herbalists recommend using peppermint externally no more than three or four times daily. We don't have the studies to either support or negate this caution.

What should you be aware of before using it?

Peppermint is on the FDA's list of spices and other natural seasonings and flavorings that are generally recognized as safe. Of course, this applies to the herb and flavorings derived from it. You can damage yourself if you use high doses of peppermint, especially of the essential oil.

Most adults can drink peppermint tea without adverse effects. The amount of menthol in the tea is negligible. Most of the problems with peppermint come when the concentrations of menthol are high as in the essential oil.[1379]

Some people get bronchospasms from peppermint.[1380] Others get stomach upset or acid reflux.[1381]

Some people are allergic to menthol (both internal and external use), getting reactions such as headache, rash, and flushing. If you get any of these symptoms from menthol, don't use peppermint.[1382]

Don't use peppermint internally if you have obstruction of bile ducts, gallbladder inflammation, severe liver damage,[1383] cholecystitis, cholelithiasis, esophageal reflux, hiatal hernia, or hepatic disorders.[1384] If you have gallstones, use peppermint medicinally only after consultation with a physician.[1385]

In animal experiments, peppermint tea inhibits the absorption of iron by the body. Children and people prone to anemic should be cautious about using peppermint tea regularly.[1386]

Preparations containing peppermint oil should not be used on the face, particularly the nose, of infants and small children.[1387] We have reports of infants collapsing after menthol preparations were applied to their noses to treat colds.[1388]

Don't take peppermint oil internally if you are taking nifedipine or a related drug.[1389]

Never take pure menthol internally. As little as a teaspoonful (over 1 g per kilogram of body weight may be deadly) can be fatal.[1390] Never exceed the recommended dose of peppermint oil if you are taking it internally.

Peppers

(see Capsicum)

Rhodiola

Scientific name: *Rhodiola rosea*

Also known as golden root, roseroot, Arctic root

Rhodiola is a plant used in traditional medicine in Eastern Europe and Asia. It is indigenous to the cold mountainous regions of Asia, Europe, and the Arctic. It also grows in the northeastern United States. At least twenty species of rhodiola are used medicinally in various parts of the world, but *Rhodiola rosea* is the most commonly used and studied species in the West.[1391] Until recently only wild varieties were available. As the demand for rhodiola has grown, however, cultivation has begun in Canada, Russia, and other cold climates.

Its species name, *rosea*, comes from the rose-like odor that emanates from the cut root. Rhodiola has been used for centuries in northern latitudes—Sweden, Iceland, Russia. Legend has it that the Vikings used rhodiola to improve endurance and enhance physical strength. The Eskimo also used an infusion of the flowers as a general medicine.[1392] In modern times, the Soviet Union used to give rhodiola to their Olympic athletes, cosmonauts, and soldiers to mitigate stress and increase stamina, and overall well-being. We don't have access to most of the Soviet studies on the herb because the Soviet government considered adaptogen research a state secret. The

Rhodiola rosea

Courtesy of Björgvin Steindórsson

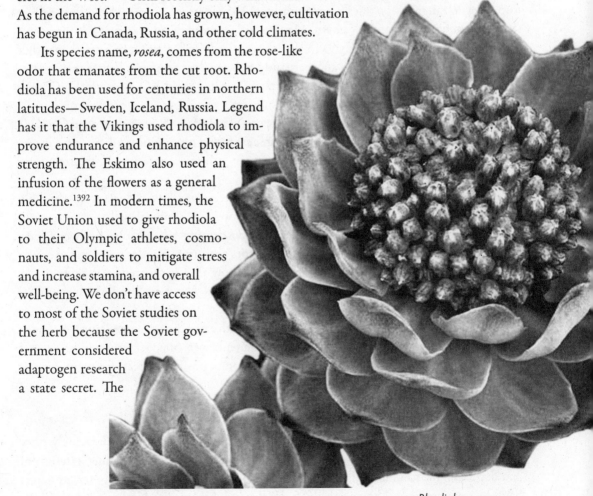

widespread use of artic root by Soviet agencies, however, suggests their researchers found some benefit.

What is it good for?

Endurance. We aren't sure what's going on, but rhodiola does seem to have some ability to protect bodies under stress. Snail larvae incubated in water extracts of *Rhodiola rosea* survived heat shock, oxidative stress, and heavy metal stress significantly better than larvae that had not been pretreated.[1393] Mice given a related species were significantly more likely to survive lethal radiation levels.[1394] This protective function may also have implications for physical endurance. Rats given rhodiola were able to swim 135–159% longer than they could without.[1395]

The adaptogenic properties of *Rhodiola rosea* are presumably due to two compounds found in its roots: p-tyrosol and rhodioloside.[1396] In a study of 161 Russian military institute cadets on night duty, researchers found that the cadets who received rhodiola extract showed significant lowering of physical fatigue as measured by an anti-fatigue index compared to those on placebo. They were also clearer headed after all-night duty than either placebo or control groups.[1397] In another study, a single dose one hour before exercise improved exercise endurance in young healthy people. It improved VO_2peak and VCO_2peak as well as time to exhaustion by 3% when subjects worked out on a cycle ergometer.[1398] However, a third study looked at the influence of a blend of *Cordyceps sinensis* and *Rhodiola rosea* on male cyclists' performance.[1399] Researchers found no significant differences in circulatory dynamics, specifically muscle tissue oxygen saturation between the treated group and the control group.

Mental performance under stress. When rats were given a water-extracted rhodiola preparation, the amount of serotonin in their body increased substantially.[1400] (Serotonin is a neurotransmitter that assists in the proper functioning of emotions, body temperature, and appetite.) In another study, young doctors performing under stress and exhausting conditions were given rhodiola. The results show that it can reduce fatigue under stressful conditions.[1401] The same was true for students who took rhodiola during final exams.[1402]

Improved learning and memory. Experiments with rats point to some improvement in memory with rhodiola use. However, the experiments were small-scale, on animals, and not unequivocal in their conclusions.[1403] It's too soon to posit any effects for people at this time.

How do you use it?

The traditional way to use rhodiola is to make a decoction of the root. Fortunately, since the herb has become trendy, one no longer has to go to the trouble of finding a fresh root and decocting it. A number of commercial formulas are available. One way that rhodiola has been standardized is known as SHR-5. SHR stands for Swedish Herbal Institute. SHR-

5 is a proprietary blend standardized to 3% rosavin and 0.8% salidroside.[1404] The Swedish Herbal Institute is a reputable company to buy from.

Dosage: How much do you use?

The optimal dose has not been determined. One study used 185.0 mg of rhodiola dry extract (standardized to 3% rosavin and 0.8% salidroside) to good effect.[1405] Another used 370 mg for one group and 555 mg for another and did not find much difference in effect between the two.[1406]

Not everyone can handle the stimulant effects of that kind of dose, however. A psychiatrist who uses rhodiola in her practice recommends that most people start on a small dose of 100 mg and increase to a maximum of 400 mg (200 mg 30 minutes before breakfast plus 200 mg 30 minutes before lunch) over a period of 1 to 2 weeks. If you are particularly sensitive to stimulants, you may want to start as low as 50 mg per day.[1407]

For chronic administration, a likely daily dose would be 360–600 mg rhodiola extract standardized for 1% rosavin, 180–300 mg standardized for 2% rosavin, or 100–170 mg standardized for 3.6% rosavin. For a single specific event—a tournament or arduous seminar—you can take up to three times the chronic dose.[1408] If you are taking it before a specific event, one hour seems to be enough time for the effects to take hold. In one study, taking the rhodiola for four weeks prior to an event did not improve performance over the single dose.[1409]

At doses of 1.5–2.0 g and above, rhodiola extract standardized for 2% rosavin may cause irritability and insomnia within several days.[1410]

What should you be aware of before using it?

No significant problems have been reported with rhodiola, but there is still much we don't know about the herb and how it works.

The governments of the former USSR and of Sweden have recognized the safety and efficacy of rhodiola.[1411]

If you experience irritability or insomnia, cut back or discontinue rhodiola use.

We don't know it rhodiola is safe during pregnancy or lactation.

Rosehip Seed Oil

Scientific name: *Rosa affinis rubiginosa*

Also known as *rosa mosqueta* oil

The genus *Rosa* contains more than a hundred different species. The one most commonly used medicinally is *rosa mosqueta*, also known as *Rosa affinis rubiginosa*, which is a wild bush of the rose family. It grows primarily in South America as a garden escapee.

All South American roses are descendents of roses introduced from Europe and North America. At least three other European species (*Rosa moschata*, *R. rubiginosa* [= *eglanteria*] and *R. canina*) are called "*rosa mosqueta*" in South America. To further complicate matters, roses that grow wild in South America have developed at least one new species and probably several new subspecies since introduction. The difference between those new roses and European ones is unclear. Rosehip seed oil from other rose species may have medicinal value as well. *Rosa rubiginosa* and *Rosa canina* are likely candidates for medicinal use, but they have not been studied.

The seeds, when cold pressed, produce an oil with a very high percentage of polyunsaturated fatty acids. Rosehip seed oil is an excellent source of topical trans-retinoic acid (a naturally-occurring form of vitamin A also known as tretinoin). Trans-retinoic acid has been researched repeatedly over many years and has been found useful in the prevention and treatment of scar tissue.

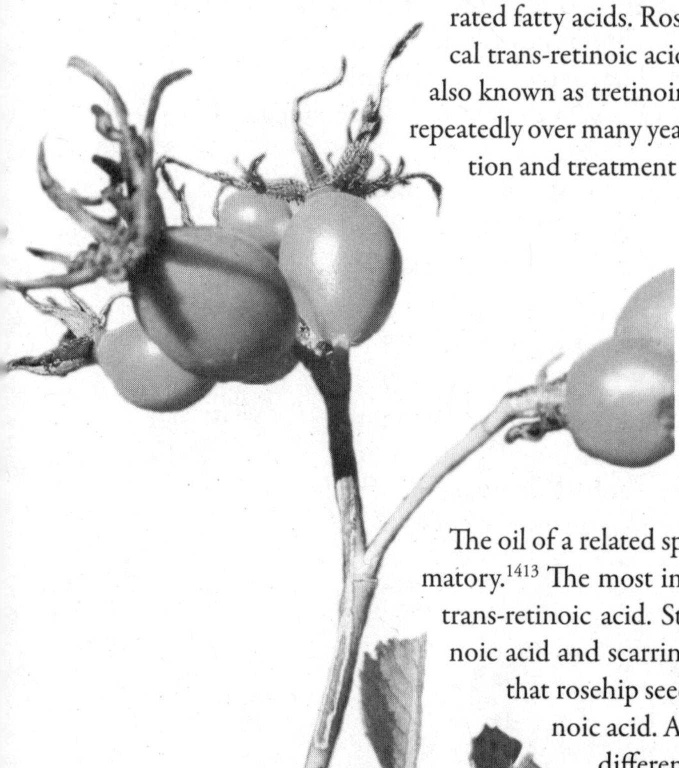

Rosa Mosqueta, *Rosa affinis rubiginosa*
Courtesy of Marcia Martinez Carvajal

What is it good for?

To reduce the appearance of scars. The Costanoan Indians used the California wild rose (*Rosa californica*) on scars, and the Paiute used the woods' rose (*Rosa woodsii* Lindl.) on sores and cuts. *Rosa mosqueta* contains antioxidant substances, a number of different carotenoids.[1412] The oil of a related species, *Rosa canina*, is a proven anti-inflammatory.[1413] The most important component of rosehip seed oil is trans-retinoic acid. Studies have been conducted on trans-retinoic acid and scarring for some time. At least one study shows that rosehip seed oil contains ample amounts of trans-retinoic acid. At least one other study shows none.[1414] The difference in the two studies might be explained by the fact that "*rosa mosqueta*" can refer to three different species. If you can be sure that you are getting a rosehip seed oil that contains trans-retinoic acid, you have something with a long track record for reducing the appearance of scars. In clinical settings, *rosa mosqueta* rosehip seed oil has been tested on post-surgery scars, sun damage scarring, skin ulcers, and acne scars with good results.[1415]

How do you use it?

Getting good quality rosehip seed oil is not a simple matter. Look for the species name, *Rosa affinis rubiginosa* rather than the common name, "*rosa mosqueta*." Buy from a reputable company. If the product is too cheap, be suspicious. Rosehip seed oil take lots of raw material and careful cold pressing to make.

Store the oil in the refrigerator; it goes rancid quickly. The essential oil is used without dilution. After the scab on the wound is gone, apply the oil every morning and evening. Don't use the oil until the scab is completely gone, because the oil can slow healing. Put two or three drops on your finger and massage them into the scar for a minute. The massage helps the oil penetrate the skin and also helps break up the scar tissue.

Dosage: How much do you use?

Use the oil twice a day, spreading just enough to cover the wound.

What should you be aware of before using it?

Rosehip seed oil (from roses of all species) is on the FDA's list of essential oils that are generally recognized as safe.

For external use only. Don't use it on oily skin or on active acne as it will compound the problem.

Note that rosehip seed oil is made from a South American plant, *Rosa affinis rubiginosa*. Rose hips, the fruit of common roses (*Rosa canina*, *Rosa gallica*, *Rosa rugosa*, etc.), are also sometimes used medicinally because of their high vitamin C content. They are not, however, interchangeable with *Rosa affinis rubiginosa*.

Rosemary

Scientific name: *Rosmarinus officinalis*

Also known as compass plant, old man, polar plant, *mi die xiang*, rosamarine

Rosemary is a small evergreen shrub, with long, needle-like leaves. It is native to the Mediterranean region, but because of its use as both a medicinal and culinary herb, it is now grown around the world. It grows wild as a garden escapee in some of the warmer parts of the United States. The above-ground parts are used medicinally. The essential oil is obtained by distillation of the leaves.

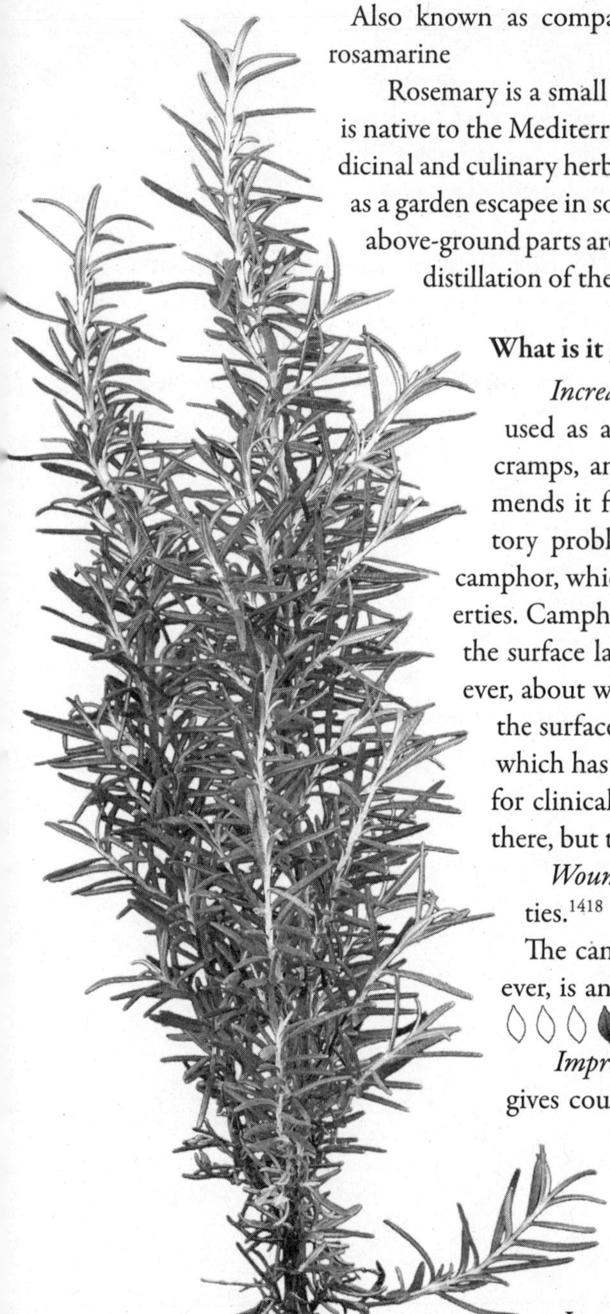

Rosemary, *Rosmarinus officinalis*

What is it good for?

Increased circulation. Rosemary has traditionally been used as a supportive therapy for rheumatic diseases, leg cramps, and circulatory problems. Commission E recommends it for rheumatic pain, bruises, sprains, and circulatory problems like varicose veins.[1416] Rosemary contains camphor, which has proven antispasmodic and analgesic properties. Camphor is also an irritant that increases blood flow to the surface layers of the skin.[1417] The question remains, however, about whether the increased blood flow extends beyond the surface of the skin. Rosemary also contains eucalyptol, which has anesthetic properties and is a counterirritant. As for clinical and animal studies, the potential for benefit is there, but the research isn't.

Wounds. Rosemary has some antimicrobial properties.[1418] The eucalyptol, especially, is an antibacterial. The camphor in the essential oil and in tinctures, however, is an irritant and may be too strong for broken skin.

Improves memory. Folk wisdom says that rosemary gives courage and optimism. Students in ancient Greece used to put sprigs of rosemary in their hair while studying. Two modern studies concur with these ancient customs. One study suggests that the scent of the essential oil produces improvements in cognitive performance and mood.[1419] In another study, the smell of rosemary was pumped into a cubicle where volunteers were given an assessment test. Subjects who had the smell of rosemary in their cubicle were more alert and had a better memory (though not as quick a memory) than controls.[1420] ◊ ◊ ◊ ◆ ◆

Flatulence. This is a traditional use for rosemary tea. Some herbalists maintain that it has a calming effect on the digestive system, especially when the upset is caused by stress. The research evidence for this use is sparse, but preliminary studies show that it might help relax the smooth muscles of the digestive tract.[1421] ◊ ◊ ◊ ◆ ◆

Athlete's foot. Tradition says that rosemary has anti-fungal properties. Studies to back up this assertion are lacking. The eucalyptol it contains is effective against bacteria, but we have no evidence that it destroys fungus. ◊ ◊ ◊ ◊ ◆

Yeast overgrowth in the intestines. Rosemary tea is a treatment recommended by some herbalists. It's not universally recognized by herbalists, and it has no research or testing to back it up. ◊ ◊ ◊ ◊ ◆

Baldness. As a counterirritant, the camphor in rosemary does increase circulation. This use, alas, has no research to back it. ◊ ◊ ◊ ◊ ◆

How do you use it?

Infusion. Infusions (of the above-ground parts) bring out the best in rosemary if you plan to take it internally.[1422] Water dissolves many of the active ingredients but dissolves very little of the camphor and eucalyptol, which are irritants. Use one teaspoon (2 g) of chopped fresh leaves per cup of water.[1423] Pour boiling water on the rosemary and allow to steep covered for 10–15 minutes. Take it hot for rheumatic pain, colds, and headaches. Soak a pad in the infusion and use for sprains or other areas of poor circulation. Alternate 2–3 minutes of hot compress with 2–3 minutes of ice.[1424]

Baths. Conventional wisdom says that a rosemary bath is good for aches and muscle spasms. Add 50 g of herb to a quart of very hot water, let it infuse for 15 minutes, and then add that infusion to a full bath. Or add 10 drops of the essential oil to a bath. The infusion will be more gentle if you have sensitive skin.

Infused oil as a massage oil. Chop the rosemary leaves finely and place them in a glass jar with a tight lid. Cover the plant material with a light extra-virgin olive oil making sure the oil completely covers the plant. Place in a dark, warm place. Infuse for 10 days to 6 weeks, then strain, bottle, and label.

Tincture. 1:5, 50%, 4–6 weeks. Note that alcohol dissolves the camphor in rosemary, so tinctures tend to be more irritating than infusions. If what you want, however, is the irritant properties, tinctures will provide that better than infusions.

Essential oil. The essential oil contains camphor and eucalyptol, both of which can irritate the skin, eyes, mouth, etc. Dilute the essential oil to no more than 10% for external use (less if you have sensitive skin). Be very cautious using the essential oil if you have a history of reaction to eucalyptus, camphor, or pine. Don't use it straight and don't take it internally.

Dosage: How much do you use?

Essential oil. If you want to use the essential oil internally, get professional supervision. Most herbalists suggest that the essential oil be used externally only.[1425]

Infusion. A typical dose is no more than 2 g of the herb as tea, 3–4 times per day.[1426] Some herbalists recommend no more than 6 g of the herb per day.

Tinctures. Tinctures are more irritating that infusions when taken internally. Use no more than ¼–½ teaspoon of the tincture three times a day.

What should you be aware of before using it?

Rosemary is on the FDA's lists, both of essential oils and of spices and other natural seasonings and flavorings that are generally recognized as safe. It is still possible to cause yourself damage if you misuse rosemary, especially the essential oil.

Commission E advises that women not use rosemary in medicinal quantities if they are pregnant.[1427] It has long been recognized as an emmenagogue (menstrual stimulant).

Rosemary contains camphor, which is an irritant. Some people are more sensitive than others. Test it on sensitive skin before using. Keep it away from your eyes and mucous membranes.

The essential oil should not be used internally without professional supervision (and perhaps not even then). Rosemary essential oil has been known to cause seizures when taken internally.[1428] Toxic reactions are possible with large internal dose.[1429]

Rosemary theoretically can lower blood sugar levels. If you are diabetic or have other blood sugar problems, exercise caution when using rosemary in medicinal doses. Be cautious when using it in conjunction with herbs known or suspected to affect blood sugar levels. (See Chapter 5 for a list.)

Sage

Scientific name: *Salvia officinalis*

Also known as broad leaf sage, garden sage, meadow sage, red sage, true sage

Sage grows wild in southern Europe, but can now be found in gardens throughout the temperate zone. It also grows wild as a garden escapee in several U.S. states. The leaves are used medicinally. The root of a related species, *S. miltiorrhiza* is known in China as *dan shen* and is used in cases of blood stagnation. The essential oil is extracted by steam distillation.

What is it good for?

Excess sweating (hyperhidrosis). Traditionally sage was used for colliquative sweats, sweats that led to exhaustion or wasting. In fact, it is best known for limiting any kind of excessive sweating. Several natural products use sage extracts topically—in soaps and lotions—on the theory that they may help sweaty, smelly feet. The Cahuilla Indians used a

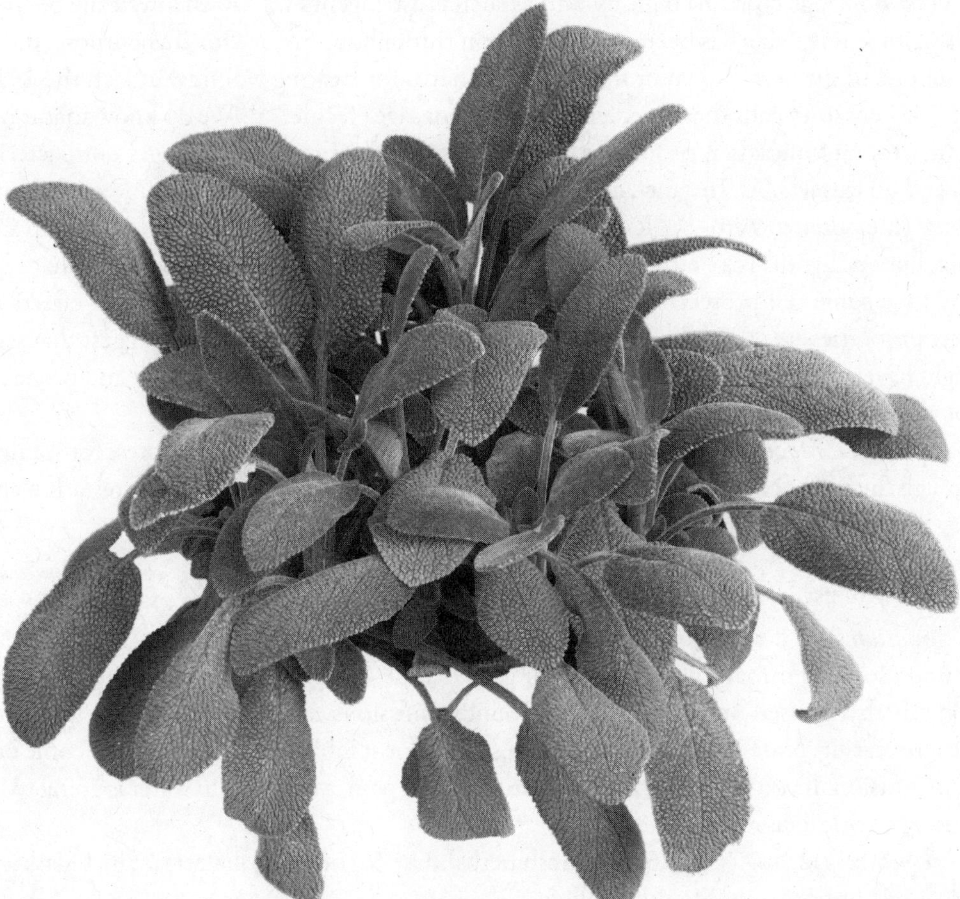

Sage, *Salvia officinalis*

related species for this purpose.[1430] The Eclectic School also recommended it for this purpose. Commission E recommends sage tea (taken internally) for excessive perspiration. As for scientific research, we have only one article. An Italian study shows good results using sage to treat secondary hyperhidrosis (abnormal and excessive perspiration) due to menopause.[1431]

Sore throat. In the early twentieth century, sage gargles were a common medical treatment for sore throats.[1432] The Eclectic School used it for this purpose. The Cherokee used it as a cold remedy.[1433] The Paiute Indians used a related species for colds and coughs.[1434] Sage tea can be used as either a mouthwash or gargle, and Commission E recommends it for inflammations of the mucous membranes of nose and throat. Sage contains tannins, which act as an astringent and increase blood flow to the area.[1435] Sage also contains compounds that fight some kinds of bacteria, including *Staphylococcus aureus*, a common bacteria implicated in pneumonia, abscesses, and septicemia.[1436] We don't, however, have any clinical studies to attest to its effectiveness.

Wounds. Sage contains tannins, and as such is astringent and can theoretically be used to stop bleeding. Sage has been used off and on throughout history for this purpose, but it is not one of the best-known or most effective herbs for treating wounds. In fact, the 1918 U.S. Dispensatory calls these medicinal qualities of sage "feeble."[1437] We do know that it has some weak antimicrobial properties, with the essential oil having a stronger antibacterial effect than extracts.[1438] The ancient Greeks used it to preserve meat. It has some antioxidant effects (measured in vitro).[1439] It contains some eucalyptol, which reduces inflammation and pain, but eucalyptus is a better source of this compound. An in vitro study shows that sage may have some cell-protective properties, but it is not clear what the practical effects of these properties are.[1440] In short, both traditional use and modern research suggest that sage might have some modest benefit for treating wounds, but that benefit is slight and probably not worth the risk of wound contamination.

Sprains. *A Modern Herbal* suggests sage boiled in vinegar used as a compress for sprains. Though the presence of eucalyptol might support this use, it has no scientific attestation and very little traditional support.

How do you use it?

Infusion. Use 2 teaspoons (5 g) per cup of water to make an infusion.[1441] Use a weak infusion for sore throats, mouth ulcers or gum disease. Gargle, or rinse and spit. The infusion can also be used on a compress for wounds. Infusions can also be taken internally for excess sweating. Note that the eucalyptol in sage is not soluble in water and won't come out in an infusion. If you're using it for inflammation and pain, a infusion in water is going to be missing a critical ingredient.

Tincture. 1:2, 40–76% (76% for fresh herbs). Use 5 g of alcoholic extract in 1 glass water. Gargle or rinse only. Do not swallow.

Honey. For a sore throat or painful cough, mix 50 g of the powdered herb with 80 g of honey and take as a syrup.

Essential oil. Don't take essential oil of sage internally. When making preparations using the essential oil, follow safe handling practices: keep it away from foodstuffs, be careful that anything that may have a residue on it (pots, strainers, spoons, etc.) doesn't come in contact with food. Label all preparations as "external use only." Better yet, get professional advice if you want to use sage oil. It's potentially very dangerous.

Capsules. .25 g, three times per day before meals can be taken for excessive perspiration. Note that sage can lose as much as a quarter of its essential oil through improper drying. Powdered sage begins to deteriorate in as little as 24 hours. Don't store dried sage for more than 18 months. Use powdered sage immediately after grinding it.

Dosage: How much do you use?

Infusions (for internal use). 4–6 g of herb per day as tea in divided doses[1442] More than 15 g of the herb per day can be dangerous.

Tincture. 2.5–7.5 g of tincture per day in divided doses.[1443] Note that thujone is more soluble in alcohol than it is in water, making sage tincture less safe for internal use than water-based sage preparations.

What should you be aware of before using it?

The Food and Drug Administration lists sage used as a seasoning as a "substance generally recognized as safe." That judgment, however, does not apply to sage used in medicinal doses or to the essential oil of sage.

Do not take sage essential oil internally. It is toxic and can cause seizures, mental and physical deterioration, and coma.[1444]

Be cautious when using sage in medicinal doses.[1445] Sage contains thujone, which is toxic. Thujone dissipates with heat, so cooking with culinary amounts of sage is generally recognized as safe. Moreover, the levels of thujone vary with the preparation. Consult a trained herbalist or naturopath if you wish to use the essential oil, if you plan to use medicinal doses or preparations of sage internally, or if you plan to use it for an extended period of time.

Topical sage seems to be fairly well tolerated.[1446]

S. miltiorrhiza root (the "sage" used in Chinese medicine) is not interchangeable with the *S. officinalis* leaves referred to here.

Don't use sage medicinally when pregnant.[1447] It may have estrogen-like effects.[1448]

Don't use sage if you are epileptic. The thujone in sage can trigger seizures in epileptics.[1449] Sage may also decrease the effects of seizure medications.[1450]

Theoretically sage could make you drowsy. It may also compound the effect of other sedative herbs. (See Chapter 5 for a list.)

Shepherd's Purse

Scientific name: *Capsella bursa pastoris*

Also known as capsella, mother's heart, shovel weed, pick pocket, caseweed, rattle pouches

Shepherd's purse is a weed. It's an annual, very hardy, very invasive, very nasty smelling. Originally found in parts of Europe, it was introduced to North America by early settlers and has since spread throughout North America and other temperate parts of the world where it is typically unwelcome.[1451] The above-ground parts are used medicinally.

Most of the names for shepherd's purse refer to the seedpods, which resemble small heart-shaped purses. The plant is in the cabbage family. It contains an oil that is very similar to mustard oil, which accounts for part of the smell.[1452] Historically, it was used to prevent scurvy,[1453] but it is best known as an agent to stop bleeding, even hemorrhages. In World War I, soldiers used it when other antibleeding agents ran out.[1454]

What is it good for?

Wounds. The anecdotal attestation for this use is strong. *A Modern Herbal* cites use in Europe as far back as the seventeenth century.[1455] In North America, the Menominee used it as a wash for poison ivy.[1456] Fyfe of the Eclectic School recommended it for hemorrhoids. It's mainly based on this traditional use that Commission E recommends topical shepherd's purse for superficial, bleeding skin injuries and for nose bleeds. The scientific basis for this recommendation is, however, quite weak.[1457] Test-tube studies show a weak antibacterial effect.[1458] Some of the active ingredients, when isolated from the rest of the plant, show more promise as antibiotics.[1459] Clinical studies and animal studies are virtually nonexistent.

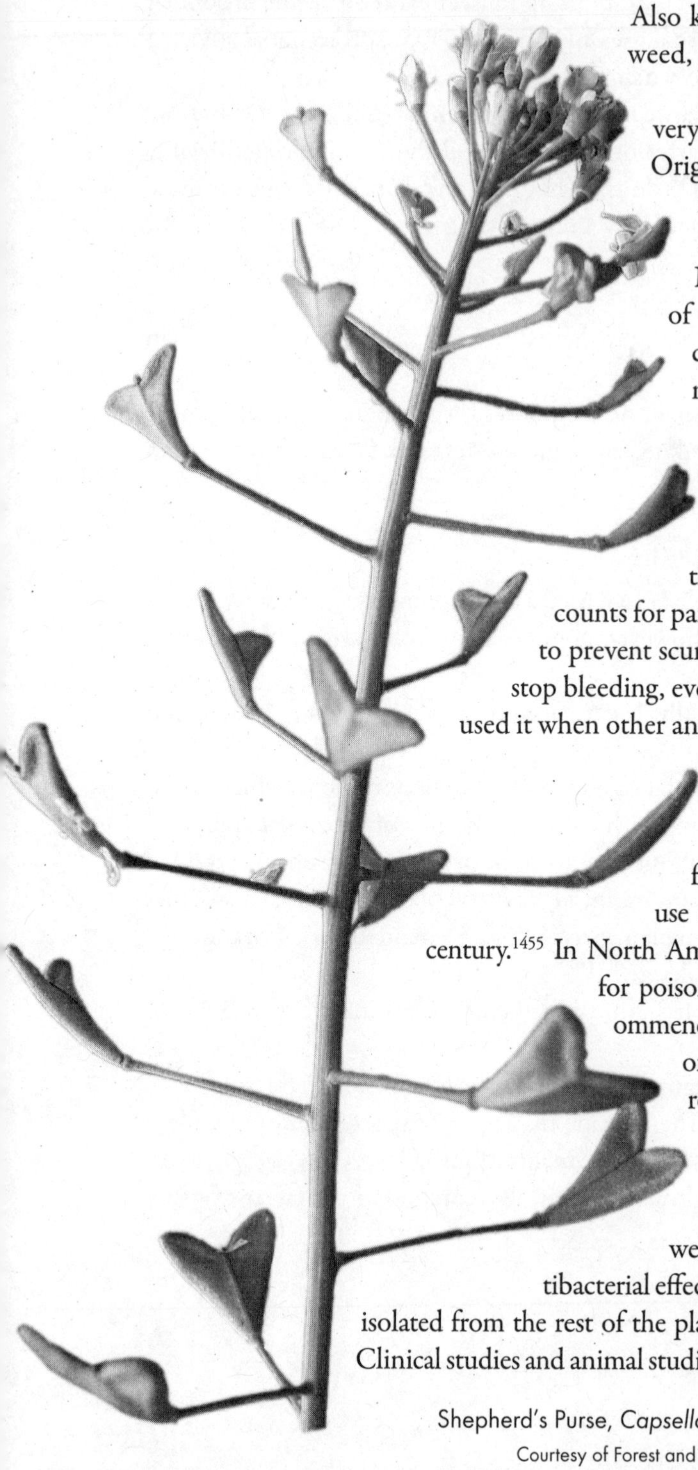

Shepherd's Purse, *Capsella bursa pastoris*

Courtesy of Forest and Kim Starr

How do you use it?

Internal use. We have no good evidence that it does any good when taken internally. We also have no safety studies regarding internal use. The active ingredients tend to break down quickly in the stomach.[1460] All that and the nasty taste of shepherd's purse suggest it's best used externally.

Infusion. The best way to use shepherd's purse is as an infusion, or, if you can get it, as juice expressed from a fresh plant. The active ingredients tend to degrade with storage, so don't buy or store shepherd's purse in bulk.[1461] Be careful, too, of the quality of your shepherd's purse. It's often contaminated by various fungi, who find it a likely host. Some of these fungi can have toxic properties. Find a reliable source of the above-ground parts. Make a standard infusion of them, and apply the infusion on a compress.

Dosage: How much do you use?

Infusion. For an infusion use 3–5 g of the herb per ¾ cup of water.[1462] The infusion can be used on a compress. Avoid using it internally.

What should you be aware of before using it?

People have been using shepherd's purse for centuries. If it has harmful effects, those effects haven't worked their way into the medical literature. Mouse studies show a low toxicity level.[1463] However, human studies are sparse.

One of the greatest dangers of using shepherd's purse is that it can cause people to delay appropriate medical attention. If you have any wound, injury, or other condition that won't stop bleeding, you need to see a doctor.

It's very easy to introduce microbes into the body through broken skin. You can infect a wound using an herbal remedy, and infected wounds can kill you. Before using shepherd's purse on open skin, consider carefully the risks and what you hope to gain using this herb rather than, say, direct pressure and an antibiotic.

If taken internally, even in low doses, it can cause high blood pressure and heart palpitations.[1464] At high doses, it may lower blood pressure to dangerous levels. Be cautious when using it in conjunction with other herbs known to affect blood pressure. (See Chapter 5 for a list.)

Avoid shepherd's purse if you are pregnant.[1465]

Avoid if you have heart arrhythmia, high blood pressure, renal stones, or thyroid disorders.[1466]

It may increase the effects of cardiovascular medications or antihypertensive drugs.[1467]

Siberian Ginseng

(see Eleuthero Root)

Slippery Elm

Scientific name: *Ulmus rubra, Ulmus fulva*

Also known as American elm, Indian elm, moose elm, sweet elm, red elm, soft elm

Slippery elm is a tree indigenous to the forests of eastern North America. A large tree, it can reach twenty inches in diameter and sixty feet in height. The inner layer of the bark is dried and used medicinally. A related species, *Ulmus davidiana*, has been more extensively studied for its anti-inflammatory properties.

Slippery elm is typically thought of as a cooling soothing herb. It's been used for inflammation and irritation. The Ojibwa prepared a tea from slippery elm and *Arctium lappa*, *Rumex acetosella*, and *Rheum officinale*. Called Essiac by the Canadian nurse that brought it into the Anglo world, this combination has been proclaimed by some to be an immune support and general tonic. Until the 1960s, slippery elm was listed in the *U.S. Pharmacopoeia* and the *National Formulary*.[1468] Slippery elms still grow in the United States because it is less susceptible to Dutch elm than most trees of its genus. If you do want to harvest slippery elm bark yourself, learn the technique from someone with experience. Girdling the tree will kill it. Also be aware that harvesting slippery elm on public lands is illegal and can result in a fine.[1469]

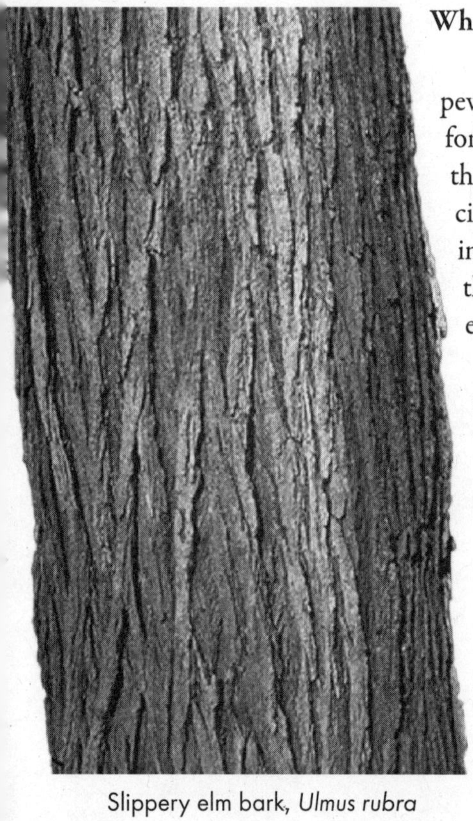

Slippery elm bark, *Ulmus rubra*
Courtesy of Ohio Department of Natural Resources

What is it good for?

Bronchitis or cough. The Cherokee used it for colds.[1470] Chippewas used it for sore throats.[1471] The Iroquois chewed raw bark for sore throats.[1472] Mohegans used it for coughs and sore throats.[1473] The main medicinal ingredient of slippery elm is mucilage. When mixed with water, it creates a coating that soothes inflamed mucous membranes. The FDA has approved it for this use, and slippery elm can be found in cough and cold lozenges.[1474] ◊ ◆ ◆ ◆ ◆

Wound healing (topical). The Cherokee used a poultice of the inside bark for old sores and wounds.[1475] The Menomini used a poultice to draw pus from a wound.[1476] The Meskwaki used it for old sores.[1477] Ojibwa Indians used an infusion of the roots for bleeding cuts.[1478] Slippery elm contains small amounts of tannins, which have an astringent property.[1479] Its main use is as an emollient due to the high mucilage content.[1480] Before the advent of modern "liquid bandages," slippery elm served much the same purpose. The mucilage in slippery elm dries over wounds to create a protective coating.[1481] ◊ ◊ ◊ ◆ ◆

Joint and bone disorders. We have some limited tradition for using slippery elm for bone and joint disorders.

The Mahuna Indians applied a poultice of the bark to fractured arms and legs.[1482] *A Modern Herbal* suggests slippery elm, bran, and vinegar for a poultice for rheumatism.[1483] However, the tannins and mucilage in slippery elm are the only components with any known medicinal properties. Furthermore, we have no experimental attestation for this use. From what we know about the herb, it seems unlikely to be of help for either arthritis or fractures. ◊◊◊◊◊◆

Minor burns. Traditionally, slippery elm was used for burns in Europe. Some modern herbalists suggest that its cooling properties can be used specifically for sunburn. The "liquid bandage" properties may help some with burns, but that's just conjecture. This use has virtually no scientific attestation. ◊◊◊◊◆

How do you use it?

Decoction. A tea for bronchitis is made by simmering 1–3 teaspoons of powdered bark per cup of water for ten minutes.[1484] For a larger batch to use topically, use 1 part of the powdered bark to 8 parts water. Bring the mixture to a boil and then lower the heat and simmer for 10–15 minutes.

Cold infusion. The Eclectic School recommended cold infusion to protect the mucilage. To make a cold infusion tie together shredded bark and suspend it in a vat of ice water overnight.

Compress. The decoction or infusion can be applied topically using a compress to wounds and burns.

Poultice. Poultice is a traditional use of slippery elm. In fact, slippery elm is one of the herbs that works particularly well as a poultice. A poultice is made by mixing the powdered bark with enough boiling water to make a paste. Cool it before using.

Commercial lozenges are available for bronchitis.

Tinctures do not work well for extracting slippery elm's mucilage.[1485]

Dosage: How much do you use?

You can use 4 g of the herb as tea (decoction) three times per day or 1 teaspoon liquid extract three times per day[1486]

What should you be aware of before using it?

Slippery elm has a good track record when it comes to safety.

Don't use it if you are pregnant. Spontaneous abortions have been reported.[1487] Reports of women using slippery elm bark to induce abortion also contain stories of severe, uncontrollable, and sometimes fatal bleeding.[1488]

Some people are allergic to slippery elm.[1489] Contact dermatitis is the most common symptom of this allergy.[1490]

Internal use of slippery elm may slow the absorption of other drugs.[1491]

A related species has some influence on the blood sugar levels of rats. Granted, that's not much evidence that slippery elm will affect your blood sugar, but if you're diabetic and use slippery elm internally, you might want to keep a closer eye on your numbers while you're doing so.

The California slippery elm is a different tree. Though its bark is reputed to have similar properties, it is not the elm covered here and may or may not work for these uses.[1492]

St. John's Wort

Scientific name: *Hypericum perforatum*

Also known as *Hypericum vulgare*, amber touch-and-heal, rosin rose, klamath weed, goatweed, hypericum

Hypericum is a large genus with roughly 400 species within it. Most are called "St. John's wort." The species most often used medicinally is *Hypericum perforatum*, usually called "common St. John's wort." A shrubby perennial, St. John's wort is indigenous to Europe. Today it grows throughout North America and Australia, where it is often considered a noxious weed. The above-ground parts are used medicinally. The leaves contain glands that produce volatile oils and resins.[1493] Just the flowers are used to make St. John's wort oil. Though the flowers are yellow, the infused oil turns a beautiful red. Little black dots on the margins of the petals contain hypericin, which is both the red pigment and one of the biologically active compounds of the plant.[1494]

It was used in traditional Greek medicine. We know that Hippocrates, Theophrastus, and Galen all used it.[1495] It's said that the name "St. John's wort" comes from the Knights of St. John of Jerusalem, crusaders who used the herb to treat wounds on the battlefield. In the Middle Ages, it was ascribed near magical powers, repelling not just disease but also evil spirits.[1496] In fact the scientific name *Hypericum* comes from the Greek for "over an apparition" and refers to its supposed power to make them go away.[1497]St. John's wort came to be used to treat mental disorders and "nerves" in fifteenth century Europe.[1498]

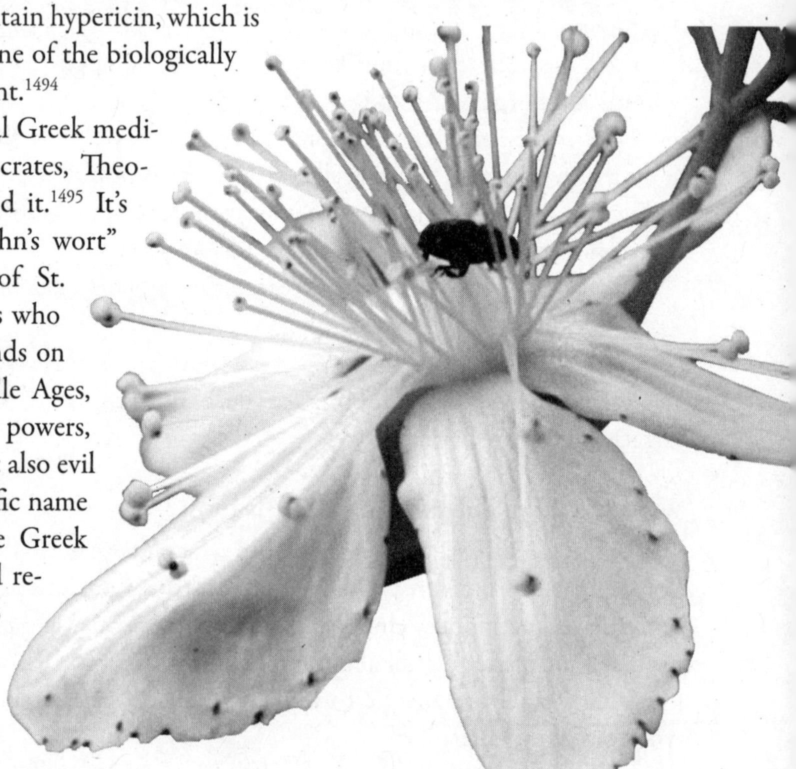

St. John's wort, *Hypericum perforatum*
Courtesy of Stanislav Doronenko

What is it good for?

Depressive moods (mild), anxiety and/or nervous unrest. The use of St. John's wort for mild depression has very strong evidence behind it. Not only has it been used for this purpose for literally millennia, it has support from in vitro studies, animal studies, and numerous studies in humans, both pharmacokinetic and clinical studies.[1499] From all of these studies, here's what we know: The use of St. John's wort for depression is more strongly attested to than the use for anxiety. Its use in lifting situational depression is more strongly attested to than its use in treating true melancholia (clinical depression). The stronger the depression, the less likely St. John's wort is to work.[1500] One study showed St. John's wort to be slightly superior to Paxil® (a prescription antidepressant) in treating moderate to severe depression.[1501] Another recent study that compared St. John's wort to Zoloft® (another prescription anti-depressant) and placebo for the treatment of major depression showed St. John's wort to be no better than the placebo in relieving symptoms of depression. On the other hand, it also showed Zoloft to be no better than placebo either.[1502] On the whole, though, we have good evidence to show the benefit in treating mild to moderate depression with St. John's wort.[1503] If your depression is accompanied by suicidal thoughts, or if it is causing you to become unable to deal with the day-to-day responsibilities of your life, you need to talk with a doctor (either mainstream or preferably a doctor of Chinese medicine) about whether you need something stronger than St. John's wort.

Injuries with nerve involvement. A lesser known use of St. John's wort is as a treatment of injuries, especially those with nerve involvement. This use is an ancient one, dating back to ancient Greek times.[1504] Commission E recommends oily hypericum preparations for treatment and post-therapy of acute and contused injuries, myalgia, and first-degree burns. One study showed that St. John's wort reduces inflammation in cases of neurodermatitis.[1505]

Wounds. The 1918 U.S. Dispensatory mentions the high regard St. John's wort has had throughout the ages as a healer of wounds. Taken both internally and externally, it has been one of the most common wound treatments for centuries.[1506] The Cherokee rubbed the sap on sores.[1507] The Miwok used a related species to make a wash for running sores.[1508] St. John's wort contains tannins that can help dry oozing sores.[1509] In Europe, it was used for black-and-blue marks. The Eclectic School recommends it for puncture wounds, especially those with considerable pain, as well as bruises, contusion, sprains, and swellings. This strong tradition has some scientific backing. Test-tube studies show that it has antimicrobial properties, and fights staph and certain viruses.[1510] Two related species (*Hypericum hookerianum* and *Hypericum patulum*) have been shown to have wound healing properties in rats.[1511] St. John's wort cream has been shown to be effective in treating dermatitis.[1512]

How do you use it?

Infused oil. Infused oil is made by putting fresh flowers in cold pressed safflower, olive, walnut or sunflower oil and letting it sit for a few weeks. (Herbalists disagree about whether the oil should sit in the sun or not. You might try it both ways. If the oil turns red and does not mold, you may consider it a success.) The oil is used for inflammations and is the most common way St. John's wort is used externally.

Infusions. Infusions (in water) is used for anxiety, irritability, and upsets. Make the infusion by pouring one cup of boiling water over the flowers (2–4 g works out to about 1–2 heaping teaspoons). Allow the infusion to steep for about ten minutes, then strain.[1513] St. John's wort tea doesn't have as good a track record for treating mood disorders as commercial St. John's wort preparations, perhaps due to inconsistent quality of the herb available, possibly due to something in the infusion process that we don't yet know about.[1514] The infusion can also be used for wounds, sores, and bruises, though it is not as well recognized as the oily preparations.

Tinctures are possible. (1:10 in 45% alcohol)

Commercial preparations. These are widely available. Standardization by a single component (such as hypericin) are somewhat less useful for St. John's wort than other herbs because research shows that several compounds work together to produce the medicinal effects.[1515] However, standardization does typically reflect a certain level of quality. Two common standardizations are for hyperforin and hypericin. If you are using it to treat depression or anxiety, buy your St. John's wort from a reputable company, one that produces "pharmaceutical grade" preparations. The commonly prescribed German brand is Jarsin®. Another widely studied preparation is LI-160®, manufactured by Lichtwer Pharma, AG in Berlin. If you don't notice an improvement in 4–6 weeks, you may need to try another option.

Dosage: How much do you use?

Dried herb. Take 2–4 g of dried herb or .2 to 1.0 mg of total hypericin daily.[1516]

Commercial preparations: Take commercial preparations according to label directions. More is not better. High doses don't work any better, and they can cause unpleasant, and sometimes dangerous, side effects. Your best bet is to find a reputable brand and to follow label directions. You will need to take the herb for at least 4–6 weeks to begin to notice the effect.[1517]

Tincture. ½–1 teaspoon (1:10 in 45% alcohol) three times daily.[1518]

What should you be aware of before using it?

Short-term side effects of St. John's wort seem to be mild and rare. They include restlessness, mild allergic reactions, and stomach upset.[1519] In general, the side effects for St. John's wort are less than those for prescription antidepressants.[1520]

In large doses, it causes photosensitivity if you take it internally. Be especially careful to avoid the sun if you are light-skinned or are also taking omeprazole or another proton pump inhibitor.[1521] Also be careful using it in conjunction with cosmetics that increase sun sensitivity (such as alpha-hydroxy acids and certain acne treatments).

Research has shown that St. John's wort has possible adverse reactions with the following drugs: immunosuppressants, digoxin, SSRI antidepressants, phenprocoumon or other drugs in the warfarin family, theophylline and related drugs, cyclosporin, and indinavir. Check with your doctor if you are taking any of these drugs and want to use St. John's wort.

Don't take it with drugs or herbs that have monoamine oxidase inhibitor (MAOI) activity or that interact with MAOI drugs. Headache, tremors, mania, and insomnia may occur.[1522] (See Chapter 5 for a list.)

Check with your doctor if you are taking hormone supplements and want to take St. John's wort.[1523]

If you have thyroid problems, check with your doctor before using St. John's wort. It has been associated with an elevation in thyroid-stimulating hormone (TSH) levels.[1524]

St. John's wort may affect a metabolic pathway used by various AIDS, heart disease, depression, seizure, cancer, and anti-rejection drugs.[1525] If you are taking any of these drugs, check with your doctor about potential drug interactions.

St. John's wort can cause some medications to be excreted from your body more quickly than they otherwise would be. It may even interact with oral contraceptives. The most prudent course of action is to check with your doctor before taking St. John's wort if you are taking any prescription medication.[1526]

We are still not sure what the side effects of taking St. John's wort over long periods of time are. If you want to take it for more than a few months, check with your doctor.

Tea Tree Oil

Scientific name: *Melaleuca alternifolia*

Also known as cajeput oil, Australian tea tree oil, narrowleaf paperbark oil

It has nothing to do with the tea you drink. The oil is an essential oil, distilled from the leaves of a small tree or shrub native to only the northeast coastal region of New South Wales, Australia. The meleuca plant is now cultivated in Florida, Louisiana, and Hawaii.

Tea tree oil is an antiseptic, one of the strongest in the plant world. Its use in Australia goes back many centuries. News of its value spread to Europe with Captain John Cook, who reported its value in healing cuts and burns.[1527] In World War II, Australian soldiers used tea tree oil as a disinfectant.[1528]

What is it good for?

Antiseptic. In test-tube studies, tea tree oil has shown itself to be a powerful antimicrobial.[1529] In vitro, it kills transient flora while maintaining resident flora.[1530] (In other words, it spares the microbes that are supposed to be in and on your body while killing invaders.) One study found that adding tea tree oil is more effective than soap alone in reducing the kinds of infections found in hospital contexts.[1531] ◊ ◊ ◆ ◆ ◆

Toenail fungus. One study used 5% tea tree oil with 2% butenafine hydrochloride (sold over the counter as Lotrimin®) in a cream. After 16 weeks, 80% of the patients were cured as opposed to none of the placebo group. It is not clear, however, how much of the effect was due to the tea tree oil and how much was due to the butenafine.[1532] Another study compared 100% tea tree oil to a prescription medicine (both applied twice a day) and found the tea tree oil worked just as well as the prescription.[1533] ◊ ◊ ◊ ◆ ◆

Acne. One study showed that a 5% solution of tea tree oil was not quite as good as benzoyl peroxide for acne, but it was better than a placebo. However, tea tree oil tended to have fewer side effects than benzoyl peroxide.[1534] ◊ ◊ ◊ ◆ ◆

Wound healing. Tea tree oil's value in healing wounds lies mostly in its antiseptic properties. In test-tube studies, it has proven itself to be a powerful antimicrobial.[1535] It contains terpinen-4-ol, a compound that weakens bacteria so the body can fight the infection off more effectively.[1536] ◊ ◊ ◊ ◆ ◆

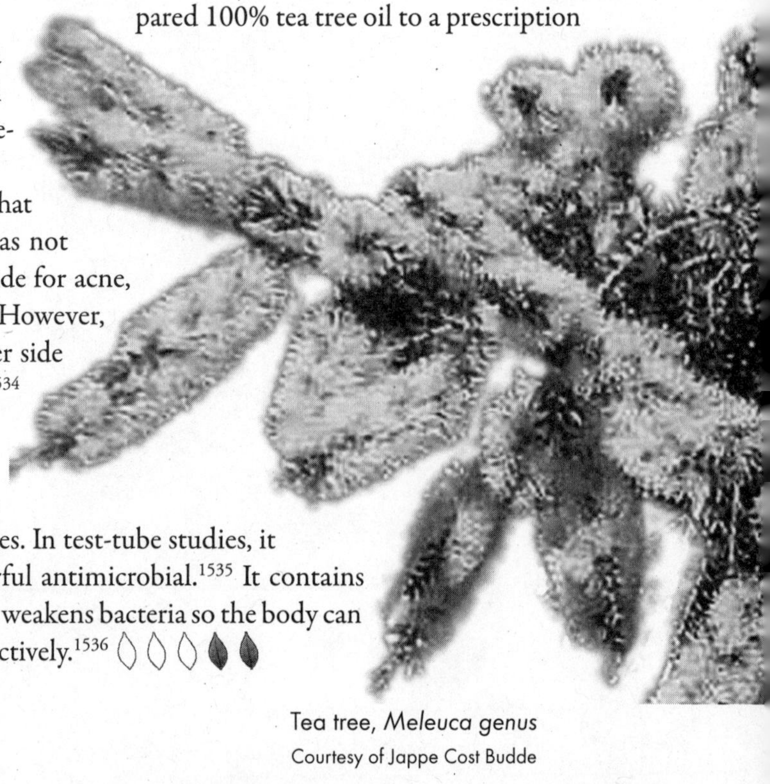

Tea tree, *Meleuca genus*
Courtesy of Jappe Cost Budde

Athlete's foot. One study found that a 10% tea tree oil cream lessened symptoms of athlete's foot but didn't actually kill the fungus very well.[1537]

How do you use it?

Use commercially distilled tea tree oil. The essential oil contains an irritant, cineole, also known as eucalyptol. Dilute the essential oil in a carrier oil such as olive oil before using it on sensitive skin.[1538]

Pure tea tree oil is pretty harsh. Ease into it slowly until you know how you react to it. Some people are allergic; others are just very sensitive. Use very small amounts (a drop or two) at first, and dilute the oil with water to about 5% (in other words, twenty drops of water to every one of tea tree oil). Even if you know you tolerate it well, you typically don't want to use it on your skin in dilution of stronger than 25%.[1539] Some studies have used tea tree oil at 50% strength on feet or full strength on nail fungus, but you need to dilute it more than that for use on anything but nails or very tough skin. Keep tea tree oil in a sealed, opaque bottle, because it tends to break down when exposed to light.

Dosage: How much do you use?

Apply the essential oil topically twice daily in dilutions appropriate to the skin it's being used on.[1540]

What should you be aware of before using it?

Don't take tea tree oil internally. Large doses can damage the kidneys. Smaller doses can cause gastrointestinal irritation.[1541] It has also been known to cause central nervous system depression when taken internally.[1542]

A small percentage of people are allergic.[1543] Others are sensitive to it. About 2% become sensitized over time.[1544]

It has been known to cause contact dermatitis especially when used at full strength. Be sure to dilute it. Try it on a small patch of skin to see how you react before using it on larger more sensitive areas.[1545]

Don't use tea tree oil on your animals as they have been known to lick it off and then get sick or die, especially when used in high concentrations.[1546] Use caution when using it on children for the same reason.

Don't use tea tree oil if you are pregnant.[1547]

Animal studies have found that undiluted tea tree oil taken internally can cause difficulty walking, weakness, muscle tremor, slowing of brain function, and poor coordination. One study applied it full-strength to the ears of animals and found that it caused hearing damage.[1548]

Thyme

Scientific name: *Thymus vulgaris*

Also known as Thymi herba, common thyme, French thyme, rubbed thyme, garden thyme

Originally a wild perennial plant from southern Europe, particularly the south of France, thyme is now widely cultivated. It can be found growing wild (as an introduced species) in parts of New England. Thyme is a member of the mint family and bears lilac or pink flowers. The dried leaves and flowers are used medicinally.

Thyme is a common culinary herb, growing in gardens and window boxes across Europe and North America. In ancient times, meats were preserved with it.[1549] Ancient Egyptians used it in embalming. The ancient Greeks considered it a symbol of courage and sacrifice. In Europe in the Middle Ages, thyme leaves were given to warriors departing for battle because thyme was thought to give courage. Today we know that the medicinal properties of the herb are due to thymol, a compound found in the essential oil. Thymol has been used widely in prescription and patent medicines as well as toothpaste, mouthwash, and cosmetics.

What is it good for?

Antiseptic, especially for gingivitis and other irritations of the mouth. The antiseptic properties of thyme have been known since the sixteenth century. Essential oil of thyme is a broad antimicrobial.[1550] Thymol, one of the active ingredients in the essential oil of thyme, is the main ingredient in Listerine® mouthwash.[1551] Before modern antibiotics, thymol was used to medicate surgical bandages.[1552] Studies show a broad antibiotic activity.[1553]

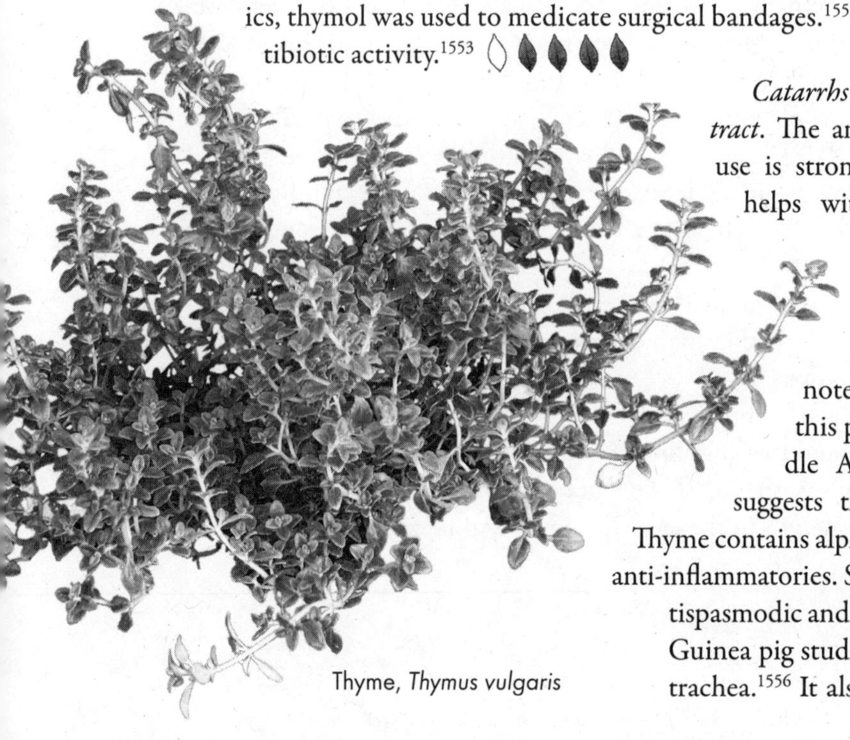

Thyme, *Thymus vulgaris*

Catarrhs of the upper respiratory tract. The anecdotal evidence for this use is strong, suggesting that thyme helps with both congestion and cough. *A Modern Herbal* recommends it for all kinds of coughs, even whooping cough and notes that it has been used for this purpose since the late Middle Ages.[1554] Modern research suggests this use may have merit. Thyme contains alpha-linolenic acid and other anti-inflammatories. Studies show that it has antispasmodic and expectorant properties.[1555] Guinea pig studies show that it relaxes the trachea.[1556] It also inhibits net nitric oxide production, which plays a role in the inflammation of bronchitis, asthma, and other respiratory diseases.[1557] Clinical studies are unavailable. Nonetheless, Commission E recommends it for this use.

Fungus. Essential oil of thyme is a broad-spectrum fungicide. Thymol, a compound found in the essential oil of thyme, has been found to kill the fungus that infests toenails.[1558] It also works against candida and can also help magnify the effect of other fungicides.[1559]

Arthritis and joint pain. One of the traditional uses of thyme is in topical preparations used to treat arthritis. Modern research doesn't show any benefit to the disease. However, if we look at the components of thyme's essential oil, we see that using it for joint pain might not be so far-fetched as the clinical research would suggest. The oil of thyme is an irritant. It increases blood flow to the skin it is rubbed on. As such it may function as a counterirritant: irritation of the skin may offset the pain of arthritic joints. It also contains alpha-linolenic acid, an anti-inflammatory and p-cymene, a mild analgesic. Nonetheless, we are still in the realm of conjecture in saying that thyme is good for this use.

How do you use it?

Infusion. An infusion is made using one teaspoon of the herb per cup of water.[1560] Pour the boiling water over the herb, steep for 10 minutes, and strain. Infusions can be taken internally, or they can be used on a compress.

Syrup. Thyme syrup can be used for coughs and colds. (See Chapter 3 for instructions on making a syrup.)

Tincture. A couple of drops of the tincture can be used externally as an antiseptic.[1561] You can also use a small amount in a large bowl of hot water. Inhale the steam to help clear bronchial passages and ease spasms.[1562]

Essential oil. The essential oil of thyme is strong, and it is dangerous. Thyme oil contains roughly 20–55% thymol. Commercial mouthwashes typically limit the amount of thymol to 0.06% or less, and they still are effective germ fighters. Dilute the essential oil in a carrier oil before using it on the skin.[1563] *Never* take essential oil of thyme internally. Even small amounts can be fatal. When making preparations using thyme oil, follow safe handling practices: keep it away from foodstuffs, don't get it near your nose or mouth, be careful that anything that may have a residue on it (pots, strainers, spoons, etc.) doesn't come in contact with food, and label all preparations as "external use only." Better yet, get professional help if you want to use thyme oil. It is not a do-it-yourself oil.

Dosage: How much do you use?

Infusion. Use 1–2 g of the herb for 1 cup of tea, 2–3 times a day as needed.[1564] Take no more than 10 g of the herb per day.

What should you be aware of before using it?

Thyme is on the FDA's list of spices and other natural seasonings and flavorings that are generally recognized as safe. In culinary quantities, thyme is quite safe, as are infusions and tinctures.[1565] The danger comes in using the essential oil. Internal use of the essential oil can be toxic and is not advised.[1566] Even in amounts as small as a teaspoon, thymol can cause nausea, vomiting, headache, dizziness, convulsions, coma, and even cardiac and respiratory arrest.[1567] When using the essential oil externally, it must be diluted.[1568] Even so, it can cause rashes, swelling, inflammation, and cracks in the skin. Suffice it to say that essential oil of thyme is *not* a do-it-yourself herb.

Be careful taking thyme preparation internally if you are prone to gastritis or have inflammatory bowel disease.[1569]

If you have thyroid problems, check with your doctor before using thyme.[1570]

Traditionally, thyme was used to alter the menstrual cycle. Though we aren't quite sure exactly what's going on there, pregnant women should probably avoid using thyme in medicinal quantities.[1571]

Some species of thyme, camphor thyme for example, are not edible. Know what you are taking before taking thyme internally.

Allergy to thyme is very rare but possible and is more likely if you are allergic to sage, mint, lavender, or basil.[1572] Thyme has a low potential for sensitization.

Turmeric

Scientific name: *Curcuma longa*

Also known as *Curcuma domestica*, *Curcuma aromatica*, curcuma, Indian saffron, red valerian, *jiang huang*, *yu jin*, Indian yellow root, yellowroot

Turmeric is a relative of ginger. The rhizome (underground stem) of this perennial shrub is used both in food and medicinally. Turmeric is native to southern Asia, but it now grows in tropical regions throughout the world. In the United States, the only state it can be found in is Hawaii though it is not native there. The rhizomes are boiled or scalded, dried, and then ground into a bright yellow-orange powder.

In India and China, turmeric is highly regarded. It is a key ingredient in curry and prepared mustard. It is used as a dye and a food coloring. In China, topical preparations are used to reduce pain and itching.[1573] In Chinese medicine, it is known as *jiang huang* and is used to invigorate the blood and promote warmth.[1574]

What is it good for?

Gas. Commission E recommends turmeric for dyspeptic conditions. In the test tube, curcumin, the compound that give turmeric its yellow color, fights the protozoan responsible for infectious diarrhea.[1575] The Chinese use turmeric in formulas that treat bloating, abdominal pains, and flatulence.[1576] In a clinical study, it proved better than placebo in reducing gas and dyspepsia.[1577] It might even have some benefit for ulcers.[1578]

Cardiovascular health. We are just now beginning to understand how turmeric can help improve overall cardiovascular health. Animal studies show a reduction in cholesterol and triglycerides in animals given turmeric orally.[1579] In animal studies, turmeric especially helps reduce serum cholesterol and triglycerides in animals fed a high fat diet.[1580] As for human studies, researchers have reported that healthy humans given turmeric for seven days showed an increase in HDL (good cholesterol) and an overall decrease in all cholesterol.[1581] It also inhibits platelet aggregation.[1582] One study shows that it might help keep the mind clear in the elderly. Singapore residents 60 or older who regularly eat curry show higher scores in cognitive function tests.[1583] One possible explanation is that it improves circulation to the brain. Another is that it breaks up plaque in the brain, like that which forms in Alzheim-

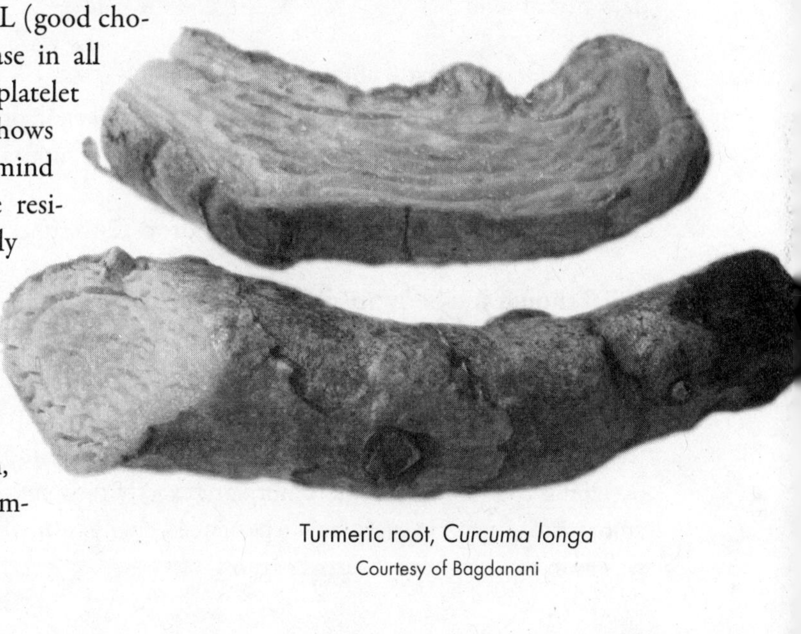

Turmeric root, *Curcuma longa*
Courtesy of Bagdanani

er's patients.[1584] A related Chinese species improved mouse maze running times.[1585] ◊ ◊ ◆ ◆ ◆

Inflammation. The native Hawaiians used turmeric as a gargle for a swollen, sore throat.[1586] In China, topical preparations are used to reduce pain and itching.[1587] In Ayurvedic medicine, turmeric is used for cuts, burns and bruises, as well as for inflammation.[1588] One clinical trial showed that it is a better anti-inflammatory agent than a placebo.[1589] The exact implications of this finding, however, are unknown. ◊ ◊ ◊ ◆ ◆

Wound healing. In animal tests, both oral and topical turmeric sped up wound healing time.[1590] In a study of mice, pretreating the mice with turmeric led to faster healing of wounds exposed to radiation.[1591] Human clinical studies are, however, unavailable. ◊ ◊ ◊ ◆ ◆

Rheumatic disorders. Rats given curcuma oil from turmeric showed improvement in arthritis inflammation.[1592] Dogs with osteoarthritis showed some modest improvement when given an extract of turmeric.[1593] ◊ ◊ ◊ ◆ ◆

How do you use it?

Powdered in capsules. Standardized capsules are available. Taking bromelain and turmeric, or fish oil and turmeric, is believed to enhance the absorption of the turmeric. However, because all three are known to increase the risk of bleeding, caution should be exercised when taking them together.[1594]

Tinctures. Homemade tinctures are not always successful, and the powder works well anyway.[1595] But if you want to try, use a 1:10 strength.

Infusions. Infusions are made by scalding .5–1.0 g of the powder with boiling water, covering and letting it infuse for five minutes. Strain out the powder before using the infusion.

Infused oil. Cover powdered turmeric with a good quality oil. Mix it well, and then add enough oil to cover the moistened powder by about an inch. Shake the mixture daily for 10 days. Strain well.[1596]

Dosage: How much do you use?

The typical daily dose is 1.5–3 g of turmeric taken in doses of 400–600 mg.[1597] It should be taken on an empty stomach[1598] One study found no toxicity when people took 8000 mg of curcumin per day for 3 months[1599]

Tincture. The tincture dose is 10–15 drops, 2–3 times daily.

What should you be aware of before using it?

Turmeric is on the FDA's list both of essential oils and of spices and other natural seasonings and flavorings that are generally recognized as safe. As a spice, turmeric has been used safely by millions of people for centuries. Not much study has been done, however, into the safety in medicinal doses. As with most herbs, it is most likely possible to hurt yourself by taking too much, but we're not sure exactly how much is "too much." Mice fed large amounts of turmeric every day experienced changes in white and red blood cell counts as well as in the weight of internal organs.[1600]

It is possible to be allergic to turmeric. If you are allergic to ginger, be especially careful as chances are good that you are also allergic to turmeric. In some people, it can cause stomach irritation and upset.[1601]

Don't take it if you have obstruction of bile passages. [1602]

Don't take it in conjunction with any other herb or drug known to affect liver function.[1603] (See Chapter 5 for a list.)

In case of gallstones, use only after consulting with a physician

Don't take it if you have ulcers.[1604]

Don't use it if you are pregnant.[1605]

Turmeric may affect blood sugar.[1606] If you are diabetic or have other blood sugar problems, exercise caution when using turmeric in medicinal doses.

Turmeric may increase the effects of cholesterol medication.

Don't take turmeric if you are taking any of these medications: antithrombotic drugs, immunosuppressive drugs[1607] If you plan to have surgery, tell your surgeon you have been taking turmeric and discontinue use. Be cautious when using it in conjunction with other herbs known or suspected of increasing the risk of bleeding. (See Chapter 5 for a list.)

Taking turmeric in conjunction with NSAIDs may increase the risk of bruising or bleeding[1608] Don't take it you have a clotting disorder without first consulting with a physician. Be cautious when using it in conjunction with other herbs known or suspected of increasing the risk of bleeding. (See Chapter 5 for a list.)

Valerian

Scientific name: *Valeriana officinalis*

Also known as all-heal, garden heliotrope, Belgian valerian, common valerian, garden valerian, blessed herb, capon's tail, *phu*, vandal root

Valerian is a tall perennial that grows in temperate regions throughout the northern hemisphere. In the United States, it grows in many of the northern states, and is considered to be a noxious or invasive weed by some of them. The genus *Valeriana* includes more than 250 species. Medicinal valerian preparations are made from the dried rhizomes (underground stems) and roots of common valerian, *Valeriana officinalis*.

There is no polite way to say this. Valerian reeks. The smell is so distinctive and so pronounced that the Greek physician gave it its own name, *phu*. Some cats are fascinated by it. Your bed partner might be less so as the smell can be very pronounced on the breath and even from the pores while you sleep. Valerian is not a reliable sedative for all people. Some get little or no effect. Some get nightmares and restless sleep. Some actually become a little hyper. But for others, it's a good occasional sedative. In fact, valerian is one of the few insomnia herbs that has been tested and found effective in large-scale trials. The quality of sleep, however, is sometimes not the best. Taking valerian in conjunction with other herbs can sometimes mitigate this effect. Check Chapter 4 for some suggestions.

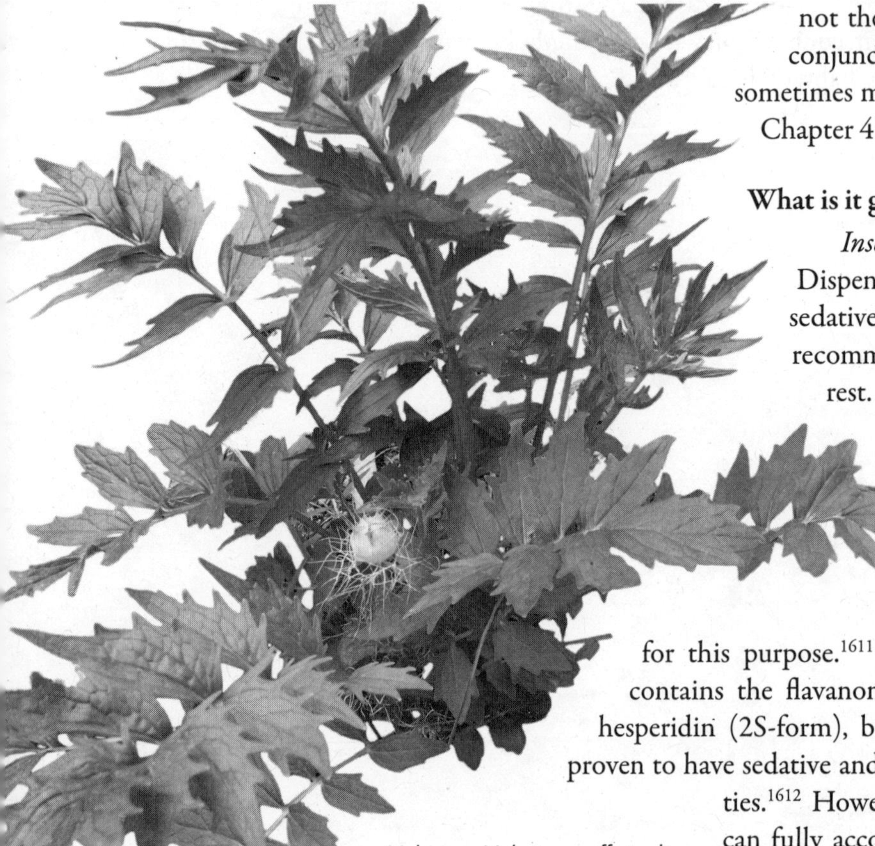

Valerian, *Valeriana officinalis*

What is it good for?

Insomnia. The 1918 U.S. Dispensatory lists valerian as a sedative.[1609] The Eclectic School recommended it for nervous unrest. This use is an ancient one. In the second century, Galen advised use of valerian for insomnia.[1610] Chinese and Ayurvedic medicine also use it for this purpose.[1611] We know that valerian contains the flavanones glycoside linarin and hesperidin (2S-form), both of which have been proven to have sedative and sleep-enhancing properties.[1612] However, no single ingredient can fully account for valerian's effects.

Researchers are beginning to believe that the active ingredients in combination make valerian an effective sedative.[1613]

This sedative effect has been shown in several Western studies. Sleep studies show that valerian is not so powerful a sedative that it interferes with REM (dreaming) sleep like some prescription sedatives do.[1614] Numerous clinical trials show that overall valerian improves both the quality and quantity of sleep. Unfortunately, studies of valerian tend to be plagued by methodological problems and sometimes bias.[1615] Yet the consensus is that valerian does indeed have value in treating insomnia.

Anxiety. During World War II, valerian was commonly used by the citizens of England, whose nerves were frazzled by nightly air raids.[1616] During World War I, it was given to shell-shock victims.[1617] A couple of small studies support this use. One investigated valerian's effectiveness in social stress situations.[1618] Another compared it to clobazapam, an anti-anxiety drug.[1619] Both found benefit.

Muscle cramps. Valerian is sometimes used for cramping muscles caused by muscle tension and stress. We know that the herb contains valerenic acid, which has spasmolytic and muscle relaxant effects.[1620] But valerian's use on muscle cramps has not been studied clinically. Furthermore, we have little or no evidence that it helps with muscle cramps resulting from exercise.

Bruises and wounds. A number of Indian tribes—Thompson, Gosiute, Menominee, Meskwaki, Okanagon—used decoctions or poultices of the roots of other plants of the *Valeriana* genus for wounds and bruises.[1621] Unfortunately, we have no experimental or clinical evidence to support this use. One study discovered that an extract of valerian stimulated the immune function of bone marrow cells, but that study did not use topically applied valerian.[1622]

How do you use it?

Infusions. Valerian root needs to be dried at a low temperature or it loses its effectiveness. Similarly, make your infusions using cool water.[1623] If you have access to fresh roots, soak 2 teaspoons of chopped roots for 8–10 hours in a cup of cold water. These infusions can be used for anxiety and insomnia. You can add peppermint oil to help disguise the flavor if you'd like. If you are taking the valerian for help sleeping, take it about a half hour before bed. The effect kicks in in about a half hour and wears off in about four hours.[1624]

Compresses. Make compresses by soaking a cloth in the tincture. They can be used for muscle cramps.

Tinctures. Tinctures are also useful for insomnia. If you are making your own tincture (1:5), use cool alcohol, not warm or hot. Some herbalists suggest that tincture of valerian is more effective than an infusion because some of the ingredients are not water-soluble.[1625] Tinctures also keep better than other valerian preparations.[1626]

Plant juice. The roots can be juiced and the juice used instead of an infusion or tincture.

Commercial preparations. These are also available. The amount of active ingredient in valerian tends to vary from year to year and from month to month within the growing season.[1627]

If you want consistency in your valerian preparation, you won't be able to achieve it with homemade preparations. You'll need to find a standardized commercial preparation.

Bath. Externally, valerian can be used as a bath additive to help with relaxation and sleep, but the smell makes the experience somewhat less than luxuriant.

Dosage: How much do you use?

Infusions. A typical dose is 2–3 g of the herb per cup, taken a half an hour to one hour before bed. Alternatively, you can use 1–2 g, 2–3 times per day.[1628]

Tincture. ½–1 teaspoon, once to several times per day. Start with the lower dose until you see how well you tolerate it. It can cause headaches at higher doses.

Plant juice. 1 tablespoon, 3 times per day is a typical adult dose.

Capsules. The recommendations for powder capsules vary widely, ranging from one 150 mg capsule to three 475 mg capsules before bed.[1629] Your best bet is to find a reputable brand and follow label directions.

Don't exceed 15 g per day if taking valerian internally. Don't exceed 100 g in a bath.

It's safe for occasional use only. Don't take it for more than 2–3 weeks without a break. Though valerian is not, strictly speaking, "addictive," you can become dependent on it. Continual use can also lead to headaches and heart palpitations.

What should you be aware of before using it?

Valerian is on the FDA's list of herbs generally regarded as safe. However, some people don't digest valerian as well as others. In them, it can cause headaches, agitation, restlessness, and night terrors. Other people get a hangover from it, especially if they take too much. Valerian also causes stomach upset in some people.[1630]

Most problems with valerian occur when people exceed the safe dose or take it for prolonged periods of time. Repeated large doses can cause headaches, heaviness, and stupor.[1631] Prolonged use can also cause restlessness and insomnia if you take enough of it or take it for too long. As with any sleep aid, you can become dependent on valerian.

Allow at least four hours between the time you take valerian and the time you need to be alert to drive, spar, or participate in any activity that requires a quick mind. Take it for the first time when you don't have to drive or operate machinery the next morning so you can see what kind of lingering effects it might have for you. One study showed that valerian caused no change in psychomotor or cognitive performance in young healthy adults.[1632] Anecdotal evidence suggests, however, it may cause grogginess.

Don't take valerian with alcohol or any other sedative.[1633] It may compound the effect of other sedative herbs. (See Chapter 5 for a list.)

If you have liver disease, don't take valerian. Don't take it in conjunction with any other herb or drug known to affect liver function).[1634] (See Chapter 5 for a list.)

Don't take it with drugs or herbs that have monoamine oxidase inhibitor (MAOI) activity or that interact with MAOI drugs. Headache, tremors, mania, and insomnia may occur.[1635] (See Chapter 5 for a list.)

Some doctors and herbalists recommend that you don't take it while pregnant or nursing.[1636] No adverse reactions have been reported officially, but the effects have not been studied. In other words, valerian has not been proven safe.

If you are prone to depression, be careful when using valerian. Large doses can bring on depression in healthy people. Even moderate doses may affect those with a predisposition. Don't take it if you are taking an antidepressant.

If you have large skin injuries, a fever, an infectious disease, cardiac insufficiency, or hypertonia, don't use valerian in a bath without first consulting a doctor.

Valerian is not the same as *Centranthus ruber*, known as red or American valerian. It is also not *Curcuma longa*, sometimes called red valerian. It is also not valium, though one of its nicknames is "the valium of the nineteenth century."

Some of the ingredients in valerian are not recommended for children. Children should take it only under medical supervision.

Willow Bark

Scientific name: *Salix alba*

Also known as white willow bark, common willow, European willow. *Salicis cortex* is willow bark.

Hundreds of different species of willow exist. The white willow, a tall tree with grey bark, is the one most commonly used medicinally. It is the dried bark that contains medicinal compounds.

The Chinese have been using the bark of willows as a pain reliever for more than 2500 years.[1637] The white willow tree was introduced to North America by colonists from Europe. In the mid-1800s, researchers discovered the active ingredient in willow bark, salicin. They refined and purified it, creating first salicylic acid and then its derivative acetylsalicylic acid, the active ingredient in aspirin.[1638]

What is it good for?

Willow bark is typically used as an aspirin substitute.[1639] The Cherokee used an infusion for fever.[1640] Commission E recommends it for fever, aches, and headache. Some people say it doesn't have the side effects of aspirin, particularly the stomach irritation.[1641] But it often doesn't have as much salicin (the active ingredient) either. Moreover, it doesn't have the effect that aspirin does on blood platelet function.[1642] That's good if you find that an undesired trait of aspirin, but it's bad if you want to take it for heart health (as in the practice of taking an aspirin a

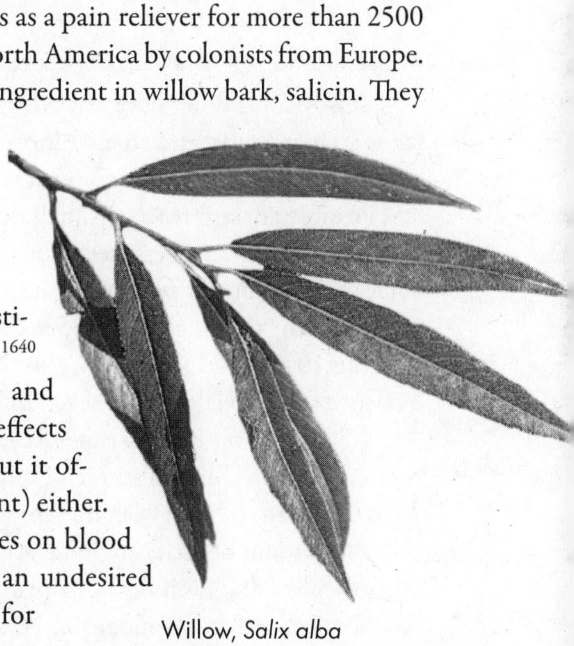

Willow, *Salix alba*
Courtesy of U.S. Department of Agriculture

day to reduce the risk of heart disease). One study found some help for low back pain.[1643] Another small, poorly controlled study showed benefit when willow bark was used in combination with feverfew for migraines.[1644] ◊ ◊ ◊ ◆ ◆

How do you use it?

Decoction. A strong decoction brings out the best in willow bark. Combine the herb with water at a 1:32 ratio. Bring the mixture to a boil slowly, boil for ten minutes, cool until warm, and strain. Pour additional water through the herb in the strainer to return the volume of the decoction to 32.[1645]

Commercial preparation. Standardized commercial preparations are available, but are much more common in Europe than in the U.S. If you can find one, look for standardization to 120 mg salicin. That's the only way you can be assured of getting the active ingredient in your preparation.

Dosage: How much do you use?

The concentration of salicin in willow bark varies widely from species to species and even from tree to tree. If you make your willow bark preparations from the actual bark, it's difficult to say exactly how much salicin will be in it.[1646] The recommended average daily dose of willow bark should contain 60–120 mg total salicin. Some commercial preparations, particularly those made in Germany, may be able to ensure that amount, but it is almost impossible to do so with your own preparations at home.

A rough dosage, however, is 1–3 g of dried bark 3 times per day as a tea (decoction).[1647] One teaspoon is roughly 1.5 g of willow bark.

What should you be aware of before using it?

Most people don't have any adverse reactions to taking willow bark. The tannins may cause stomach upset in a small minority of people.[1648]

Don't take willow bark if you are taking antithrombotic drugs.[1649]

Possible adverse reactions include bleeding, asthma, renal toxicity, and dermatitis.[1650] If you plan to have surgery, tell your surgeon you have been taking willow bark and discontinue use. Be cautious when using it in conjunction with other herbs known or suspected of increasing the risk of bleeding. (See Chapter 5 for a list.)

The 1918 U.S. Dispensatory lists willow bark as a sexual depressant.[1651] The modern evidence for this claim is, however, lacking.

We don't know if it can cause Reye Syndrome, a potentially fatal disease associated with aspirin intake in children with chickenpox or flu symptoms. Until we know more, don't give willow bark to children with flu symptoms.

The amount of active ingredient has been known to vary widely between different species of willow and even between plants within the alba species. Don't lean too heavily on anything other than a standardized commercial formula.

Witch Hazel

Scientific name: *Hamamelis virginiana*

Also known as *Hamamelidis Cortex*, snapping hazel, spotted alder, tobacco wood, winter bloom, hamamelis, hamamelidis aqua, hamamelis water, hamamelis bark, winterbloom, striped alder, spotted alder

Witch hazel is a small tree or shrub that grows in North American forests. The name *Hamamelis* is from the Greek word for apple, so called because the plant resembles an apple tree. Twigs from the dormant tree, harvested in the autumn, are soaked and softened in water, and then steamed distilled to produce witch hazel.

The name witch hazel refers not to a witches brew, but to the use of witch hazel sticks as divining rods or "witching sticks," a tool of dowsers searching for water or precious metals. Before the steam distillation process was invented, decoctions of leaves and twigs were used on sores and achy muscles and joints. Native Americans introduced witch hazel to settlers, and before long it was being used for ailments of all kinds.[1652] The steam distillation process came on the scene in the 1900s. Though it made making witch hazel preparations easier for manufacturers, it didn't extract the tannins in the twigs nearly as effectively as decocting. The result was a watered-down product with significantly less medicinal value.[1653]

What is it good for?

Minor skin injuries and inflammation. The Cherokee used witch hazel on scratches and sores.[1654] The Chippewa used an infusion for skin troubles.[1655] The Iroquois used a poultice of the bark for bruises and as an astringent.[1656] The Mohegans used it for cuts, bruises, and insect bites.[1657] Traditional North American herbalists used a poultice of the fresh leaves or bark for bleeding and inflammations.[1658] The Eclectic School recommended it for inflamed or wounded skin as well as for sprains and sunburn. Fyfe of the Eclectic School recommended it for bruises and wounds. It was a part of several patent medicines in the nineteenth century. Even today, over-the-counter medicines, especially those for hemorrhoids, can contain witch hazel. The FDA recognizes its external use "for relief of minor skin irritations

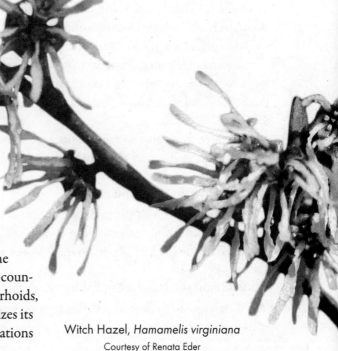

Witch Hazel, *Hamamelis virginiana*
Courtesy of Renata Eder

due to. . . insect bites, minor cuts, minor scrapes."[1659] Commission E recommends it for minor injuries of skin and local inflammation of skin and mucous membranes.

The leaves of the witch hazel tree contain up to 10% tannin and the bark up to 3%. The tannin is a powerful astringent. It is also an anti-inflammatory and hemostatic (stops blood from cuts).[1660] It has a drawing effect that helps with insect stings and bites. Witch hazel was common in most home medicine chest before the advent of modern antibiotics and was used not just to stop bleeding, but to sooth burns and general inflammation of the skin.[1661] It can help with inflammation that comes with a sunburn, and it might have some ability to undo some of the damage caused by UV radiation.[1662] It is a powerful antioxidant and protector against cell damage.[1663]

As a carrier for other herbs. Witch hazel can be used as a carrier to dilute other herbs. For example, witch hazel can be combined with arnica, goldenseal, myrrh, or chamomile. It can be made into an ointment either alone or in combination.

Muscle aches. Ellingwood recommended witch hazel for "soreness of muscles, muscular aching, a bruised sensation, soreness from violent muscular exertion, soreness from bruises and strains."[1664] His is a lone voice for this use.

How do you use it?

Distilled. If you purchase water steam distillate ("witch hazel water"), you can use it undiluted or diluted 1:3 with water. Be aware, however, that some commercial steam distillate witch hazel contains little or no tannin. The astringent property comes from the added alcohol.[1665] The bark contains 31 times more astringent tannins than the leaf extract.[1666]

Infusion. Traditional wisdom says that cold infusion brings out the best in witch hazel. Wrap the herb in cheesecloth, pre-moisten it and suspend it in tepid water at room temperature, overnight. Use a 1:32 ratio. Squeeze out the herb into the infusion in the morning.[1667]

Decoction. A strong decoction also works well. Combine the herb with water at a 1:32 ratio. Bring the mixture to a boil slowly, boil for ten minutes, cool until warm, and strain. Pour additional water through the herb in the strainer to return the volume of the decoction to 32.[1668]

Tincture. You can also make a tincture, though the result should be diluted with two parts of water to one part tincture before use and should not be used around the eyes.[1669]

Dosage: How much do you use?

Externally, witch hazel produced by either steam distillation or infusion or decoction seems to be safe enough that we can simply say "use occasionally, as needed." The wording suggested by the FDA is, "Apply to the affected area as often as necessary."

What should you be aware of before using it?

Witch hazel can cause dermatitis in some people.

Note that witch hazel is an astringent and anti-inflammatory but it is *not* a proven antiseptic. It can take down swelling, stop minor bleeding, and tighten the skin, but it does nothing to reduce the chance of infection.

Some would suggest that extended use of tannin-rich herbs increases the chances of cancer.[1670] At this point, we don't know enough to say definitively whether or not that's true.

Taken internally, it can cause nausea and stress the liver.[1671] Some people do take certain commercially produced extracts of witch hazel internally, but that practice is not advisable. Be aware that historically some commercial witch hazel preparations have been made with methyl alcohol and/or may contain formaldehyde, both of which are extremely toxic.[1672]

Yarrow

Scientific name: *Achillea millefolium*

Also known as nosebleed, milfoil, wound wort, achillea, bloodwort, soldier's herb, soldier's woundwort, thousand weed, thousand-leaf, green arrow, and yarroway

Yarrow is a perennial that grows wild in every state in the United States as well as in Europe and Asia. The stems, leaves, and flowers are used medicinally. It is used both dried and fresh, and is most potent when harvested while in flower.

Yarrow was used to treat wounds during the Trojan War. If you'll look at the Latin name, you'll see it's named after Achilles, the mythical hero of that war, who used the herb to staunch the bleeding of his soldiers.[1673] Its Latin name was *Herba Militaris*, the military herb, because of its use as a wound treatment.[1674] In the Middle Ages, yarrow was known as a treatment for nose bleeds.[1675] Chinese medicine uses a related plant *Achillea sibirica* Ledeb for abscesses, traumatic falls, and bleeding. Incidentally, yarrow stalks are the traditional way to cast the *I Ching*, an ancient Chinese oracle.

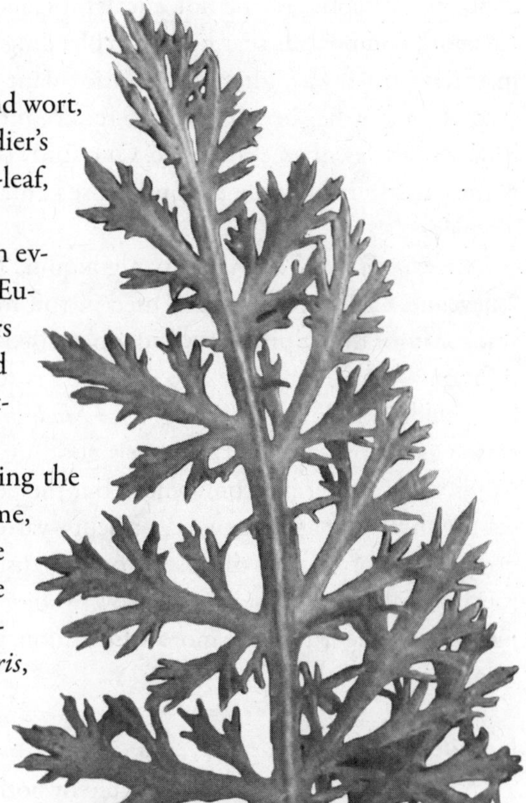

Yarrow, *Achillea millefolium*

What is it good for?

Wounds. The herb has substantial tradition for this use that extends across three continents and three millennia. The Blackfoot and Flathead Indians used an infusion on sores.[1676] The Bella Coola and Crow used a poultice on burns, the Carrier on swellings, and the Gosiute on bruises.[1677] Highland Scots made an ointment that they applied to wounds.[1678] Because the leaves encourage clotting, they were once inserted whole into the nose to stop nosebleeds. We now know, however, that this use can irritate the nose and actually *cause* nosebleeds. European herbal tradition says that a decoction is very good for chapping.[1679] The Eclectic School used it as an astringent.

All this tradition is not without merit. The test-tube studies on yarrow have been extensive. The essential oil contains camphor (up to 20%) and eucalyptol (up to 10%). It contains antiseptics (terpeniol, eucalyptol, and tannins) and pain relievers (camphor and eugenol), compounds that help stop bleeding (achilletin, achilleine) and are anti-inflammatories (azulene).[1680] It also has antioxidant and antimicrobial properties.[1681] In animal studies, yarrow has been proven to reduce inflammation.[1682] Clinical studies in humans, however, are less than conclusive. One study showed it no better than placebo in treating dermatitis.[1683] In another, a mouth rinse containing yarrow showed no benefit in treating gingivitis.[1684]

Colds and flu. The Abnaki, Algonquin, Bella Coola, Blackfoot, Carrier, Cherokee, Cheyenne, Clallam, Flathead all used yarrow for colds, flu, and related symptoms.[1685] Some smoked it for throat problems, and others used various other preparations, most commonly infusions. The flowers were also used for hay fever. Conventional wisdom says that yarrow helps colds by inducing sweating.[1686] *A Modern Herbal* suggests yarrow tea for colds for this reason as well. It says that yarrow is good in cases of "obstructed perspiration," in other words when a fever has commenced but the perspiration needed to cool the body has not yet begun.[1687] On at least two continents, yarrow is used to treat colds. No research exists, however, to corroborate this use. Moreover, using yarrow to treat colds involves taking yarrow internally, and considering yarrow's thujone, camphor, and beta-pinene content, internal use is problematic. (For more information, see the "What should you be aware of before using it?" section.)

How do you use it?

The active ingredients are extracted by both water and alcohol.[1688]

Infusion. An infusion is made of 1–2 teaspoons of dried yarrow in a cup of water.[1689] Steep for 10–15 minutes and strain. It can be used on a compress.

Decoction. To make a decoction of yarrow root, simmer one ounce dried or two ounces fresh yarrow root (chopped) in 3 cups of water for about 30 minutes.[1690] The decoction can also be used on a compress.

Ointment. Yarrow used to be mixed with butter or lard to make an ointment. You can make your own ointments using methods two or six for making creams and salves in Chapter 3. Commercially prepared ointments are available but difficult to find.

Essential oil. The essential oil, extracted from the flowers, is used as a chest rub for colds or flu. How much of the essential oil to use in a wound wash is a matter of debate. Most herbalists recommend somewhere between 4 and 30 drops of the essential oil in ½ cup of water as an antiseptic compress or to wash wounds.[1691] It's possible to be allergic or just sensitive to yarrow. Start with the higher dilution first to see how you tolerate it. Store the essential oil in glass, not plastic.

Poultice. Use a poultice of fresh leaves on a cut or scrape.

Baths. You can use yarrow in a bath by adding 100 g of yarrow to five gallons of water.[1692]

The amount of the active ingredients in yarrow varies widely from plant to plant, even in the same habitat.[1693] This fact, plus the presence of thujone (see "What should you be aware of") is a good argument for using only standardized yarrow with the thujone removed if you want to take it internally.

Dosage: How much do you use?

Externally, yarrow is used mostly for first-aid purposes. For that reason, we don't know much about how people tolerate it long term.

If you plan to use yarrow internally, contact an herbalist or naturopath for both dosage and supervision because it contains ingredients that can be dangerous. For internal use, yarrow is not a do-it-yourself herb.

What should you be aware of before using it?

Yarrow has traditionally been considered to be a safe herb, though recently it has been found to contain some thujone, which can cause muscle spasms and convulsions when taken internally. Moreover, the essential oil also contains camphor and beta-pinene, both of which are harmful if swallowed in sufficiently large doses. The 1918 U.S. Dispensatory notes that 2–5 g causes marked irregularity of the pulse.[1694] The FDA approves the use of use of yarrow in beverages only if the thujone in it is removed.[1695] The safest course of action is to use yarrow only externally.

Using any herb on an open wound can be risky. Any contamination of the herb or the carrier can cause infection, and infections can become dangerous.

Some people are allergic to yarrow.[1696] It is in the same family as ragweed and chamomile. If you have allergies to plants in that family, avoid taking yarrow internally and take precautions when using it externally for the first time.[1697]

Avoid skin contact with the undiluted essential oil.

If you are on an anti-coagulant or blood pressure medicine, check with your doctor before using yarrow internally.[1698] If you plan to have surgery, tell your surgeon you have been taking yarrow and discontinue use. Be cautious when using it in conjunction with other herbs known or suspected of increasing the risk of bleeding. (See Chapter 5 for a list.)

Yarrow can cause photosensitivity.[1699] Be extra careful about sun exposure while using it.

Yarrow is a mild diuretic. If you use it internally, make sure to take it with water.[1700] Be cautious when using it in conjunction with other herbs that have a diuretic effect. (See Chapter 5 for a list.)

Yarrow may make some people sleepy. It may compound the effect of other sedative herbs. (See Chapter 5 for a list.)

It also can cause miscarriage in higher doses. Avoid taking yarrow internally if you are pregnant.[1701]

In animal studies high doses of yarrow cause abnormal sperm.[1702] We don't know if it has similar effects in humans, but men would do well to avoid exceeding the recommended doses when taking yarrow internally.

Chapter Three

Preparing the Herbs

It's possible to use herbs without making your own preparations. A wide variety of commercial preparations are available. Many of them, however, are quite expensive, especially if you are buying from overseas. Fortunately, many preparations can be made with dried herbs which are becoming increasingly available in health food stores, vitamin stores, and online. You can also find some fresh herbs online. The "Further Resources" Chapter at the end of the book can give you some ideas about where to look.

Generally, when working with herbs, glass, ceramic, enamel, or pottery containers are best. If you don't have a glass or enamel pot you can use on the stove, stainless steel or copper is a decent second choice. Avoid aluminum, iron, or tin. Stir with wooden spoons. Store the resulting mixtures in glass or ceramic. Your best bet is to have pots dedicated just to working with herbs. In fact, if you are going to work with herbs that are toxic, it's a good idea to dedicate some of your pots and utensils exclusively to topical and/or toxic preparations. Sure, you'll clean them well after each use, but there's always the chance of a bit of herb-impregnated wax sticking to the inside. The last thing you want when you're making a nice stew is bits of arnica or menthol getting into it.

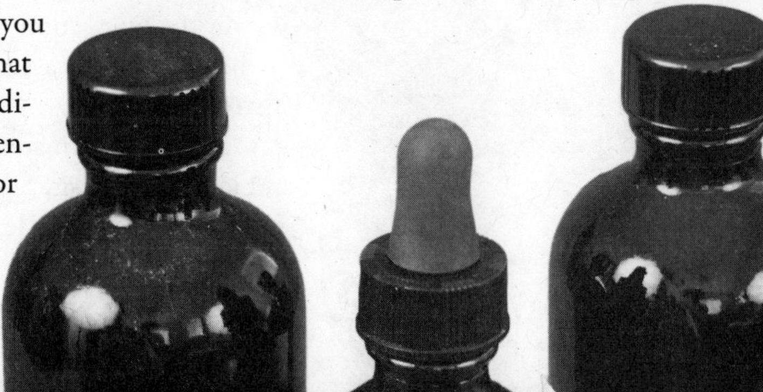

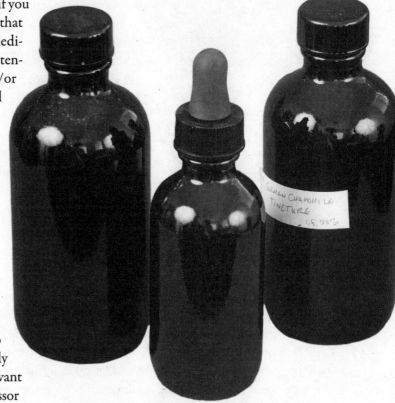

Dark glass storage bottles for storing herbal preparations

In addition to pots, you'll also need a gram scale—herb weights are typically given in grams—and various measuring spoons and cups. If you plan to crush herbs, you'll need a sturdy mortar and pestle. You *don't* want to use an electric food processor or grinder to crush herbs because you want to keep the heat due to

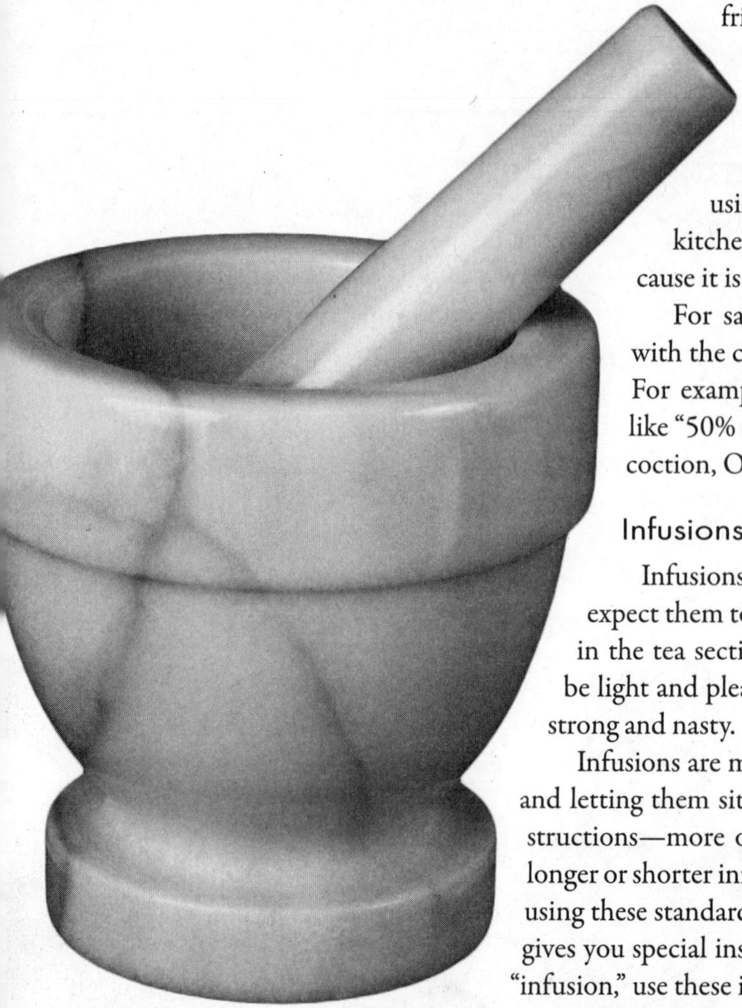

Use a mortar and pestle for crushing herbs

friction to a minimum. That kind of heat changes herbs. For decoctions and infusions, you'll need a strainer, maybe some cheesecloth or coffee filters. Again, exercise caution when using kitchen utensils. Don't use your kitchen strainer for toxic, topical herbs because it is very difficult to get completely clean.

For safety's sake always label your bottles with the contents, the procedure, and the date. For example, your label might say something like "50% cinnamon, 50% fresh ginger root, decoction, October 21, 2009."

Infusions

Infusions are essentially teas. However, don't expect them to be the wimpy herbal brews you find in the tea section of your grocery store. Some may be light and pleasant tasting, but others can be quite strong and nasty.

Infusions are made by pouring hot water over herbs and letting them sit. Some herbs will require special instructions—more or less herbs, hotter or cooler water, longer or shorter infusion. Most, however, can be infused using these standard instructions. Check the herbal. If it gives you special instructions, follow them. If it just says "infusion," use these instructions.

Note: If the tap water in your area is heavily laden with chemicals and fluoride, you would do well to consider filtered or distilled water for your infusions.

Standard infusions

1 ounce (30 g) dried herbs or 2 to 3 ounces (75 g) fresh herbs

2 cups water

If you are making an infusion with seeds like anise or fennel, bruise the seeds lightly. Put the herbs in a pot with a secure lid. Ideally the pot should be nonmetallic. A teapot works well. Boil the water in a separate kettle. Cool it a few seconds, just long enough to stop the boil. Pour the water over the herbs and let them infuse covered for ten to fifteen minutes. After they've steeped, pour the resulting infusion through a strainer or coffee filter. What you don't use immediately can be stored in the refrigerator for up to a day. Infusions should

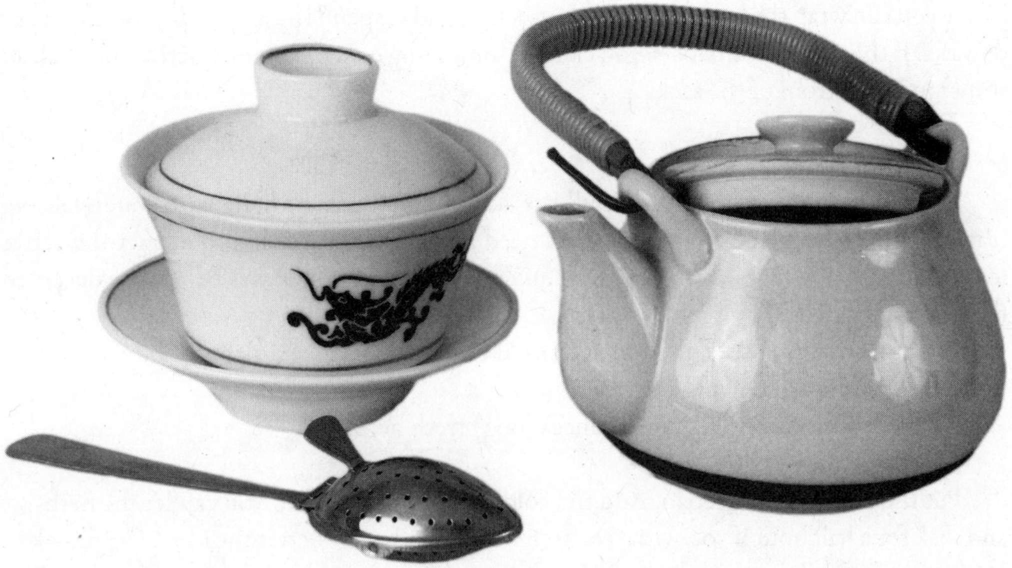

A nonmetallic teapot can be used to make infusions.

be made fresh daily. Note that many herbalists recommend that you *not* use the microwave to reheat herbal decoctions and infusions.

Cold Infusions

Some herbs need cold infusion as heat degrades their active ingredients. Here's how you make a cold infusion:

1 ounce (30 g) dried herbs or 2 to 3 ounces (75 g) fresh herbs

2 cups cool or cold water

Put the herbs in the bottom of a pot with a secure lid. Add the water. Put the lid on tight to prevent the essential oils from evaporating any more than necessary. Let the infusion sit for eight to twelve hours. Strain before using. Alternatively, if you are making a larger

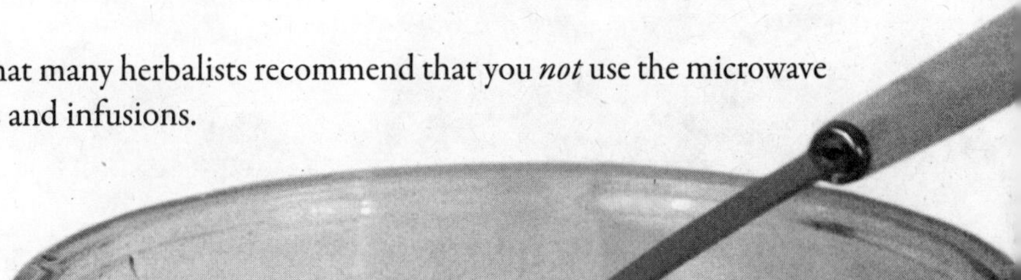

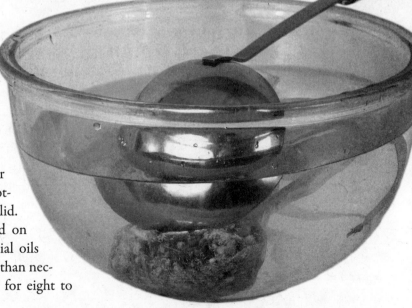

Make cold infusions by tying the herbs in cheesecloth and suspending them in water. You may have to weight the herbs to keep them submerged.

batch, you can wrap the herbs in some cheesecloth and suspend the cheesecloth sack in a pot of water. If the cheesecloth floats, you can put something heavy and nonreactive (like a clean stone) in the bottom of the sack.

Decoctions

Like infusions, decoctions also pull the active ingredients of herbs into water. Decoctions, however, are made from herbs that need a bit more processing to extract the active ingredients. Roots, twigs, bark, tough stems and seeds, and sometimes berries are decocted rather than infused.

If you aren't given specific instructions about how to make a decoction, you can use these standard measurements and procedures:

1 ounce (30g) dried herbs or 2 ounces (60g) fresh herbs

3 cups of water

Put the herbs in a saucepan. Add the cold water. At this point, you can let the herbs sit and soak for a half hour if you wish. The tougher the herbs, the better the idea of a presoak is. Bring to a boil, and then reduce to a simmer. Simmer uncovered at least thirty minutes. You can decoct herbs for an hour or more. A good guideline is to remove the herbs from the heat when the liquid has been reduced by about one third to one half. Pour the liquid through a non-metal strainer or coffee filter. What you don't use immediately can be stored in the refrigerator for up to a day. Decoctions, like infusions should be made fresh daily. Alternatively, they can be frozen in ice cube trays and then stored in cubes in labeled bags in the freezer. The herbs may lose some potency when stored in this way, but decocting the herbs in advance does allow you to keep a decoction on hand for emergency use. Note that many herbalists recommend that you *not* use the microwave to reheat herbal decoctions and infusions.

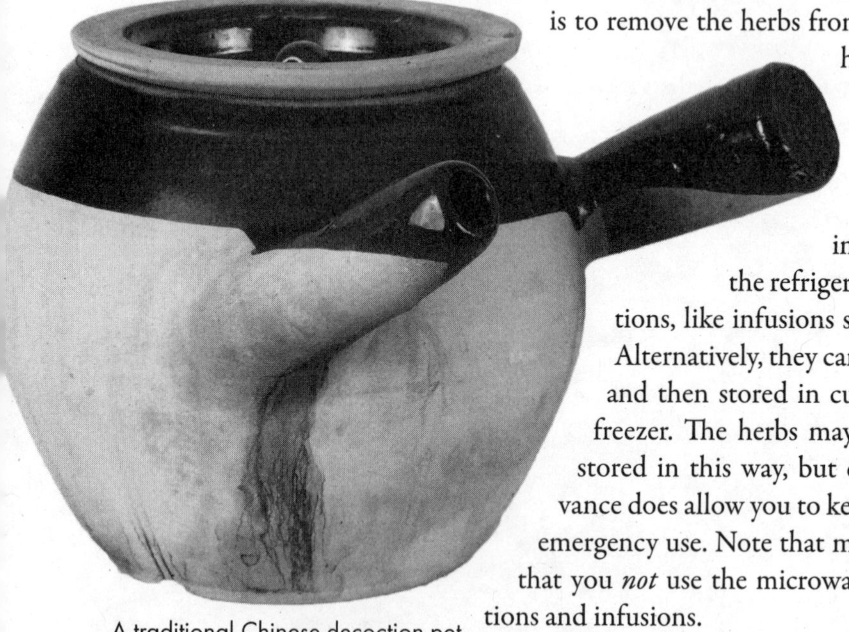

A traditional Chinese decoction pot

Syrups

Syrups are one way to preserve infusions and decoctions. The sugar acts as a preservative in much the same way as it does in jams and jellies. Syrups are especially good for cough formulas as the honey or sugar syrup can be soothing for a raw throat.

Be aware, however, that some herbalists recommend that you not use sugar in your herbal preparations. They cite sugar's harmful effects and its nutritionally "empty" calories. At the very least, try to stay away from refined sugar.

From an infusion or decoction

one part infusion or decoction
one part honey or unrefined sugar
Heat the infusion or decoction. Add the honey or sugar.

From dried herbs

2 ounces herbs
1 quart water
2 ounces honey or glycerin (minimum—you may use more)
Add the water to the herbs. Heat to a boil, reduce to a slow boil, and cook until reduced by about half. Strain. Add honey or glycerin.

From powdered, dried herbs

8 ounces powdered herbs
24 ounces honey, maple syrup, or sugar syrup
Add the herbs directly to the syrup, heat gently for 30 minutes.

For all three versions, allow the syrup to cool, and then pour it into a dark glass bottle with a cork or stopper. The stopper is important because syrups sometimes ferment. A bottle with a tight lid can explode. If you take exception to fermentation and or alcohol, make only enough syrup to use within a few weeks and store it in the refrigerator.

Tinctures

Infusions and decoctions are made with water. Tinctures are made with alcohol or a mixture of alcohol and water (such as can be found in vodka and other liquors). Until about fifty years ago, tinctures were common in the U.S. Pharmacopoeia, the list of medicinal preparations offered by commercial pharmacies. Today the U.S. Pharmacopoeia recognizes few or none.

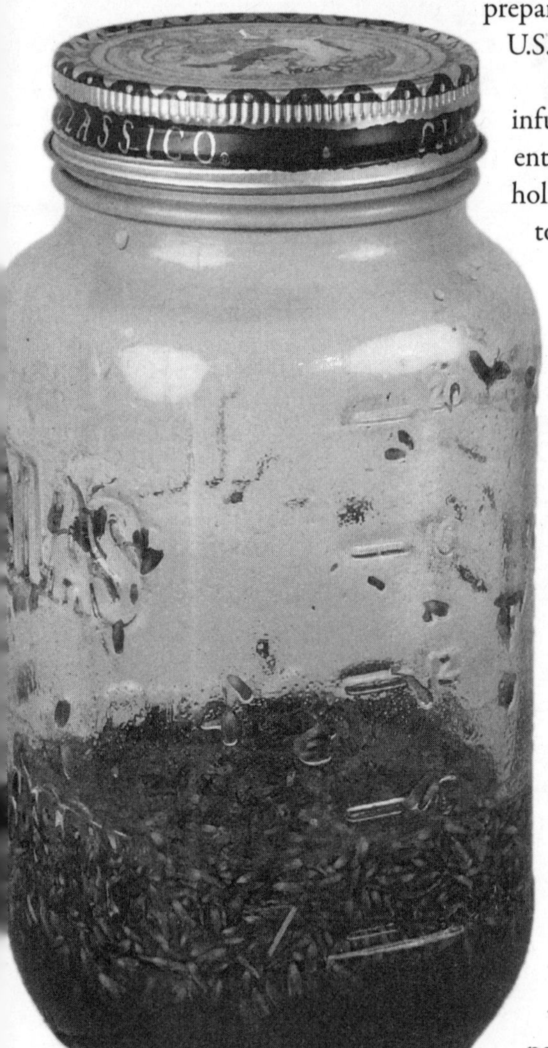

A tincture macerating in a Mason jar.

Why would you want to use a tincture rather than an infusion or decoction? Some herbs have active ingredients that aren't soluble in water but are soluble in alcohol. Tinctures are also particularly good when you want to capitalize on the antimicrobial properties of an herb. Alcohol is a disinfectant, and it also enhances the antimicrobial properties of the chemicals dissolved in it.[1703] If you want to capitalize on this property of alcohol, use an alcohol water mix that is 60–90% alcohol.

If you wish to go beyond the basics, to fine-tune your tinctures, I suggest Richo Cech's *Making Plant Medicine*. He gives the optimal ratio of herb to alcohol and also discusses the fine points of making tinctures. There are advantages and disadvantages, for example, in making tinctures from fresh vs. dried herbs (and those advantages and disadvantages change with the herb). Cech goes into these matters in detail.

Tinctures are formulated by weight. A 1:5 tincture is one part herb to five parts liquid. For a rough calculation, you can say that one fluid ounce of liquid (water or alcohol) weighs one ounce. A 1:5 ratio would then be about one ounce (by weight) of herb to five fluid ounces of liquid.

When you see instruction for tinctures, they will typically look like this: 1:5, 60%. That means use one part herb to five parts alcohol (by weight), and use an alcohol blend that is 60% alcohol to 40% water (or 120 proof). For each herb, follow the instruction in the herbal chapter. If that chapter gives no specific instruction for a given herb, you can use a standard tincture recipe.

Alcohol tincture

For a standard tincture with dried herbs, use a 1:5 ratio and 60% alcohol (though you can get by with 40–50%). For a tincture with fresh herbs, use a 1:2 ratio and 90–95% alcohol. The difference between the two is due to the greater amount of water in the fresh herbs. In the end, both kinds of tinctures end up containing roughly 60% alcohol.

Vodka works fine for dried herbs, but if you want to boost the alcohol percentage beyond 50% (100 proof), you'll need to get a hold of some pure grain alcohol. Caution: NEVER use any kind of industrial or topical alcohol, including methyl alcohol, isopropyl alcohol, or wood alcohol in making tinctures you plan to take orally. They are extremely toxic and could kill you.

If you're using fresh herbs, you can chop them coarsely or you can leave them whole. If you are using dried herbs, crush them with a mortar and pestle. Pour the vodka over the herbs in a large jar with a lid. Allow plenty of headroom. Let the jar stand at room temperature (or slightly warmer), out of direct sunlight. Once a day shake the jar. Tinctures should macerate for roughly two to six weeks. The length of time depends on how tough the herb is. Fresh blossoms are sometimes finished in a week or less. Tough roots can take six to eight weeks.

Tinctures get stronger the longer they macerate. You can tell a tincture is finished when the alcohol has taken on the color, smell, and (for nontoxic herbs) taste of the herb. Pour the liquid through cheese cloth or a jelly bag, or if you have one, you can use a wine press. Once the liquid has run through, squeeze the herbs to get the last of the liquid out. Let tinctures sit for a few days until the sediment settles to the bottom. Then pull the clear liquid off and discard the sediment. Alternatively, a coffee filter can catch a lot of the sediment. Store tinctures in dark glass bottles. Some people like dropper bottles for tinctures because they allow easy measurement of the proper dosage.

Alternative tincture

If the alcohol in the tincture troubles you—if you have religious, health, or personal reasons for avoiding it—you can use the tincture in very hot water. Add the recommended number of drops to near boiling water. Most of the alcohol will evaporate in a few moments, but you will still need to have alcohol around the house. If that's a problem, it's possible to substitute cider vinegar or glycerin for the vodka. These solvents don't work quite the same way as alcohol, and they don't keep as well either, but they are viable alternatives for some herbs. Alternatively, you could simply skip the tinctures. Though tinctures extract more of the plant's active ingredients than water, and though tinctures have a longer shelf life than infusions and decoctions, they are by no means an essential way to use herbs. Most herbs can be used successfully relying on just infusions and decoctions.

Vinegar tincture

1 ounce of dried herb per 5 ounces of vinegar

Follow the instructions for the alcohol tincture, but be aware that the vinegar does not keep as well as alcohol.

Glycerin tincture

Glycerin is sweet, an added benefit when you're making a tincture for a child. It also doesn't dry the skin like alcohol, a benefit for topical preparations being made to treat dry or battered skin. Glycerin has a shelf life of up to a year, not quite as long as alcohol, but longer than vinegar.

Use a 1:4 ratio of herbs to glycerin. Heat the herbs and glycerin until near the boiling point. Then let the mixture macerate in glass, ceramic or clay, not metal. The tincture is ready in about 20 days. Strain it as you would an alcohol tincture.

Infused Oils

Sometimes called infused oils or extracted oils to differentiate them from essential oils, these are plant oils extracted into a carrier oil. Olive, almond, canola, safflower, and sesame are common carrier oils.

Standard infusion

2–4 ounces of dried herbs or twice that if using fresh herbs

1 pint of oil

Crush the herbs with a mortar and pestle. Add the oil. Let the mixture stand in a warm place out of direct light for between three days and a week. Tradition says that oils are best made at the new moon, but we have no known scientific basis for that tradition.

Note that fresh herbs will tend to go bad while infusing more readily than dried herbs. Also, though warmth will help the herbs infuse into the oil more quickly, it will also increase the chances of the herbs in the oil rotting.[1704]

Hot infusion

Hot infusion is good for herbs with coarser, tougher leaves. It's also an alternative if you don't want to wait three days to a week for your infused oil.

Mix the herbs and the carrier oil in a heat-resistant pot. What you want to do is heat the oil gently for 2–3 hours instead of letting it sit. The best way to do this is to warm the oil in a double boiler. Watch it carefully to make sure it doesn't begin to bubble. You want to keep the oil just below a simmer. If the oil is allowed to become too hot, you will be deep-frying your herbs. If you do end up with fried herbs, throw them out and start again.

Alternatively, you can pour oil over herbs in a glass casserole or heat-proof bowl. Put the casserole in a 150-degree oven for 4 hours. Check and stir once an hour. Pour through the oil gauze or a muslin strainer.[1705]

Once the oils have infused, either through the hot or standard method, strain them through cheese cloth and store them in dark glass containers. Some people like to add a 500 I.U. capsule of vitamin E to each cup of oil to help preserve the oil. The more oils are exposed to oxygen, heat, and light, the faster they will go rancid. Unrefined oils go rancid faster

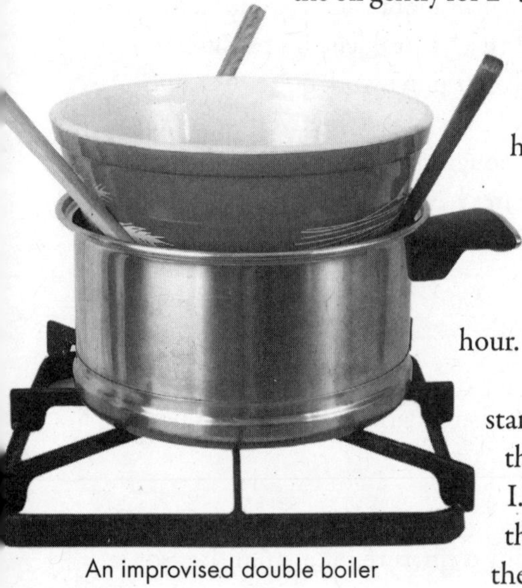

An improvised double boiler

than refined oils, and oils high in polyunsaturated fats go rancid faster than those high in monounsaturated.

Oils for infusion

Almond. A good all-purpose oil for all skin types, it leaves a thin film but penetrates well. It has a light, nutty aroma. It is a good emollient, and consequently it is good in lotions and ointments. Almond oil is also a good massage oil, but it can stain sheets and clothes. It has a high smoke point and so is suited for the hot infusion method.

Avocado. Avocado oil is especially good if you are making an infusion to treat problem skin (eczema, dry skin, etc.). It leaves a fatty layer on the skin. It can be used as a massage oil and is also good in creams and butters. Unrefined avocado oil contains more nutrients than refined, but it's thick and heavy and consequently works best in combination with a lighter oil. Avocado combines well with grape-seed oil. It has a very high smoke point and is suited for the hot infusion method.

Grapeseed. Grapeseed, is light, and has very little odor. It is, however, often refined or partially refined and so may have solvent residues in the oil. It has a high smoke point and so is suited for the hot infusion method. Grape-seed oil will go rancid fairly quickly and needs to stored in a cool, dark place.

Olive. Olive is a good all-purpose oil. It is a common oil in salves and infusions. It leaves a thin layer but still allows the skin to breathe. It may also have some wound healing properties. Be aware that some olive oils have more aroma than others. Get cold-pressed to avoid solvents in the oil. It does not have as high a smoke point as most oils and may not be as well-suited to the hot infusion method.

Sesame. Sesame is a relatively stable oil with good nutritional qualities. It's a good bath oil and massage oil. It's also a good moisturizer. It generally doesn't stain clothes and sheets. It has a high smoke point and so is suited for the hot infusion method. Look for pure, expeller-pressed sesame oil, *not* the toasted sesame oil used in some Asian cooking.

Soybean. Soybean has good healing properties. It has very little odor, but some people are sensitive to it. It's a good bath oil. It does not have as high a smoke point as most oils and so may not be as well-suited to the hot infusion method.

Sunflower. Sunflower has good nutritional properties and doesn't leave much of a residue. It's better for bath oils and lotions than massage.

Essential Oils

Essential oils are made commercially using a steam distillation process. Many pounds of plants are distilled into tiny bottles of essential oil, which is the essence of the active ingredients of those herbs. Essential oils can be *very strong*. They are almost always used in very small quantities (drops or fractions of milliliters) and are diluted in water or oil. If you choose to use essential oils, you should know what the maximum safe dose is for that oil, and you should begin by staying well under that dose.

Essential oils can be mixed into creams and salves. They can be included in carrier oils for use in massage. Those few essential oils that are safe for internal use can be mixed into carrier liquids. How they are used depends a great deal, however, on the individual oil, its toxicity and its potential for skin irritation.

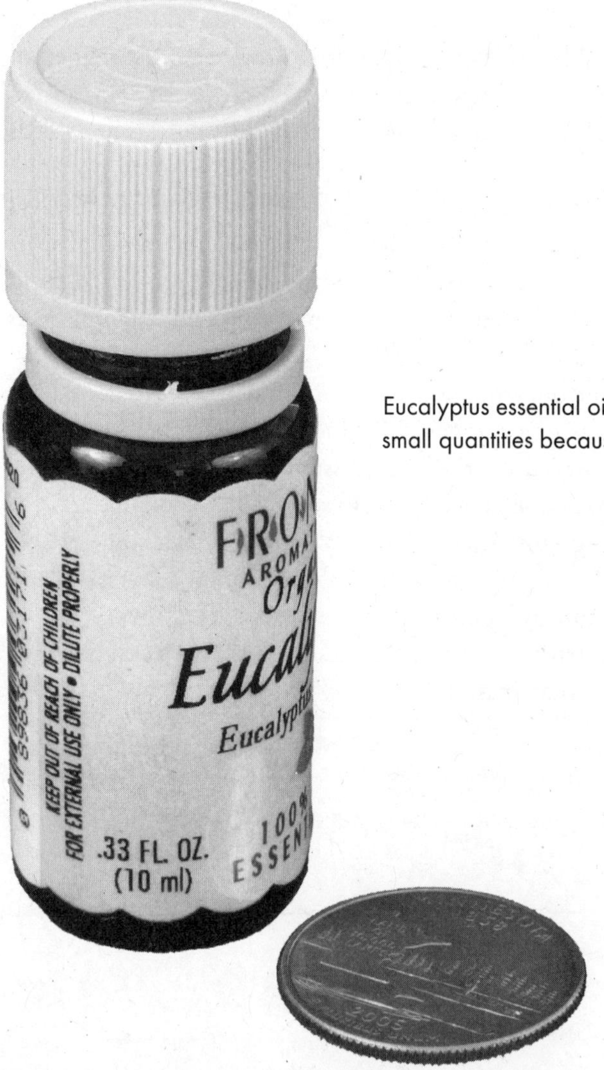

Eucalyptus essential oil. Essential oils are typically sold in small quantities because they are so highly concentrated.

Creams and Salves

Creams and salves are ways of thickening herbal preparations for ease of use. Oils tend to run off before you can work them into the skin. Infusions and decoctions require a compress. Creams and salves, however, will stay where you put them more easily.

Choosing a method for making a cream or salve depends on several factors. First is the question of how easily you want the preparation to absorb. In general, creams are made to be worked into the skin. Ideally, a cream will blend with the skin and not leave much of a discernable trace. Salves, by contrast, are not supposed to blend into the skin, but are supposed to stay as a thin layer on the surface of the skin. Salves, sometimes called ointments, provide a layer of protection against moisture or dehydration. Practically speaking, however, the difference between creams and salves is not always so pronounced. Some creams leave a residue. Some salves can be worked partially into the skin.

Second is the issue of how long you would like the preparation to keep. In general, homemade creams and salves don't last as long as store-bought ones. If you begin with fresh herbs or if you use a recipe with water in it, you have a much greater chance of your salves and creams becoming moldy. Sometimes you will choose to use water in a cream anyway because water increases the absorbability. If you're willing for the cream or salve to be a bit greasier to decrease the chance of mold, you need to make sure the oils you start with contain no water at all.[1706] Furthermore, there is the question of whether you would rather have a salve that keeps well but contains some petroleum-based ingredients, or would you prefer all vegetable oils and waxes, knowing that they won't keep as long? Oils go rancid. It's their nature. You can do a few things to retard that process, but you can't stop it. On the other hand, if you have sensitive skin, oils and waxes may be less irritating than petroleum jelly. If you need the preparation to be absorbed into the skin, vegetable oils will work better than petroleum jelly. Also petroleum jelly is *not* recommended for burns or for frequent use near or in the nose.

Third is the issue of which preparation best dissolves the active ingredients of an herb. Some herbs infuse well into oil, which can then be made into a salve. Others, however, like witch hazel, nettles, and marshmallow, give up their active ingredients best when infused or decocted in water. For herbs like this, method two, in which the active ingredients are infused into water and then transferred into oil, has the best chance of yielding a good result. Still other herbs, like myrrh and peppermint, need alcohol to dissolve some of their active ingredients. For them you'll want to use method six, in which a tincture is added to a cream. For herbs that work best as a cold infusion, use method five. For those that work best with a hot infusion method, methods one, two or four should work.

Method one: for herbs that infuse into oil

1 ounce emulsifying wax
½ cup infused oil
1 ounce vegetable glycerin
1 cup distilled water

20–30 drops essential oils (optional)

1 capsule vitamin E

In a double boiler, combine the wax, oil, and glycerin. Heat slowly until the wax has melted and everything is combined. Try to avoid heating the wax over 150 degrees. Cool to about 110 degrees. Heat the water to 110 degrees and slowly pour it into the oils. Beat with either a whisk, a mixer, or a stick blender for a few minutes (2–3). Add the essential oils and vitamin E, and beat for another two minutes. Pour into containers and label.

Emulsifying wax and glycerin are products that can be purchased at soap and lotion making supply houses. (See Chapter 6 for places where you can get them.) Emulsifying wax helps keep the oil and water in the lotion from separating. Glycerin is an emollient, which means it helps soften the skin. In this recipe, you can use just the infused oil and skip the essential oils, or you can use plain oil (in other words, not herb infused) and add the herbal ingredients via the essential oil, or you can use both.

Method two: for herbs that infuse into water

1 cup herbs

3 to 4 cups water

5 ounces sesame or olive oil

2 ounces beeswax

Simmer the herbs and water in a non-metallic container for about 15 minutes for aerial (i.e., aboveground) parts (herbs you would normally infuse), 30 minutes (at a stronger boil) for roots and twigs (herbs you would normally decoct). Strain the herbs out and return the liquid to the pot and reheat. Add the oil to the water and continue to simmer over low heat until all of the water has evaporated. Be careful that the oil doesn't heat past the smoking point. Melt 2 ounces of beeswax in a separate container. Try to have the wax and the oil mixture at the same temperature. Stir the wax into the oil mixture. Stir to combine as quickly as possible. After the mixture cools a bit, you can mix in 2 teaspoons of Vitamin E oil as a preservative. Store in small air-tight containers.

Some herbs have active ingredients that are best extracted via infusion or decoction. This cream works best for those kinds of herbs. However, any water in the final ointment increases the chance of the ointment separating and/or going moldy. You need to simmer the water and oil together until *all* of the water is evaporated. If you want to help ensure that no water gets into the final salve, you can let the oil sit for a week. The water will settle to the bottom. You can then skim or siphon off the oil and reheat it to use in your cream.

Method three: herbs in petroleum jelly

10 parts petroleum jelly or soft paraffin wax

1 part dried herb

Melt the wax or petroleum jelly in a double boiler. Add the herbs. Heat for about two hours or until the herbs become crisp. Pour the mixture through a cheesecloth or jelly bag.

Squeeze the remainder out of the bag. Quickly pour the mixture while still warm into clean air-tight storage jars.

Method four: for herbs that infuse into oil

3 ounces powdered herbs (as fine a powder as possible)

7 ounces cocoa butter or another pure vegetable butter (shea butter, sal butter, mango butter, etc.)

1 ounce beeswax, more or less, depending upon the consistency desired and the consistency of the butter you choose.

1 capsule vitamin E

Mix the herbs, cocoa butter, and beeswax and heat in a small covered pot over low heat for one to two hours, stirring frequently. If you like, you can add some vitamin E oil toward the very end of cooking. Blend the mixture thoroughly and pour it into small air-tight containers.[1707]

Method five: for herbs that infuse into oil

For a large batch, 1 to 1 1/3 quarts infused oil and 6 ounces of beeswax

or for a smaller batch, 1 cup infused oil and 1 ounce beeswax

For this method, you must start with oil that's already been infused. You can use a single infused oil for this salve, or you can combine appropriate oils. Heat the oil to about 150 degrees F in a double boiler. Melt the wax until fluid over low heat. Warning: wax left unattended on the stove for too long will ignite. Stir the wax into the warm oil and keep stirring (still over heat) until they are combined. Pour into small air-tight containers.[1708]

Method six: for herbs that infuse into alcohol

Some herbs only yield their active ingredients to alcohol, not to oil or water. For those herbs, use this method to produce the salve.

Add ½ to 1 teaspoon of tincture to each ounce of either commercial skin lotion, cocoa butter, or homemade salve. Note that you can use a homemade salve that already contains an herbal preparation.

Method seven: for essential oils

Add essential oil to prepared salve, vegetable butters, or commercial lotions. Note that the simpler the formula, the less likely the essential oil is to have a nasty reaction to another active ingredient.

Mastering Creams and Salves

Here are a couple of tricks to make the process of making homemade creams and salves simpler: The ratio of oil to wax is approximate. After the wax and oil have melted together, drop a bit of the hot mixture into ice water. The mixture should set up as a small soft glob. If it spreads over the surface like oil, you need more wax to make an salve consistency. If it sets up closer to candle-like consistency, you need more oil. Note that if you plan to rub the salve into the skin over a large area, you want it thinner. If you want it to stay on a smaller area, you want it thicker. With practice you'll be able to tell from the consistency of this glob how thick the final salve will be.

Even with cold water testing, your final product might be too hard or too soft. If that's true, you can always melt it and try again. Add a bit more oil to make it softer, a bit more wax to make it harder.

Water will decrease the storage time of your cream or salve. If you used fresh herbs in your infused oil, let the oil sit for a week to separate. The water will settle with the muck at the bottom. Skim or siphon off the oil and use it in your salve.[1709]

To delay deterioration, you can keep salves and creams in the refrigerator. Adding a single drop of mint essential oil for each ounce of salve may also help slow this process as well as protect against mold. Mint oil may, however, increase the chance of you or someone else being allergic to your salve. Alternatively, you can add a bit of vitamin E to the salve (roughly one part vitamin E oil to 100 parts salve).[1710]

Note: for all of these salves, clean your pans while they are still warm with paper towels or cloths. Once they cool (or once you pour water into them), the remaining salve will set up and the pans will be more difficult to clean.

Powders and Capsules

It's preferable to get powdered herbs in that form from commercial suppliers. Grinding your own herbs with a coffee grinder or even a mortar and pestle can generate heat, which can change the properties of the herb.[1711]

Powders can be stirred into water, sprinkled on food, or they can be made into capsules. Capsules come in 4, 3, 2, 1, 0, 00, and 000 sizes, with 000 being the largest, and 4 being child or pet size. The best all-purpose size is 00, though you will need to check the volume of your brand of capsule and compare it to your needs. Capsule fillers are available and make filling capsules quicker. You can, however, simply scoop, fill, and fit the two halves of a capsule together by hand. Unless you plan to make a lot of filled capsules, the hand method works just fine.

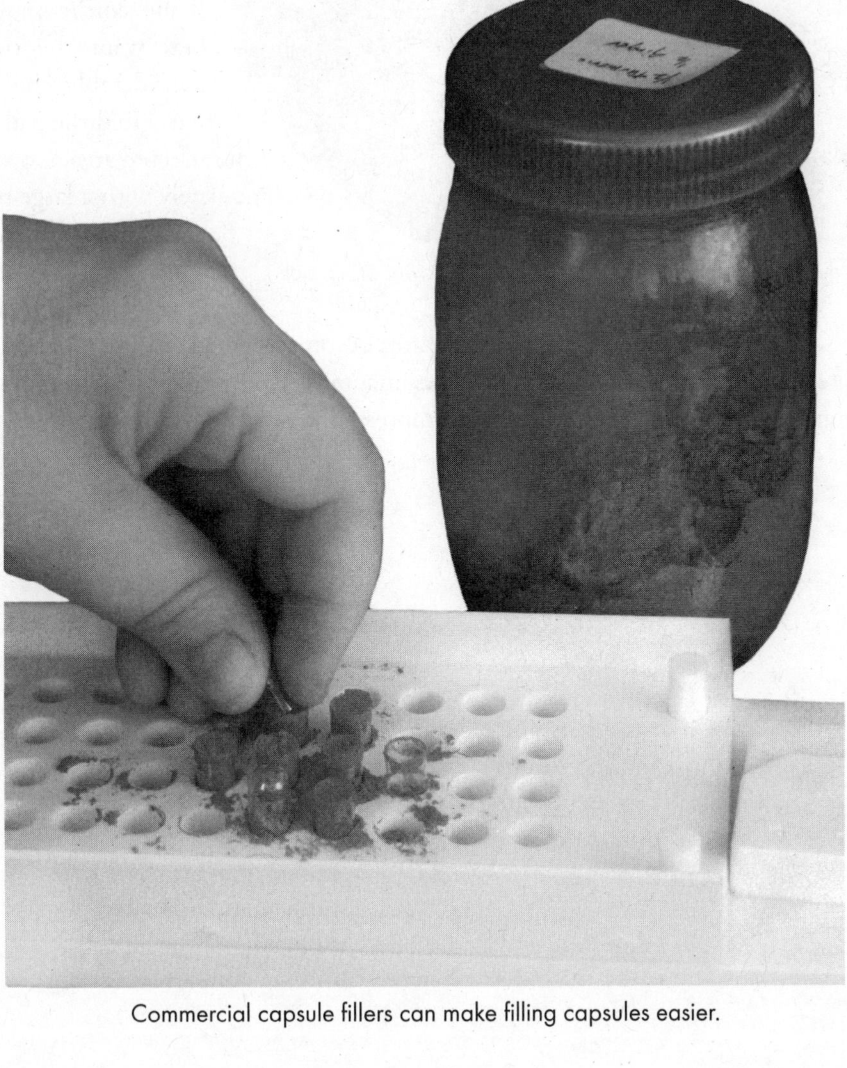

Commercial capsule fillers can make filling capsules easier.

Compresses

Compresses are used to accelerate healing of wounds or muscle injuries. Compresses can be any temperature and can apply either water- or alcohol-based preparations to the skin.

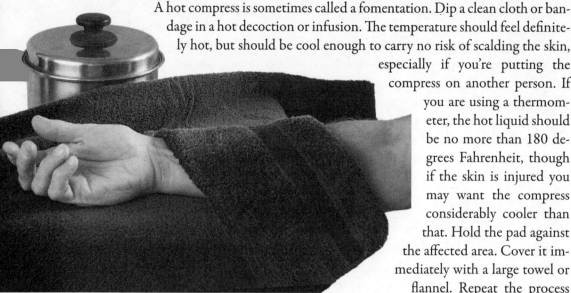

A hot compress is sometimes called a fomentation. Dip a clean cloth or bandage in a hot decoction or infusion. The temperature should feel definitely hot, but should be cool enough to carry no risk of scalding the skin, especially if you're putting the compress on another person. If you are using a thermometer, the hot liquid should be no more than 180 degrees Fahrenheit, though if the skin is injured you may want the compress considerably cooler than that. Hold the pad against the affected area. Cover it immediately with a large towel or flannel. Repeat the process when the compress cools or dries. Keep the area under compress for no more than 30 minutes. If the area becomes flushed or tingles, that's good. If it becomes red or painful or itches or becomes uncomfortable, remove the compress.

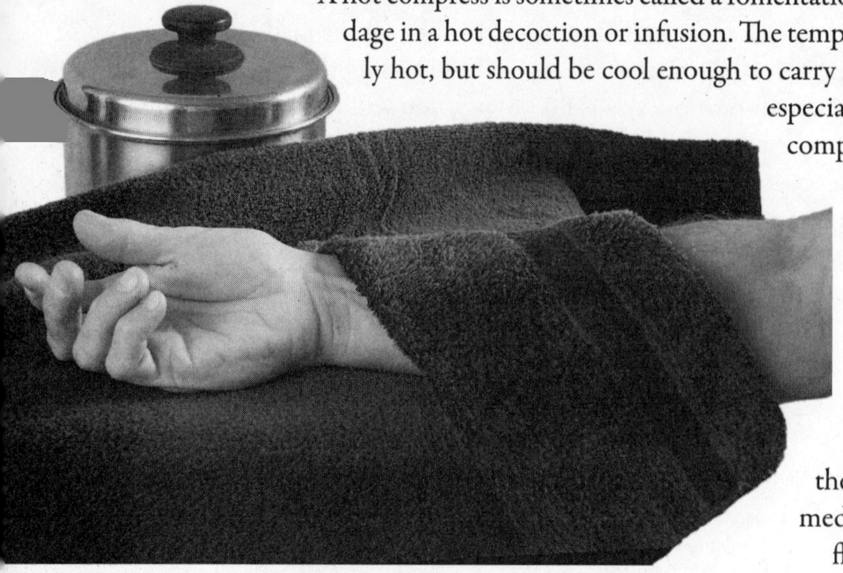

Place the compress over the affected area and cover with a towel or flannel.

If you can't insure the sterility of your compress, don't use it on an open wound.

Poultices

Poultices are used much like compresses, but poultices employ solids rather than liquids. If using powders, add enough water to make a paste. If using fresh herbs chop them coarsely and boil them in a little water for 2–5 minutes. Drain off the excess water and cool the herbs until they are still hot but not scalding. Apply a little oil to the skin to keep the herbs from sticking. Then spread the herb mixture over the affected area. Secure the mixture to the skin with a gauze bandage or cotton strips. Some people secure a poultice with kitchen plastic wrap. Doing so can be less messy than using cloth strips, but it also changes the environment inside the poultice. Air can't pass through the plastic. Neither can the fluids from the poultice or perspiration from the body.

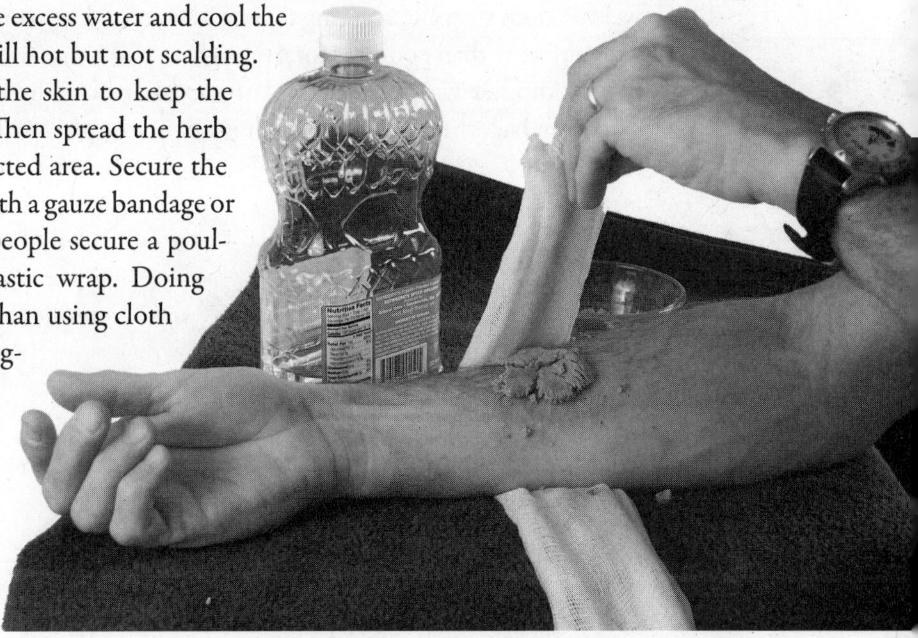

To make a poultice, make a paste of the herbs and secure them to the skin with a bandage or strip of cloth.

Note that this treatment is too intense for very hot, very active herbs such as mustard or capsicum. These herbs can cause burns and blisters when used as a poultice.

Historically, poultices have been used on wounds, even open wounds. Though some herbalists still follow this practice, its safety is questionable. It's almost impossible to control the cleanliness of poultices. Contaminants on the herbs can be introduced to the wounds. When dealing with open wounds, diluted tinctures made of alcohol tend to be a safer choice (and even then, you run some risk of infection and/or irritation from the alcohol). Always make sure that dressings, bandages, and cloth strips used in poultices are sterile.

Plasters

Plasters are like poultices, but they are more appropriate for sensitive skin. To make a plaster, put a fine layer of oil over the affected area. Put a strip of cotton cloth over that. Then proceed with the instructions for a poultice, layering herbs over the cloth strip and securing them with a second strip or a gauze bandage. Plasters are safer than poultices for overnight use.[1712]

Another way to make a plaster is to enclose the herbs in a lightweight cotton bag, then moisten it with water or vinegar and lay it over the effected area. It can be strapped down with a bandage for longer-term or nighttime use. Note that plasters have many of the same sterility issues as poultices.

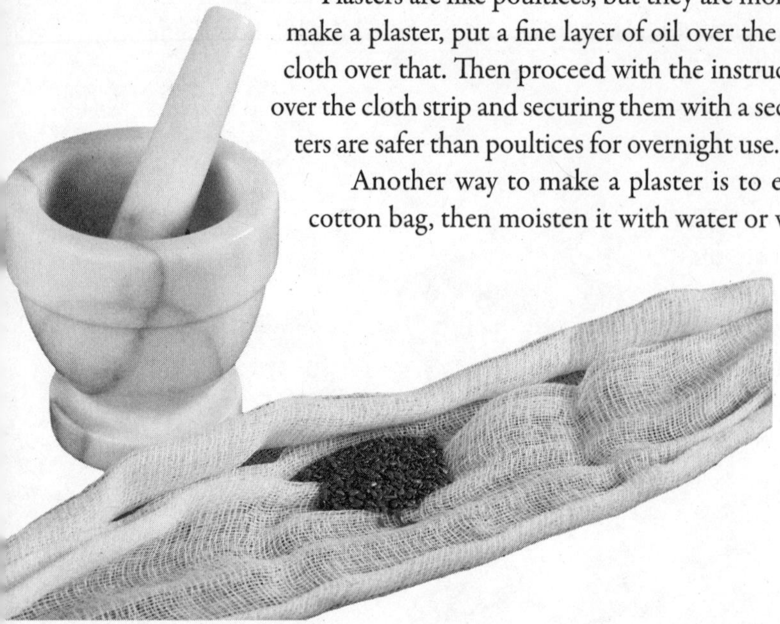

Herbs can also be folded into lightweight cotton fabric for use as a plaster.

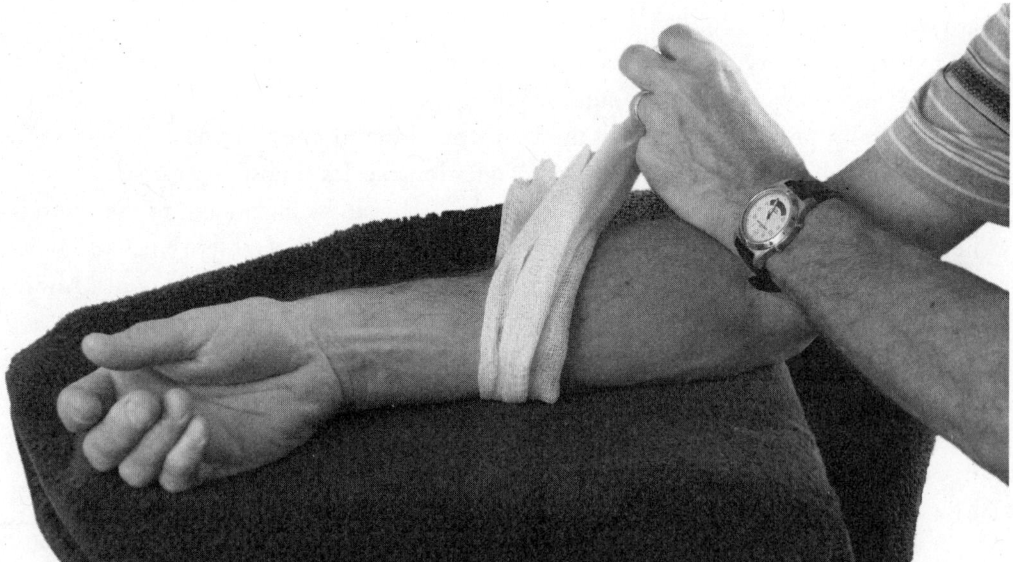

Moisten the plaster and wrap it around the affected area.

Liniments

Liniments are watery concoctions rubbed on the skin to soothe the aches and pains of sore muscles and joints. They are typically rubefacients. The word "rubefacient" comes from the Latin word "to make red." Liniments are typically counterirritants that provide a minor irritation that depletes the sensory neurons of neurotransmitters. That depletion means pain sensations can no longer be transmitted through the body to the brain. The injury that causes the pain is still there, but the pain of the injury is lessened.

Liniments are usually rubbed on the surface of the skin but not worked in too vigorously.

Surface application increases circulation to the area[1713] and blocks pain. Working them in too vigorously can increase the chance of unwanted irritation and even blisters.

Peppermint, camphor, rosemary, and cayenne pepper are common ingredients in liniments. Infused oils, infusions and decoctions, essential oils added to a carrier—all these can function as a liniment. If you wish, you can make your liniment into a cream or ointment to help it stay where you put it, thus making it easier to handle. Ben-Gay, Tiger Balm®, Atomic Balm®, and other sports rubs are essentially liniments made into ointments or creams.

Inhalants

Inhalants combine tinctures or essential oils with steam so they can be inhaled. As you might expect, you can use more tincture in an inhalant than essential oils. For most tinctures, you can use about a tablespoon of the tincture to each pint of water. For essential oil, use 3–4 drops in a pint of water. Heat the water until steaming, add the tincture or oil, and stir. Inhale the steam slowly and deeply for ten minutes, keeping your head and the bowl of water covered with a towel to trap the steam. If you feel a bit dizzy while inhaling the steam, uncover your head for a moment.

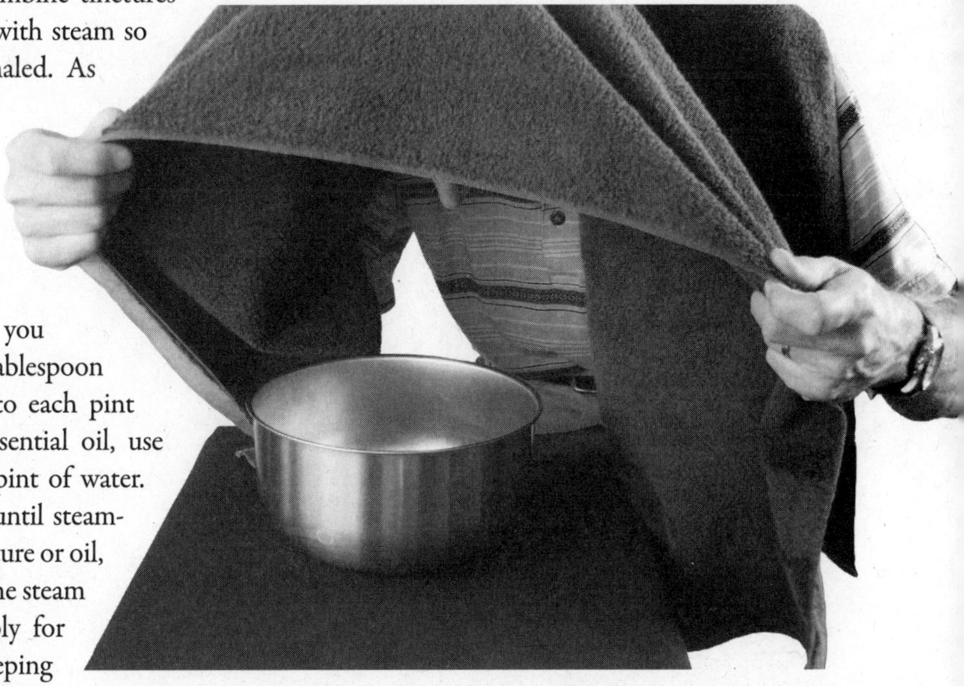

A steam tent can be made using a bowl and large towel

Massage Oils

Massage oils are made by mixing essential oils with a carrier oil. Almond, wheat germ, and sunflower oils are the most common, but if you want to experiment, here are some possibilities:

Normal Skin. Almond, canola, corn, grapeseed, peanut, sesame, safflower

Dry Skin. Almond, canola, cocoa butter, grapeseed, olive, peanut

Oily Skin. Soy

The active ingredients in essential oils begin to break down when they are mixed with the carrier oil, so only make up enough oil for your immediate use.

Infused oils can also be used for massage. Make sure, though, that the oils are matched to the condition. Most infused oils that are appropriate for strains or sprains, for example, would not be appropriate for a relaxing massage.

Chapter Four

Applications and Uses

First of all, it bears saying: use your head. Some injuries require a doctor. Get professional help to stitch cuts, assess the severity of breaks or severe bruising, and render an opinion on chronic problems. Then if the doctor sends you home saying something along the lines of "it's just a sprain; stay off it," herbal remedies give you an option that may help decrease the time you need to baby the injury before returning to training. These remedies are not to be used instead of standard medical care. They are not intended to replace commonly accepted first aid procedures. Their purpose is to give your body some herbal help while it goes about healing injuries and illness.

Secondly, know your body. If you tend to have sensitive skin, don't just slap an unknown poultice on a new injury. Test the herb first on healthy skin. Start to use it slowly to see how well you tolerate it. Some herbs have powerful effects, not all of them pleasant. Some people react more strongly to herbs' effects than others. Assess your past history with herbs and your willingness to take risks before using any herb.

Thirdly, know the herb before you use it. Before mixing up one of these remedies, read the information about the herb in this book and in a couple of other books or Web sites as well. No one book or teacher can tell you everything. If you have any questions or concerns, talk to an herbalist, a naturopath, or a doctor with training in herbal medicine. It is your responsibility to educate yourself about what you put into and on your body.

Fourthly, when combining herbs, less is more. Simples (remedies using only one herb) are common and appropriate for many uses. Adding smaller amounts of a second or third herb can enhance the effect of the first or cancel it out if you don't know what you're doing. Adding several different herbs will sometimes just give you mud. Until you know what you're doing, get your combinations from trained herbalists. Though I have not used all these combinations myself, I have gotten them from what I consider to be reputable sources.

Joint Pain and Inflammation

If you have joint pain in multiple joints, or if the pain lasts longer than you would expect for a minor injury, you need to be evaluated by a doctor. If you are already being treated for joint pain, talk to your doctor about whether one of these remedies complements the treatment you and she or he have already agreed upon.

Many of the herbal remedies for joint pain operate on the principle of counterirritation. "Counterirritation" is when you apply an irritant to treat an irritant. For example, let's say you have a mosquito bite. It itches, so what do you do? You scratch. You purposely irritate the skin and by doing so relieve the itch of the bite. Part of counterirritation is simply creating a diversion.[1714] The sensations on the skin take the mind away from pain deeper in the body. The effects, however, go beyond diversion to the neurological. When the body is continually exposed to a counterirritant, sensory neurons are depleted of neurotransmitters. The cause of the pain remains, but the pain signal no longer reaches the brain because of the lack of neurotransmitters. This leads to reduction in sensation of pain. When the exposure is discontinued, the neurons recover.[1715]

This deadening of pain is both the good news and the bad news. On the one hand, it makes you feel better until you can heal. On the other hand, it also deadens the body's natural warning system, the system by which pain persuades you to stop doing something that is hurting you. What a counterirritant doesn't do is fix the underlying problem. You don't heal yourself using a counterirritant; you simply take the pain or itch down a notch.

Here are a few formulas for joint pain. Most operate on the principle of counterirritation.

General joint pain, including arthritis[1716]

Make a massage oil of
10–20 drops eucalyptus oil
10–20 drops rosemary oil
½ tablespoon almond oil
Make a liniment of :
¼ teaspoon powdered cayenne (red pepper)
1 cup grain alcohol

Joint pain from minor injuries

Make a massage oil of

5–10 drops of yarrow oil (essential oil) in 1–½ tablespoon of infused St. John's wort oil.[1717]

If the injury is still swollen, don't massage deeply but rather spread the oil lightly over the surface of the skin.

Joint pain from exertion

Make a massage oil of
5–10 drops of ginger essential oil
1-½ tablespoons almond oil.
1–2 drops of eucalyptus oil (optional)

Joints inflammation

Other herbs can actually go to the root of the pain and inflammation, and help heal joint inflammation. These herbs are taken internally. Note that you should not be combining these herbs without professional supervision.

Bromelain: especially knee pain, both from swelling and arthritis.
Cat's claw: for both swelling and inflammation.
Evening primrose oil: for use in joint pain due to arthritis.

Ginger: for use in joint pain due to arthritis.

Fish oil: for reduction of pain and swelling due to arthritis.

Sprains

If you're sure you're dealing with a garden-variety sprain, a couple of herbs may be able to decrease the time you need to spend away from training. Sprains have two stages: the initial swelling and the subsequent repair of damaged tissue.

Western medicine typically recommends R.I.C.E. for the initial stages of a sprain. R.I.C.E. stands for rest, ice, compression, and elevation. Not all herbalists agree with this recommendation, however. Some, particularly traditional Chinese herbalists, agree with the importance of rest and elevation, but note that ice and compression decrease the circulation to the injured area. Limiting the circulation also limits the body's ability to bring resources to bear upon the healing process as well as the ability to remove waste products away from the injury. Instead of ice, these medical personnel recommend an herbal anti-inflammatory. Chinese medicine has *san huang san*, so-called "herbal ice." (See Tom Bisio's *Tooth From a Tiger's Mouth* for more information about *san huang san*.) Western herbal medicine doesn't have a formula nearly as sophisticated as *san huang san*, but it does have arnica and comfrey. Arnica excels at taking down swelling. Comfrey excels at rebuilding.

Arnica works best as a simple (not in combination with other herbs). Apply cream to the affected area, or soak a pad in diluted tincture and use it as a compress. Commercially prepared arnica cream or arnica tincture can be kept in a first aid kit. Arnica helps reabsorption of internal bleeding in sprains. Note that you should never do deep massage on any new sprain. Rub the arnica liberally onto the surface of the affected joint and let it work its way into the joint on its own.

Comfrey is perhaps the best herb for sprains. You can use it after a few days of arnica, or you can begin using just comfrey right away. Studies show that a 10% active ingredient cream, made from 25 g of fresh herb per 100 g of cream is very effective.[1718] You can also use a comfrey decoction. The decoction is made from the roots, which contain more allatoin, so it's better for deep injuries than the leaves.[1719] The leaves contain more tannins and are better for surface injuries where skin tightening is an issue. [1720] For sprained fingers, toes, or ankles, you can use the decoction as a soak, submerging the entire joint. For larger joints, you can use a compress soaked in the decoction. For those times when you have whole-body, fallen down a flight of stairs style injuries, you can add the decoction to a bath. Avoid using the comfrey bath, however, if you have any broken skin on your body.

Infused comfrey oil (made by the hot infusion method) can be used for sprains. The oil is especially good as a massage oil when sprains are in the recovery stage. (Don't massage injuries that are still in the inflammation stage.)

Comfrey poultice for general use on sprains[1721]

Grind the comfrey roots. Add water to make a thick paste. Spread the paste to a thickness of about one inch. Secure with bandages. It's best to leave it on overnight and wash it off in the morning. Leave the injury untreated during the day, and then reapply the next night until the injury is healed.

Use "Comfrey Plus" massage oil[1722] for sprains after the swelling and tenderness has subsided and mobility has begun to be restored.

Comfrey (encourages cell regrowth in the tissues)

Thyme (stimulates blood flow)

Lavender (anti-spasmodic)

Make an infused oil from the comfrey, then add 4 drops each of the thyme and lavender essential oils to 1 1/2 tablespoons of the infused comfrey oil. Don't use this oil long-term (for more than three weeks).

Jammed fingers and other joint injury with nerve involvement

Two parts comfrey

One part St. John's wort[1723]

Make an infused oil of two parts comfrey, one part St. John's wort. This oil can be applied as a liniment, or it can be made into a salve using any of the methods that work well for infused oils. (*Don't* massage the oil in deeply when the injury is still in the inflammation stage.)

Injuries that require regeneration of joint or connective tissue

You might also consider using horsetail. Horsetail decoctions contain silica, calcium, and minerals, in a form that's accessible to the body. Your body needs all these nutrients to heal connective tissue injuries.[1724] A decoction of horsetail taken orally may help speed healing of connective tissue injuries. (Make sure you read the information about thiaminase in the "What should you be aware of" section of the herbal before using horsetail internally.)

We also have one study that shows that bromelain may help with the pain during recovery from ligament damage.

Fractures

If you suspect a fracture, get professional medical help. Western herbal medicine doesn't have a very good track record when it comes to helping broken bones heal. It does, however, have one herb that may have some benefit: horsetail.

Horsetail decoctions contain silica, calcium, and minerals in a form that's accessible to the body. Your body need all these nutrients to heal fractures.[1725] A decoction of horsetail taken orally may help speed healing of fractures. (Make sure you read the information about thiaminase in the "What should you be aware of before using it" section of the herbal before using horsetail internally.)

Tradition says that hand and foot baths containing horsetail decoction may also help speed fractures in those areas. Alternatively, you can make the powder into a paste and use it as a poultice on fractures.[1726] The scientific recognition of that use, however, is lacking.

Bruises and Contusions

"Contusion" is simply another name for a bruise. Impact of something blunt upon the body causes a bruise when that impact damages capillaries and blood seeps into the surrounding tissue. The state of the body at the time of impact makes a difference in the amount of bruising. Various herbs can cause increased chance of bruising. So can dietary deficiencies. The older you get, the more likely you are to suffer a bruise from an impact. Blood vessels get more fragile with age, so capillaries are more likely to be injured and cause bruising. Consequently, if a child has a moderate to large bruise, it is more likely to be serious and require medical assistance than if an older person has the same size bruise.

The location of the bruise also makes a difference in the size of the bruise. If tissue is crushed into the underlying bone, for example, damage to the capillaries is likely to be more severe and the bruise is more likely to be large and visible. If the impact crushes the underlying muscle as well as the skin, a deeper bruise is the result.

If the bruise is on your head and of a significant size, have it checked out by a doctor. You may have injured something more than just skin.

Again, Western medicine recommends ice for bruises. And again, some herbalists take exception to this recommendation. (See the section on sprains in this chapter for more information about the controversy.) If you do chose to use an herbal remedy instead of the ice, use a light touch when applying it. Massaging fresh bruises typically worsens the injury.

Bromelain taken orally either before bruising or as soon as possible after bruising can help the bruise heal more quickly. If you are taking bromelain, you should take it instead of NSAIDs like ibuprofen or aspirin (not in addition to). Doing so may not be as great a sacrifice as it would first appear. Questions are beginning to arise as to whether NSAIDs help or hinder healing of soft tissue. A quick Internet search on "NSAID, healing, bruises" will acquaint you with the debate.

Basic bruises

Arnica is probably your best bet for garden-variety bruises. You can use it on a compress, or you can buy a commercially prepared cream.

Horse chestnut. We have one study showing that horse chestnut may be useful for treating bruises when applied topically. Ten grams of 2% aescin gel applied in a single dose within five minutes of bruising reduced the tenderness of the bruise.[1727]

Trauma salve (not for use on broken skin)[1728]

Make an infused oil using

4 parts calendula dried flowers

4 parts arnica dried flowers

2 parts St. John's wort fresh flowers (or 1 part dried flowers)

Use ointment method three in Chapter 3 to assemble the salve.

Bruises with blood stagnation. Use an arnica cream or compresses to help disperse stagnant blood.

Light bruising all over. After a hard day of training, to relax and help promote healing, add chamomile and Epsom salt to a hot bath. The Epsom salt helps with bruising, and the chamomile relaxes and helps reduce capillary fragility.[1729] Note, however, that Epsom salt shouldn't be used more than three days each week.

The morning after a hard day's training. Run a bath, add eight to ten drops of the essential oil of rosemary (or a quarter of a cup of the infused oil) and some Epsom salt (if you didn't use it the night before). The rosemary helps decrease the stiffness in your joints and muscles and improve your circulation, and the smell of the rosemary oil helps you wake up and get moving again. Note, however, that Epsom salt should not be used more than three days each week.

Old bruises. Try rosemary oil. Bruises that have died back to green or yellow can be treated with rosemary massage oil, which increases the circulation and helps clear out the stagnant blood. Finely chop the fresh rosemary leaves and place them in a glass jar with a tight lid. Cover the plant material with a light extra-virgin olive oil making sure the oil completely covers the plant. Place in a dark, warm place. Infuse for 10 days to 6 weeks, then strain, bottle, and label.

Complex bruises

Bruises with nerve involvement. Try St. John's wort. Use the infused oil of St. John's wort full strength. Soak a gauze pad in the oil, place it on the affected area, and secure it with a bandage.[1730] Leave the pad on overnight. (Note: If you suspect nerve involvement, that's a good time to get a professional medical opinion.)

Bruises that leave a hard lump. In rare cases, a bruised muscle may try to repair itself using bone cells rather than muscle cells resulting in a traumatic myositis ossificans, a hard lump in the muscle. Not applying immediate therapy can increase the chance of this happening. So can massaging the bruise before the inflammation goes down. Some of these lumps go away on their own. Others don't. Wait until the bruise has completely healed before trying to treat the lump. Massaging a bruise before it's healed *causes* these lumps; it doesn't cure them. One clinical experience shows that acetic acid, the acid in vinegar may help with these lumps.[1731] If you've talked to your doctor, and she says, "There's not much we can do short of surgery," you might try massaging vinegar into the lump for a few weeks to see if it helps. It's a long shot, but Western herbalism and medicine don't have much beyond surgery for these kinds of lumps. Chinese herbalism, however, does have some possibilities, but they require you to seek the help of a Chinese herbal or herbalist.

Black eye. Arnica has an excellent herbal track record when it comes to treating bruises. For some people, however, it's too strong to use on the face, especially the sensitive area around the eye. If you don't want to use arnica for a bruise on the face, try this: Start out with ice. Put a cold pack on the bruise for about ten to twenty minutes at a time, then taking a break for an hour or two. You can repeat this (on for twenty minutes, off for two hours) as often as you'd like for the first twenty-four hours or until the bruise has fully developed (in other words, your body has stopped bleeding into the tissue). At that point, switch to

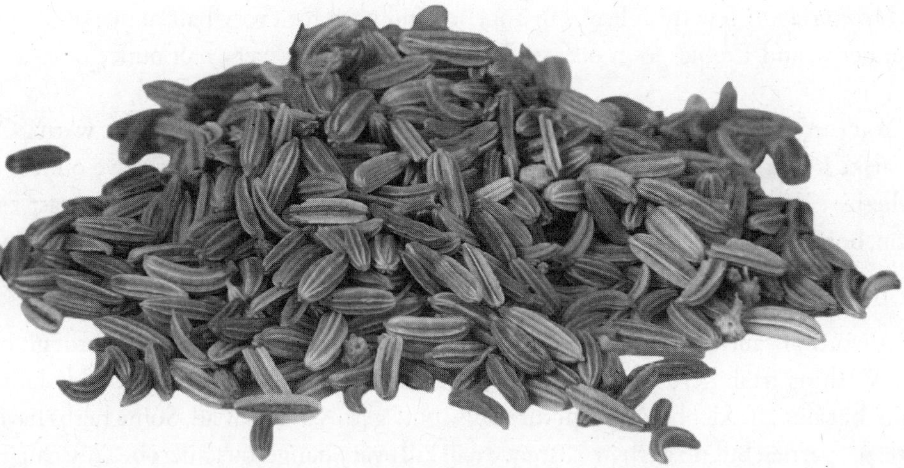

Fennel Seeds

heat. Brew up a fennel decoction (1–2 teaspoons of the seed to each cup of water). Let the mixture cool to a comfortable temperature (but still hot). Then use it to soak a compress. Keep the hot compress on the bruise for 20 minutes at a time, three times a day until the bruise fades. The heat helps improve circulation. The fennel is a mild anti-inflammatory and analgesic. Keep the eye closed, and avoid getting the decoction in the eye itself.

A tendency to bruise easily. If you tend to bruise easily, first check with your doctor to make sure your bruises aren't a sign of a more serious problem. Then you might try bilberry. We have one study that shows that it might help with the problem.

Battlefield bruises

Arquebusade Water (Eau de Arquebusade).[1732] This is an all-purpose liniment and remedy that dates back to at least the fifteenth century. It gets its name from the arquebus, a kind of gun. Arquebusade water was a battlefield remedy used for musket wounds and other cuts, bruises, and injuries from battle. I include it here not because I recommend it but because it is one of the few classic herbal remedies of the Western martial tradition.

It could be called a "shotgun remedy" (no pun intended) in that it throws fifteen different herbs at a problem, hoping at least one of them might be what the body needs. In doing so, it also (1) increases the chances of odd, unknown interactions between the herbs, and (2) increases the chances of the body getting something it doesn't want. If you want to try some, read up on all the different ingredients, including the warnings. Most are in this book. Some you'll need to look up elsewhere. It would also be wise to run the recipe past a professional herbalist. Anytime you combine herbs like this and throw them at a problem, you need more knowledge and expertise than you can get from a book.

Mix equal parts of

Dry herbs. Agrimony, calamint, fennel, hyssop, lemon balm, marjoram, peppermint, rosemary, sage, savory, thyme, wormwood.

Fresh herbs. A few fresh leaves of angelica and basil for every half ounce of each of the other herbs, and 1 tablespoon of fresh lavender flowers for every half ounce of each of the other herbs.

You can make arquebusade water as a standard decoction and apply it warm. Or you can make it as a tincture. Combine 1 quart of 100 proof alcohol per twelve ounces of the dry herbs. (That works out to one half ounce of each dry herb.) Allow to sit at least 14 days. Strain, bottle, and label.

Wounds

A word of caution: It's very easy to introduce microbes into the body through broken skin. Washing fresh herbs gets rid of some germs, but not all. Boiling a remedy kills some germs, but not all. Alcohol in a tincture kills some germs, but not all. Some herbs have antiseptic properties, but no herb in existence will kill every dangerous microbe. You can infect a wound using an herbal remedy, and infected wounds can kill you. Before antibiotics, herbal remedies were common. So was losing limbs and life to infection. If you begin to have signs of infection, or if you have a wound that isn't healing right, don't mess with herbs. Go to the doctor and take full advantage of twenty-first century medicine. Before using an herbal preparation on open skin, consider carefully the risks and what you hope to gain using an herb rather than, say, an over-the-counter antibiotic ointment.

While the wound is healing, make sure you are getting enough vitamins A (as beta carotene), C, and E. Each plays its own role in healing.[1733]

Wounds with bleeding

If you have a wound that's bleeding, put direct pressure on it using a bandage or clean cloth. If direct pressure isn't working or if the blood loss is severe, get emergency medical help immediately. The last thing you want to do if you're bleeding is to take pressure off the wound to go prepare an infusion. When the bleeding has stopped, and you have just a bit of oozing here and there, that's when herbs might be a help.

Wounds oozing blood

Several herbs have been traditionally used as simple for light bleeding (for example, agrimony, goldenrod, horsetail, and especially shepherd's purse, and yarrow). If you want to use an herbal remedy for light bleeding, consider mixing it into a prepared commercial antibiotic ointment.

Puncture wounds

Check to make sure that no part of the object making the puncture remains in the wound. If you see (or suspect) something remains deep in the wound, have it professionally removed. Then clean the wound. The standard first aid recommendation is to rinse the wound under running water for five minutes. Wash it with a mild soap and rinse well.[1734] An herbal alternative is to follow the rinse by soaking the wound in a basin with water, Epsom salt, and calendula or chamomile tincture. The water helps further clean the wound. Calendula contains anti-inflammatory compounds, and chamomile helps attract the cells that rebuild tissue. The Epsom salt helps with the inflammation and pain. Apply antibacterial ointment and cover the wound with a bandage. When the wound has closed up, the swelling and pain has subsided, and any trace of infection is gone, you can use comfrey to help rebuild normal tissue. If you use comfrey too soon on deep wounds, it can close up the surface and not allow proper drainage, thereby trapping infection and contaminants beneath the skin.[1735]

Itchy sores

Chamomile wash or ointment is a good alternative to try before you go to hydrocortisone cream.[1736] [1737] Chamomile creams are available. Or you can make a chamomile compress (infusion on a cloth), put it in the freezer, and use it cold. A few drops of lavender essential oil added to infusion may help boost the effect.

Calendula and rosemary make a good combination for itchy sores.[1738] Use one part calendula to one part rosemary. The calendula has a soothing effect and helps with inflammation. The rosemary contains camphor and eucalyptol, both of which are counterirritants. Both infusions in water and infused oil work. Infusions in water will be milder because camphor and eucalyptol are not very soluble in water. (Note that calendula itself can itself cause an allergic reaction. See the herbal in Chapter 2 for more information about contraindications)

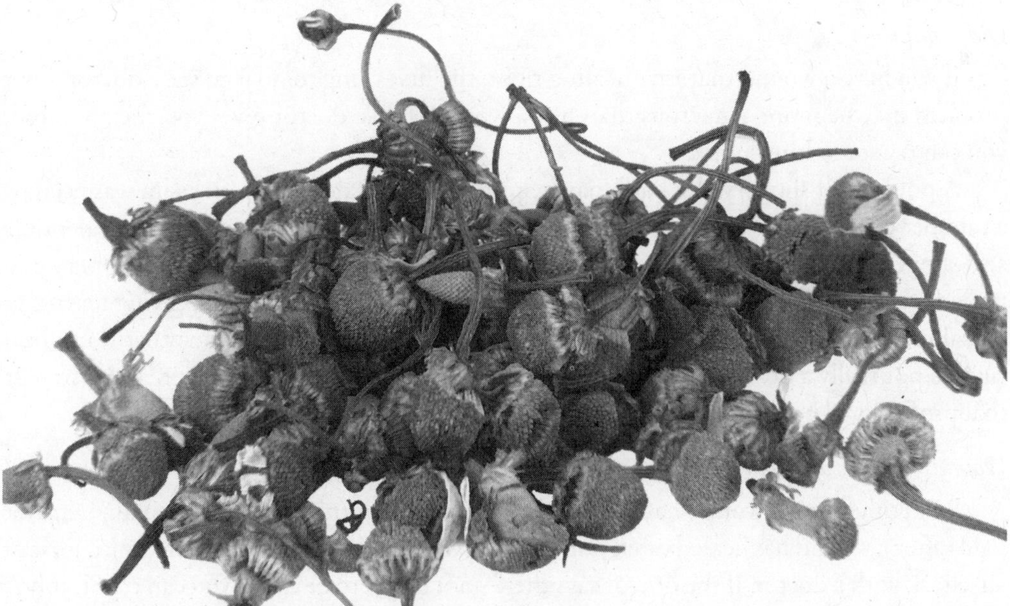

Dried chamomile flowers

If your eczema is chronic, you might consider evening primrose oil taken orally. You may also get some benefit from fish oil supplements if you suffer from chronic itching.[1739]

Oozing abrasions

Chamomile works well for abrasions.[1740] Make an infusion of chamomile and use it on a compress. Or you can mix a few drops of the essential oil into water, witch hazel, or a carrier oil and use it as a compress.

Or you can take a chamomile bath. Mix 10–12 drops lavender essential oil and 10 drops of chamomile essential oil in one or two tablespoons almond oil. Add it to a bath, pouring the oil under running water as you fill the tub (to help avoid "hot spots" of unmixed oil). The tannins in the lavender help stop the oozing. The chamomile soothes the irritation. The oil will form a protective layer. And the lavender smell will help you sleep.

Calendula is also an option for abrasions. It soothes and has mild antibiotic properties.

Another option for mat burn is aloe. Aloe also has the benefit of providing a thin protective layer over the wound.

Abrasions and chapping

Add two droppers full of black elderberry tincture to a cup of cold water. Apply it using a compress.[1741]

Or you can use eucalyptus oil well diluted.

Yarrow root is also a possibility. An infusion is made of 1–2 teaspoons of dried yarrow in a cup of water.[1742] Steep for 10–15 minutes and strain. It can be used on a compress.

Old wounds

If you have a wound that isn't healing right, the first thing to do is to see a doctor. Your problem may be more dangerous than just a wound. If the doctor gives you the go-ahead, you can try something herbal.

A poultice of slippery elm bark may help speed things along. Slippery elm was used by a number of American Indian tribes for this purpose. Alternatively, you can mix calendula and slippery elm. The calendula soothes the wound because the mucilage in slippery elm provides a coating. If the wound is an open one, however, be aware that applying herbs can actually contaminate the wound and make it worse. Treating old wounds that don't heal right is not really a do-it-yourself proposition. Get professional help and run all herbs past that professional before using them.

Wounds with nerve damage

Sometimes after a wound has healed, it leaves behind burning or stabbing pain. Leftover pains after a wound has healed often points to nerves that haven't healed quite right. First of all, check with a doctor. If the doctor says there's not much to be done, you can try St. John's wort infused oil applied to the area.[1743] If you wish you can also add lavender to the infusion. Note that this is not a long-term solution. Use it only short-term or occasionally.

Compression wounds to the mouth

Make a tea of one teaspoon of agrimony in a cup of water, cool it to a temperature that can be held in the mouth, and then swish it in your mouth to tighten the tissue and reduce bleeding and oozing.[1744] A decoction of agrimony takes longer to make, but it is a bit stronger. It is also used as a rinse or gargle.

Goldenseal has traditionally been used for a split lip. You can use a tincture either full-strength if you have a fairly good tolerance for the herb and for the alcohol in tinctures, or you can use a diluted tincture if you don't.

Goldenrod can also be used for swelling of the mouth. A commercial preparation, Urol mono, has been shown to be effective against inflammation in animal studies.[1745] It isn't, however, widely available outside Germany.

Mouth wounds with bleeding and swelling

If bleeding is severe, get professional help. If bleeding is light or oozing, you might try goldenrod. Goldenrod infusion acts as both an astringent and an anti-inflammatory. To help reduce the chance of infection, an infusion of thyme can be swished in the mouth.

Bruised or scraped gums

Rub a little infused or diluted clove oil onto the affected area once every few hours. Alternatively you can dilute the essential clove oil in some water and swish. (See the herbal for more information about safety with cloves.)

Canker sores

You can use a rinse made from tincture of myrrh.[1746] Or you can combine myrrh and echinacea tinctures to make a rinse (five drops of myrrh tincture and 10–20 of echinacea in a glass of water).

Throat irritation

For mouth and throat irritation caused by training hard in dry or cold air, gargle and rinse with a cold infusion of marshmallow.

Most injuries to skin and joints

All-purpose skin salve
Calendula
Comfrey
Echinacea
St. John's wort [1747]

Use equal amounts. Infuse in oil. Use method two to make the salve. You can use this one on sprains, irritations, just about any injury except those to the mucous membranes or open wounds, especially deep or puncture wounds.

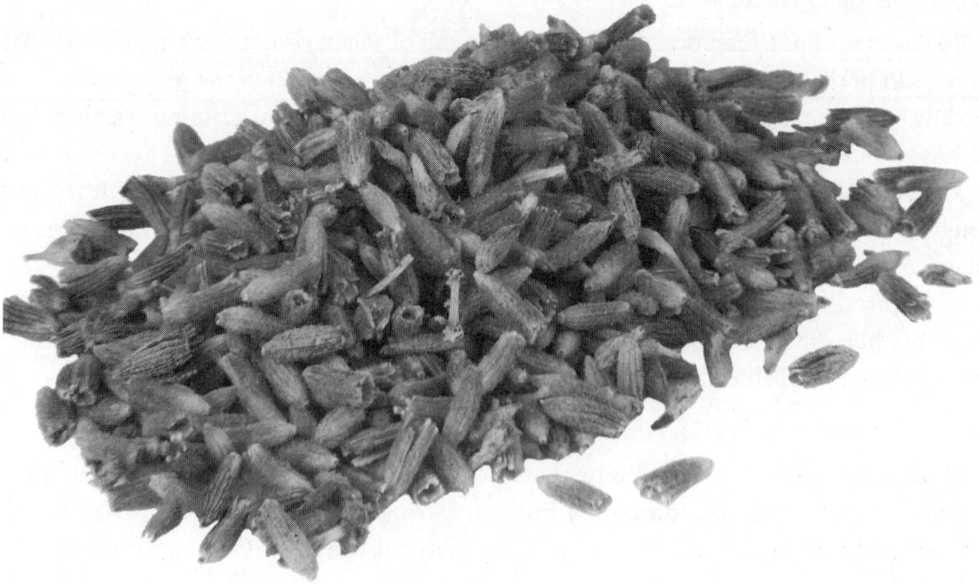

Dried lavender blossoms

Muscle Cramps

Sometimes cramps are due to too little calcium or potassium in the diet. You might try some supplementation if you are having regular problems.

You can also try lavender in a bath. Sew a cup or two of lavender flowers into a muslin bag. Put it under the spout of the tub and run the bath, or put a few drops (1–5) of the essential oil in the water.[1748] You can also add some Epsom salts to the bath (not more than three times per week).

A massage oil with oil of peppermint can help improve circulation and might help loosen muscle cramps.

Aching muscles

For muscle aches, several different liniments will help dull the pain. These liniments help with the pain by acting as counterirritants. A counterirritant irritates the skin slightly. This irritation might be felt as a warm, cool, or tingling sensation. The irritation distracts the mind from the pain and also depletes the neurotransmitters so less of the muscle pain reaches the brain. Counterirritants don't, however, necessarily speed healing.

Aching muscles due to exertion

Homemade Tiger Balm[1749]

3 tablespoons wintergreen oil

3 teaspoons camphor oil
1 ½ teaspoons eucalyptus oil
1 teaspoon lavender oil
1 ½ teaspoon peppermint oil
1 ½ tablespoon almond oil

Use the herbs straight for a liniment. Add some aloe vera gel or petroleum jelly to help it stay where you put it. Or heat the oils and add roughly a half an ounce of beeswax to make a salve. As is, this is a pretty potent balm. If you want to decrease the potential for skin irritation, cut back on the camphor and eucalyptus, and/or increase the amount of almond oil. Either way, you do not want this balm anywhere near your eyes or nose. Patch test it before using it on a more extensive area.

Peppermint. Use a peppermint liniment. Use either peppermint tincture or dissolve a teaspoon of peppermint oil in a tablespoon of grain alcohol.

Aching muscles with bruising

Make a decoction of comfrey leaves and sage leaves and add it to a bath. Be sure you don't have any broken skin before soaking in comfrey. (See "What should you be aware of before using it" in Chapter 2.)

Backache

For backache in general you can use capsicum in any of a number of different formulations. Mix it with alcohol to make a liniment. Or use it in infused oil, a decoction, tincture, vinegar tincture, or commercial preparation. Apply it topically.

Devil's claw may also help with back pain. Studies show that it might benefit both inflammation and pain.

Scars

While the wound is healing, make sure you are getting enough vitamins A (as beta carotene), C, and E. Each plays its own role in healing.[1750]

Preventing scars

After a wound has scabbed over, you can begin to use a gotu kola ointment or compress. We have animal studies that say that gotu kola helps heal wounds. Unlike rosehip seed oil, it can be used before the scab is completely gone. If you're using it on an unhealed wound, however, make sure you have a sterile preparation.

Reducing the appearance of new scars

Try rosehip seed oil. The essential oil is used without dilution. After the scab on the wound is gone, apply the oil every morning and evening. Don't use the oil until the scab is completely gone because the oil can slow healing. Put two or three drops on your finger and massage them into the scar for a minute. The massage helps the oil penetrate the skin and also helps break up the scar tissue.

Healing scars with damaged nerves

Sometimes wounds leave a patch of skin around them that feel "dead" when touched. If the wound was not too large, this nerve damage will generally heal on its own, but an herbal treatment may help speed the process.

Make a thin cream of St. John's wort infused oil using method one. When the cream has cooled, stir in a bit of rosehip seed oil and vitamin E oil. Note that rosehip seed oil breaks down when it becomes warm. You therefore want to make the cream fairly thin and stir the vitamin E and rosehip seed oil in when it is as cool as possible. Keep the cream in the refrigerator. Use it only after the scab on the wound is completely gone.

Plantar Warts

Plantar warts are bumps on the soles of your feet. Sometimes they have a cauliflower appearance. Sometimes they are a lump with a small crater in the center. Sometimes they have small dark speckles on the surface. Generally, they interrupt the normal lines and ridges of the sole of your foot. When you walk on plantar warts for a time, they develop calluses, which then get pressed into the skin of your foot by your weight. Consequently, walking on a plantar wart can be like walking with a stone in your shoe.

Plantar warts are caused by direct contact with human papillomavirus (HPV). HPV passes into the environment through flecks of skin or small drops of blood from an existing wart. HPV likes warm, moist environments. Given an environment like that, it can live outside a human host long enough for other people to pick it up on their feet. However, exposure does not mean that you will get warts. The virus is not highly contagious. Most people will not become infected by the virus when exposed to it. Others can carry the virus but never develop actual warts. Some people, however, are very susceptible.

The best thing you can do is to avoid the virus. Wear shower shoes or sandals in public showers or pools. If you train barefoot, tape over any existing warts to avoid spreading them to other people. If you know you're susceptible, tape over any cuts or scrapes on your feet as well; wart virus enters the body more easily through broken skin. Duct tape or a good quality athletic tape has the best chance of staying put through a workout. Be careful, however, because tape tends to have a different traction than a bare foot.

When should you see a doctor: If you aren't positive that you're dealing with a plantar wart, see a doctor for a positive ID. Also see a doctor if

The warts change in appearance or color.

The wart grows larger than a penny.

Home treatment doesn't seem to be having an effect.

You have diabetes or circulation problems in your feet.

Your gut tells you something's not right here." [1751]

How do you treat a plantar wart? The good news is that warts generally go away on their own eventually. The bad news is that sometimes they take years to do so, and sometimes they don't go away at all. The other bad news is that modern medicine doesn't have a great track record when dealing with warts. Most doctors will begin by using a conservative treatment,

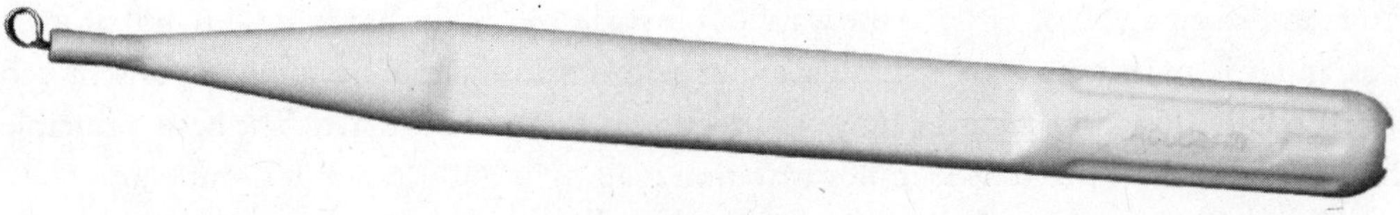

A dermal curette

salicylic acid or freezing. If the warts don't go away, they may proceed to cutting or burning the wart. If that doesn't work, they may go to antiviral medications.[1752] But, in general, an herbal approach that you might try at home is not much less sophisticated than the first line of defense in a doctor's office.

If your wart is small and you've had good luck getting rid of warts in the past, you're a good candidate for home remedies. Getting rid of a wart has two facets: you have to get rid of the callus, and you have to stimulate an immune reaction to get rid of the virus.

The most common way to get rid of the callus is to soak your feet in hot water once a week and then take a pumice stone, emery board, or dermal curette to the callus to reduce its size. Don't try cutting or burning the wart yourself. Doing so, beyond being just plain dangerous, often ends up spreading the virus and making the wart bigger.

One word of caution: Touch the wart as little as possible during treatment. If you do have to touch it, wash your hands with soap and water as soon as possible. Doing so helps avoid spreading the wart.

As for stimulating an immune reaction, that's where people get really creative. Most treatments involve either direct treatment with ointments or tinctures or covering the wart with some kind of poultice.

The best-studied treatment is not strictly herbal. In a 2002 study, duct tape got rid of more warts than cryotherapy (freezing) did. Here's how it works: Cover your wart with a piece of duct tape. Leave the tape on for a week. If the tape falls off, cut another piece of tape and put it over the wart as soon as possible. The goal is to keep the wart covered at all times. It's enough to cover the wart, the callus, and a bit of a margin on all sides. Some people, however, find they need more tape to get a tight seal on all edges or to keep the tape in place during workouts and showers. Once a week, take the tape off. Soak the wart in hot water. Then gently rub the callus down with pumice stone, emery board, or dermal curette. Immediately put on more duct tape. The treatment can take two months. A variation on the theme is to treat the wart with over-the-counter salicylic acid before putting on the duct tape.

Many untested anecdotal treatments can used with or without the tape. Calendula ointment is said to soften the callus to make the wart easier to remove. Aloe vera gel has the ability to increase blood flow to an area and it may have some antiviral properties. Goldenseal tincture has mild astringent and antiseptic properties. All these can be used with or without the tape. If you use them with the tape, remove the tape daily (maybe more often at first until you see how you react to the herb), check and clean the area, and reapply your treatment.

You can also tape a bit of garlic to the wart, or use garlic oil. Garlic has some antiviral properties, and it is an irritant. It may stimulate your body to produce an immune response. Keep an especially close eye on garlic, however, because it can be a bit harsh. The basic principle for treating warts is that a little minor irritation is all right but not out-and-out pain.

Some people also like taking something internally to help boost the immune system to fight off the virus. Andrographis, astragalus, and echinacea are possibilities, but frankly we have no evidence at all to suggest that they can help fight off the HPV virus specifically.

Coughs, Colds, Breathing Problems

The ability to breathe freely is crucial to the practice of the martial arts. Here are some combinations that can help with breathing problems due to a recent cold or hayfever. Note that a commonly accepted guideline for exercise during a cold or the flu is the "neck up or neck down rule." If your symptoms are above the neck and include a runny nose, mild headache, mild cough, you are probably okay for a light workout. If you start having problems breathing, back off. If your symptoms include anything from the neck down, bronchitis, chest cough, fever, body aches, you would do better to rest. Inflammation of the lungs or bronchial passages is aggravated by exercise.[1753]

Cold tonics

Cold tonics are remedies you take at the first sign of a cold or flu. The idea behind them is to boost the immune system and hopefully shorten the duration of the symptoms.

Echinacea. The earlier you can catch a cold and start treating it with echinacea, the more effective the herb will be.

A commercial blend of echinacea, elderberry, propolis, zinc, and vitamin C is available under the name Sambucol®. (Propolis is a resinous substance that honeybees gather from tree buds to seal cracks or open spaces in the hive. It is alleged to have antibiotic properties.). Sambucol has been shown to be effective against influenza viruses in vitro.[1754] Small-scale studies show that it reduces the severity of symptoms and shortens the duration of the influenza.[1755]

Andrographis. One study shows that a commercial blend of andrographis and eleuthero called Kan Jang® (Kold Kare®) shortened the duration of a cold and decreased post-cold complications.[1756] In fact, studies also show that it may work better at taking down a cold than echinacea.[1757] Again, the sooner you take andrographis when you suspect a cold is coming on, the better it will work for you. Note that there are two kinds of Kold Kare®—one with eleuthero and one without. The Kare-N-Herbs® brand, the brand most commonly found in the United States, does not have eleuthero. If you want the eleuthero (and the blend used in the studies mentioned above), you need to get Kan Jang, sometimes called Kold Kare, from the Swedish Herbal Institute. From the perspective of Chinese medicine, andrographis is more appropriate for the flu (with a fever, red eyes, and sore throat) than it is for a cold with lots of congestion and no fever.

General virus tea. Make a decoction of echinacea root, cool it in the refrigerator. Add garlic and dried cayenne pepper (2 parts echinacea, 2 parts garlic, 1 part peppers), and let it cold infuse overnight. The amount you can take is limited by the cayenne. You should not be taking more than 30–60 mg of cayenne per day.

Peppermint tea can also help with the general symptoms of a cold. It will make you feel a bit better, and it may help kill off some of the virus as well.

Inflammation of the mucous membranes

Chamomile. After a cold or flu has progressed some and the mucous membranes of the nose are red and inflamed, inhaling chamomile steam can also be helpful.[1758] Use a tincture of chamomile (1 ½ tablespoons in a quart of hot water). Heat the water until steaming, add the chamomile tincture, then inhale the steam slowly and deeply for ten minutes, keeping your head and the bowl of water covered with a towel to trap the steam. The effects peak after around a half hour and last for two to three hours. If you feel a bit dizzy while inhaling the steam, uncover your head for a moment. Dizziness is less pronounced with lower doses of chamomile.

Irritated cough

Anise. For dry, irritated coughs try anise tincture.[1759] Stir ¼–½ teaspoon of tincture into a glass of water. Drink or gargle three times day.

Marshmallow. For those times when you're coughing because your throat is irritated, and your throat is irritated because you're coughing, try marshmallow. Marshmallow relaxes and soothes the throat while coating the throat to offer a bit of extra protection. If you have the time, a cold infusion of the leaves works best. Otherwise, you can make a decoction of the leaves. Cold infusion of marshmallow is also good for those times when your throat is sore and it hurts to swallow.

Congested cough

For a congested cough, make an infusion of licorice root, sweet fennel, and thyme.[1760] Use deglycyrrhizinated licorice extract (preferred) or commercial licorice juice sticks.

For a cough with congestion (with or without swollen throat), try anise. Anise acts as an expectorant, making coughs more productive. It can also decrease swelling. Make an infusion of freshly crushed anise seed to use as a tea or a gargle.

Cough that keeps you awake at night

Combine a tincture of valerian (sleep) with licorice (expectorant). Use deglycyrrhizinated licorice extract (preferred) or commercial licorice juice sticks.

Cough with bronchitis

Combine tinctures of anise with deglycyrrhizinated licorice extract for bronchitis.[1761]

Cough with a "twitchy," tight throat

Try a tea made from fennel. Use 1–2 teaspoons of the seeds per cup of water, bruising the seeds lightly before decocting them.

Or try gargling or drinking an infusion of thyme.

Cough with excess phlegm

Use three parts elder to one part other herbs (a *total* of one part), which could include yarrow, goldenrod, or agrimony. You can make this remedy as either an infusion or tincture[1762] Gargle and spit.

Sore throat

You might try one part powdered sage to two parts honey.

Or you can try a tea made of fenugreek. Soak a tablespoon of the seeds in cold water for three hours. Strain and use.

If the sore throat is an irritated sore throat, try a cold infusion of slippery elm.

Laryngitis

First make an infusion using ½ teaspoon of cayenne chilies to one cup of water. Let the mixture infuse for ten minutes, and then use one tablespoon of this syrup with five drops of myrrh tincture in a cup of water to make a gargle. Cayenne and myrrh can also be used for sore throat.

A tendency toward strep throat

If you already have the symptoms of strep, go see your doctor. If you tend toward strep and have just gotten a cold and want to avoid further infection this time, one of these might help you fight it off. Note: the fresher the garlic the better. Drink these remedies cool, as heat tends to break down the active compounds. If you want to use a garlic remedy for more

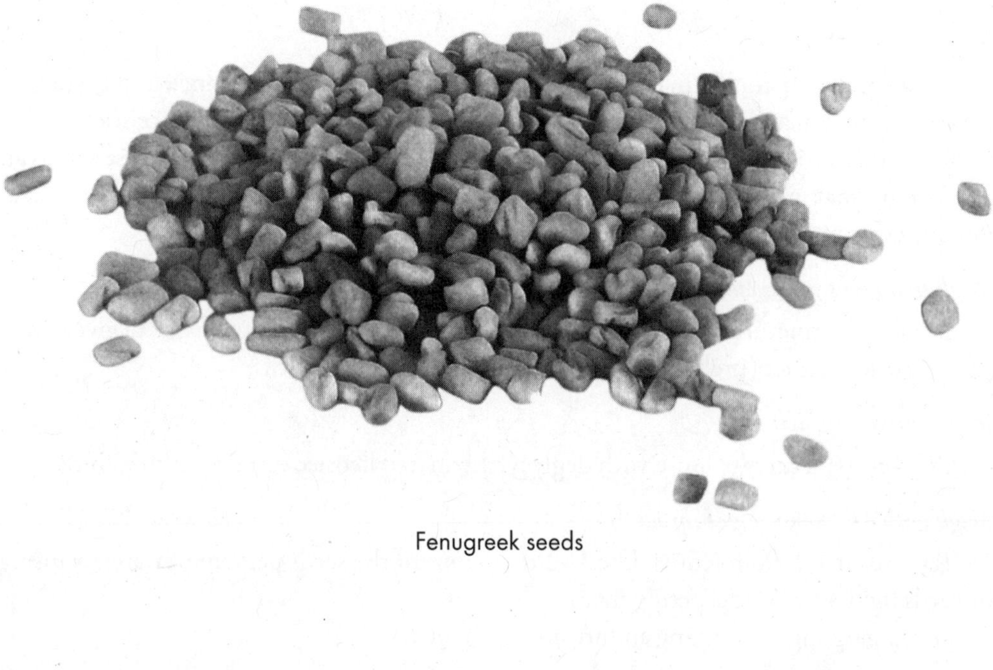

Fenugreek seeds

than one day, make up a fresh batch each day for maximum potency. Take them at the first sign of a cold.

Garlic wine. Chop or press a few cloves of garlic and cover them with red wine. Let it sit several hours before drinking[1763]

Garlic lemonade. Chop or press a few cloves of garlic and cover them with freshly made honey lemonade. Let it sit for several hours before drinking.[1764]

Clogged sinuses

Try an inhalation of eucalyptus. Use a standard inhalation method with two drops of the eucalyptus essential oil to a quart of hot water. Because eucalyptus has some virus-fighting properties, it might also help you fight off the cold as well as unplug your sinuses.

Clogged nasal passages

For clogged nasal passages unrelieved by blowing your nose, try horseradish. Grate a bit into a hot drink (a cup of tea or some chicken soup). Or you can try some cayenne instead of the horseradish. Both will produce a minor irritation that will cause your nose to run (and hopefully unplug).

Allergic asthma

Use the essential oil of roman chamomile added to a chest rub. Put a few drops of the essential oil in a half ounce of a carrier oil.

Or make a steam inhalant from the chamomile tincture.

An all purpose "cold blaster"

If you need to bring out the "big guns" to clear out the effects of a cold, make a vinegar tincture[1765] with

1–2 cloves of chopped garlic
¼ cup of grated horseradish root
½ of a finely chopped onion
¼ cup grated ginger
1 cayenne pepper pods with seeds and membranes removed

Put all in a pint bottle and fill with apple cider vinegar. Cover with a tight lid. Leave to infuse for 10 days. Strain. You can freeze the infusion, thawing it to use as needed. Use 1 tablespoon or less, twice daily, mixed into water or another liquid. This is strong stuff. Before taking it, read the precautions in the second chapter and then try a small amount to see how you handle it before taking the full dose.

Note that because of the time it takes this cold blaster to infuse, it can't really be made to order for each new cold. You also can't use a hot infusion method because doing so would lessen the potency of key ingredients. You can, however, make it and freeze it with some effect on the potency but less than you would experience with heat.

Athletic Performance Enhancement

Trying to find endurance in a bottle of herbs is an iffy thing. On the one hand, some herbs do seem to have an effect on endurance. On the other hand, the benefit you get from herbs will not be as great as the benefit you get from steady training, proper nutrition, and a good night's sleep. If you still want to try herbs in the hopes of getting that little bit of an extra edge, here are some possibilities.

Improved endurance under stress

Ashwagandha may help you improve your endurance under stress. Though this herb shows promise in animal tests, it has no conclusive scientific backing for human use.

Astragalus is used in China by young people wanting to increase performance and endurance. Though this herb shows promise in animal tests, it has no conclusive scientific backing for human use.

Rhodiola, on the other hand, has some human clinical trials backing it. A couple of studies seem to show that it helps bodies under stress, both protecting them from wear-and-tear, and increasing endurance. It may also help memory and mental performance under stress.

Improved recovery from stress

Eleuthero can help the body deal with stress. It might also be useful when convalescing from injuries.

Fish oil may help the body deal with the wear-and-tear of training. It can also help with mental focus and the regulation of emotions.

Improved exercise recovery

We have one study that suggests that fenugreek might help with exercise recovery, speeding up the time the muscles take to refuel.

Improved metabolism of carbohydrates

Cayenne. We also have a couple of studies that link cayenne to improved use of carbohydrates within the body. In other words, using a bit of cayenne supposedly helps your body get more energy from the carbohydrates you eat. The studies we have, however, are far from conclusive. If you incorporate some cayenne into your diet before an athletic event, you might get some benefit from the experiment, but you probably should not expect a magic bullet.

Improved reaction time

Eucalyptus. We have some minimal evidence that the smell of eucalyptus can help with reaction time. It also may have benefits for the speed of mental processing.

Peppermint. The smell of peppermint oil also might help improve reaction time. The evidence is scant, but combined with visualization, it might help.

Improved focus and memory

Ginkgo may help with memory and mental focus. Studies would seem to indicate that this effect is more profound in the elderly.

Ginseng may help with mental focus and with endurance.

Regulation of the Fight-or-Flight System

In the martial arts, we play with aggression, experiment with high-pressure situations, purposely get ourselves worked up and settled down. Such experiments are valuable, but more than a few martial artists have found themselves wide awake at two in the morning after a heavy class, staring at the clock and wondering what the upcoming day is going to be like after so little sleep.

In this section, we look at herbs that interact with the fight-or-flight system: herbs that help quell anxiety and its physical consequences, help you sleep when you're keyed up, and for good measure a few herbs that can help with depression. Most prescription anti-anxiety medicines make you drowsy or impair your reaction time, not a good thing if you are heading off to a sparring class. Here are a few milder herbal alternatives.

Before I discuss the herbs commonly used for anxiety and insomnia, let me just say that one of the best habits you can adopt if you suffer from anxiety is to set up a regular habit of meditation. Meditation is a great help in regulating the fight-or-flight system. (But that's beyond the scope of this section and a topic for another book.)

Nervous stomach

Try caraway tea. A couple of drops (no more than four) of peppermint essential oil can be added if you're also having heartburn. Note, however, that peppermint helps heartburn in some people and causes heartburn in others. Avoid trying it for the first time in a "high stakes" situation.

Nervous tension

Try chamomile tea. Drink 2 or 3 cups of tea a day, at least one of them before bed.[1766] See how you react to chamomile before trying it before class or any other situation where you have to be alert. It can make you groggy.

If you don't want to take something orally, the scent of lavender might help you relax. It may also help decrease aggression. Put a couple of drops of the essential oil on a handkerchief and inhale the smell.

Generalized anxiety

Hops tincture might help. Take up to ½ teaspoon three times as day.

Or try passionflower tincture (½–1 teaspoon up to three time per day.[1767])

Anxiety with trouble sleeping

Valerian has a reputation for helping people deal with nighttime anxiety. During the Blitz in England during World War II, citizens used valerian to help them deal with the nightly bombing raids. Valerian is, however, a nighttime herb, not a daytime one.

Depression with anxiety

Try St. John's wort for mild to moderate depression, especially depression with anxiety.

Mild insomnia

One bedtime tea used in Germany for children as well as adults contains 30% lemon balm leaf (*Mellissa officinalis*), 30% lavender flower, 30% passionflower herb, and 10% St. John's wort.[1768]

A passionflower infusion is also good for helping you sleep.[1769] Make an infusion with 2–3 teaspoons of the herb per cup. You can also add lavender and/or chamomile to the infusion as desired. Passionflower is especially good when you can't sleep because of a fever.

Valerian is also a common insomnia remedy. Add passionflower if valerian makes you sleep restlessly or have nightmares.[1770]

Insomnia caused by worry or anxiety

Use hops tincture (one dose of 1 teaspoon per day only before bed). You can also add to the hops a combination of valerian and passionflower tincture (one or the other, or both) combined to total 1 teaspoon. Or if you are taking your hops in capsule form, use 300 to 400 mg of hops extract combined with 240 to 300 mg of valerian extract. Don't take this one if you are prone to depression[1771]

Insomnia with indigestion

Chamomile is good for both anxiety and indigestion.

Catnip is a good herb for those days when you have something on your mind that's giving you a headache, making your stomach do flip flops, and keeping you from sleeping. Tradition has it that catnip is good for all three of those problems. It can be combined with chamomile, passionflower, and hops.

Insomnia with muscle tension

You might consider rubbing a bit of peppermint oil in ethanol (or a tincture of peppermint) into your forehead and/or temples.

Lavender is also good for insomnia with headache. You can rub a little bit of the diluted essential oil or tincture into your temples, and the smell will help deaden your perception of the headache pain.

Insomnia with pain

Mix a couple of drops of the essential oils of ginger and lavender in a carrier oil such as almond oil. Massage it into the painful area before bed. Be cautious not to use it near the eyes.[1772]

Chronic insomnia

You might consider a combination of valerian and St. John's wort. Note, however, that neither of these herbs should be used every day, long term. Short-term use, however, may help you break a chain of poor nights' sleep.

Alternatively, you might consider visiting an acupuncturist or Chinese herbalist. Both have a good track record in treating chronic insomnia.

Battered Feet or Hands

Chinese herbalism has herbs specifically for hands that have been doing a lot of punching. The martial tradition of herbalism has herbs that help condition hands as well as herbs that help heal hands and feet that have been overused. Western herbalism has no similar tradition, but it does have herbs for swelling as well as herbs that help heal banged up skin.

Swollen hands or feet

An infusion of elder flowers used as a compress or soak is good for hands or feet that have taken too much pounding and are swollen and tender.

Another good soak for scuffed up feet is either a quart of strong chamomile tea or one teaspoonful of chamomile tincture added to hot Epsom salt water. The chamomile is an anti-inflammatory and fosters healing. The Epsom salts help take down the swelling.[1773]

A decoction made from 5 ounces of fresh ginger root in 2 quarts of water is a good foot or hand bath.[1774] Ginger is an anti-inflammatory and has been shown to be particularly effective if you have some arthritis or joint inflammation. It is also an antifungal.

One traditional remedy for battered feet is ½ ounce of arnica tincture in hot water used as a footbath.[1775] Arnica is especially good for bruises.

Cracked feet

Cracked heels are made worse by a build up of calluses and dead skin. This skin is not as flexible as healthy skin, so when you step down on your heel and the weight spreads the heel out, the skin cracks rather than expands. To help avoid a build up of dead skin, soak your feet in hot water for ten minutes or so and then take a fine pumice stone to them to polish off the hard outer layer. When you've finished pumicing, coat them with something to kill any stray microbes—thyme, tea tree, eucalyptus—and then with something to soften and heal the skin.

If you have chronic problems with cracked feet, you may have a deficiency in your diet. Consider taking GLA (in evening primrose oil or by itself) or getting more omega-3s (fish oil or for women fish or flaxseed oil). You should begin to see results in two to six months.[1776]

Feet that have been exposed to bacteria and fungus

(See also "fungal infections" in this chapter.)

If you've been training hard in your bare feet on questionable surfaces, wash your feet thoroughly as soon as possible. When you get home, infuse some thyme for a foot bath. The thyme is an antibiotic and also kills some of the kinds of fungus that tend to infest feet.

Tea tree oil has been found to be useful in softening calluses. It is also useful in preventing and treating athlete's foot.[1777] You can put a few drops into hot water for a foot soak, or you can add 2–3 drops of tea tree oil to a carrier oil such as sesame and massage it into your feet.

Cold, stiff feet

One of the problems with training barefoot is cold, stiff feet. For those of you who get back from the dojo on a cold winter evening, wondering if your feet will ever be warm again, this salve is for you:[1778]

2 tablespoons ginger powder
2 tablespoons cayenne
1 tablespoon dry (powdered) mustard (*Sinapis alba*)
10 ounces vegetable oil

Heat the herbs in the oil in a double boiler for about an hour and a half. Let it cool. Then line a strainer with a large coffee filter. Pour the oil into the filter and let it drip. When you've filtered all your oil, let it sit overnight and it should be through the filter by morning. Measure the oil and add beeswax 1:8 (wax to oil). Pour into jars and label. If you have sensitive skin, try just a little bit the first time. It's potent, and the heat also tends to build over time. Massage a little into your feet, and then cover them with some warm socks. Until you know how you react to it (and each time you make a new batch), wash it off before going to bed. Also wash your hands after applying.

Massage oil for feet

1 cup sesame oil
20 drops eucalyptus essential oil
a few drops of rosemary essential oil
one or two vitamin E capsules

Eucalyptus helps kill bacteria and fungus. It also has the property of making your skin more porous so anything else you rub into the skin penetrates more easily.[1779] Rosemary helps circulation.

Fungal Infections

Some of these herbs—tea tree oil, eucalyptus oil, thyme oil, and others—can be irritating. If you have a fungal infection in a sensitive location, try the least irritating herbs first, and always test a little bit on a very small area to see how you respond.

The best regimen for stifling a fungal infection is to keep the area clean and dry as much as possible. Use powder to absorb moisture. Change socks (or other relevant clothing items) when they get sweaty.

Athlete's foot

Cinnamon and ginger combine well. Both have possible use for athlete's foot. Cinnamon is a broad antimicrobial and has considerable traditional evidence for use on athlete's foot. Ginger has been shown to be effective against a wide range of fungi in vitro.[1780] Make a decoction of 8–10 cinnamon sticks and a thumb-sized piece of fresh ginger in a quart of water. Simmer for five minutes, then take it off the heat, cover it, and let it steep for an hour. Add additional water to make a footbath.

Toenail fungus

Thyme has been shown effective against the fungus that infests toenails.[1781] Thyme oil may work synergistically with cinnamon oil. The two combine well in agricultural and food preservation applications.[1782] Dilute the essential oils in a carrier oil. One formula is as follows:

12 parts carrier oil
2 parts thyme essential oil
1 part cinnamon bark essential oil

Note that this is a strong formula. Use it only on toenail fungus, and avoid getting it on nearby unaffected areas of skin. Don't use this strong a formula on anything more sensitive than a toenail. Also be aware that essential oil of thyme is dangerous. Read the "What you should know before using it" section.

Miscellaneous fungus

Eucalyptus diluted in a carrier oil or ointment has proven value against athlete's foot, jock itch, toenail fungus, and ringworm. Use about two drops eucalyptus oil in a teaspoon of the carrier.

Garlic oil has been shown to inhibit fungus in vitro.[1783] Apply it to the affected area twice a day.[1784] Note that garlic oil is very strong and can cause burns in some people. Don't apply it if you won't be able to keep an eye on it. If the garlic is too strong applied straight, consider using a plaster instead. (See Chapter 3 for instructions on making a plaster.) Be aware that even topical garlic use can cause you to have garlic breath. This may not be the best treatment if you have a date or job interview.

Calendula doesn't have anti-fungal properties, but it has a good track record for making fungal infections feel better while you're trying to get rid of them.[1785] Make a salve (method 5) of ½ cup hot infused calendula oil. When the beeswax has dissolved, just before pouring it into jars add a ¼ cup aloe vera gel and a 1/3 teaspoon tea tree oil. Or you can start with commercial calendula cream and add 10 drops tea tree oil in 2 tablespoons of calendula cream.[1786]

Tea tree oil may work on toenail fungus. Some people use it on athlete's foot. Though it can help with the symptoms, it doesn't actually kill the fungus.

Flatulence and Other Digestive Problems

Here are a couple of remedies for those who kick or grapple after supper (enough said).

Flatulence

For flatulence, caraway combines well with chamomile.[1787] Combine about a half-ounce of the caraway seed, a teaspoon or two of the chamomile, and a pint of water. Bruise caraway seeds and make a tea using the standard infusion method.

Or make a tea of rosemary. Rosemary works especially well if your digestive problems are due to stress and include cramping.

For flatulence with indigestion, make a tea using a spoonful of peppermint leaves and a half spoonful of caraway seeds. Infuse them using the standard method.

Or you can try a couple of drops of ginger oil on a sugar cube.

Gas pains

For gas pains, you can mix a half teaspoon each of anise, caraway, and fennel seeds. Lightly crush the seeds just before infusing to release the volatile oils. Pour one cup of boiling water over the seeds and let them stand covered for 5 to 10 minutes. Take one cup three times daily.[1788]

For gas with bloating, try turmeric in a capsule, or you can add turmeric to your meal.

Motion Sickness

If every time you roll or are thrown, it hits your stomach with a burst of motion sickness, here's a tea that may help keep your supper inside where you put it.

Ginger cinnamon tea. In a small saucepan bring to a boil: 1 cinnamon stick (i.e., a 2-inch long curl of bark) and a thumb-sized piece of ginger root, peeled and thinly sliced, and two cups of water. Reduce the heat and simmer covered for twenty minutes. Add honey to taste.

Massage Oils

Many infused oils aren't appropriate for massage. Either they stain badly, are too irritating, smell terrible, or don't have the right friction properties. Here are a couple of herbal oils that work well for massage.

For achy muscles

Add ¼ teaspoon rosemary essential oil to 1 ½ sunflower or almond oil.

For back pain

Make an infused oil of St. John's wort and use it as a massage oil.

CHAPTER FIVE

Herbal Contraindications

Herbs that may increase the risk of bleeding[1789]

Increased risk of bleeding supported by reports or studies:

Ginkgo biloba, garlic, saw palmetto.

Increased risk of bleeding theoretically possible:

alfalfa, American ginseng, angelica, anise, *Arnica montana*, asafetida, aspen bark, birch, black cohosh, bladderwrack, bogbean, boldo, borage seed oil, bromelain, capsicum, cat's claw, celery, chamomile, chaparral, clove, coleus, cordyceps, *danshen*, devil's claw, *dong quai*, evening primrose, fenugreek, feverfew, flaxseed or flax powder (not a concern with flaxseed oil), ginger, grapefruit juice, grapeseed, green tea, *guggul*, gymnestra, horse chestnut, horseradish, licorice root, lovage root, male fern, meadowsweet, nordihydroguairetic acid (NDGA), onion, papain, Panax ginseng, parsley, passionflower, poplar, prickly ash, propolis, quassia, red clover, *reishi*, Siberian ginseng, sweet clover, rue, sweet birch, sweet clover, turmeric, vitamin E, white willow, wild carrot, wild lettuce, willow, wintergreen, and yucca.

Herbs that affect blood sugar levels[1790]

Aloe vera, American ginseng, bitter melon, burdock, fenugreek, fish oil, gymnema, horse chestnut seed extract (HCSE), marshmallow, milk thistle, Panax ginseng, rosemary, Siberian ginseng, stinging nettle, and white horehound.

Herbs that may lower blood pressure[1791]

aconite or monkshood, arnica, baneberry, betel nut, black cohosh, bryony, calendula, California poppy, coleus, curcumin, eucalyptol, eucalyptus oil, ginger, goldenseal, green hellebore, hawthorn, Indian tobacco, jaborandi, mistletoe, night blooming cereus, oleander, pasque flower, periwinkle, pleurisy root, shepherd's purse, Texas milkweed, turmeric, and wild cherry.

Herbs that may have a laxative effect[1792]

alder buckthorn, aloe dried leaf sap, black root, blue flag rhizome, butternut bark, *dong quai*, European buckthorn, eyebright, cascara bark, castor oil, chasteberry, colocynth fruit pulp, dandelion, gamboges bark, horsetail, jalap root, manna bark, plantain leaf, podophyllum root, psyllium, rhubarb, senna, wild cucumber fruit, and yellow dock root.

Herbs that may make you drowsy[1793]

calamus, calendula, California poppy, capsicum, celery, cough elecampane, German chamomile, goldenseal, hops, *kava*, lemon balm, sage, sassafras, shepherd's purse, Siberian ginseng, skullcap, stinging nettle, valerian, wild carrot, wild lettuce, and yerba mansa.

Herbs that contain pyrrolizidine alkaloids

borage, comfrey, boneset (*Eupatorium cannabinum*), coltsfoot.

Herbs that may affect liver function[1794]

ackee, bee pollen, birch oil, blessed thistle, borage, bush tea, butterbur, chaparral, coltsfoot, comfrey, DHEA, *Echinacea purpurea*, *Echium* spp., germander, *Heliotropium* spp., horse chestnut (parenteral preparations), *jin bu huanly* (*Lycopodium serratum*), *kava*, lobelia, L-tetrahydropalmatine (THP), mate, niacin (vitamin B-3), niacinamide, Paraguay tea, periwinkle, *Plantago lanceolata*, pride of Madeira, rue, sassafras, scullcap, *Senecio* spp., groundsel, tansy ragwort, turmeric, *tu san chi* (*Gynura segetum*), *uva ursi*, valerian, and white chameleon.

Herbs that may affect heart function[1795]

adonis, balloon cotton, black hellebore root/melampode, black Indian hemp, bushman's poison, cactus grandifloris, convallaria, eyebright, figwort, foxglove or digitalis, frangipani, hedge mustard, hemp root or Canadian hemp root, king's crown, lily of the valley, motherwort, oleander leaf, pheasant's eye plant, plantain leaf, pleurisy root, psyllium husks, redheaded cotton bush, rhubarb root, rubber vine, sea-mango, senna fruit, squill, strophanthus, uzara, wallflower, wintersweet, yellow dock root, yellow oleander. Notably, bufalin or *chan suis* is a Chinese herbal formula that has been reported as toxic or fatal when taken with cardiac glycosides.

Herbs that may have a diuretic effect[1796]

artichoke, celery, corn silk, couchgrass, dandelion, elder flower, horsetail, juniper berry, *kava*, shepherd's purse, *uva ursi*, and yarrow.

Herbs that have monoamine oxidase inhibitor (MAOI) activity or that interact with MAOI drugs[1797]

Headache, tremors, mania, and insomnia may occur if ginseng is combined with supplements. Some examples are 5-HTP (5-hydroxytryptophan), California poppy, chromium, DHEA (dehydroepiandrosterone), DLPA (DL phenylalanine), ephedra, evening primrose oil, fenugreek, *Ginkgo biloba*, hops, mace, St. John's wort, SAMe® (S-adenosylmethionine), sepia, tyrosine, valerian, vitamin B6, and yohimbe bark extract.

In theory, ginseng can increase stimulatory effect of caffeine, coffee, tea, cocoa, chocolate, guarana, cola nut, and yerba mate.

Chapter Six

Further Resources

Finding Herbs

Because for medicinal herbs you will generally be using larger quantities of herbs than you would be for cooking and because you will be steeping out oils and other active ingredients, you might consider using organic herbs, even if you generally don't go organic. Growers of organic herbs in the United States will generally be certified by the National Organic Program (http://www.ams.usda.gov/nop/indexNet.htm).

Here are two sources of herbs that I've used:

Frontier Natural Products Co-op
http://www.frontiercoop.com/index.html

Frontier is a high-tech, highly reliable outfit. They test each lot of herbs for safety and potency. If you go to their Web site, you'll see that they pride themselves on their formally-trained staff and high-tech equipment. They are a member of AHPA, Co-op America, National Cooperative Business Association, and are certified USDA organic. Minimum order is a pound, but you can sometimes find Frontier products in bulk bins at your local health food store if you want smaller quantities.

Mountain Rose Herbs
http://www.mountainroseherbs.com

In business since 1987, they offer all organic herbs including bulk herbs, essential oils, grape alcohol tinctures, supplies for making herbal preparations, seeds, etc. They also carry some ready-made balms and salves. They are scrupulous about freshness. You can order herbs in smaller quantities from them. Furthermore, just about everything mentioned in this entire book—herbs, supplies for making preparations, bottles—everything is available from this one supplier. They offer a print catalog or online ordering. Mountain Rose herbs bears the following seals: AHPA, Co-Op America, Bio-Dynamic, Fair Trade certified herbs, and Oregon Tilth Certified Organic. Their chemical-free facility is powered by 100% renewable energy.

Finding Herb Seeds

Horizon Herbs
http://www.horizonherbs.com/

This is the one of the major sources for seeds, rootstock, and potted plants.

Mountain Rose Herbs
http://www.mountainroseherbs.com
A limited retail selection of Horizon Herbs.

Finding an Herbalist

In the United States

In the United States, the most recognized organization of professional herbalists is the American Herbalists Guild. They are a peer-reviewed educational organization for herbalists specializing in the medicinal use of plants. If herbalists have "RH (AHG)" after their name, that means they are a member of the American Herbalists Guild, have at least four years of training, and meet the AHG minimum professional requirements.

American Herbalists Guild, 141 Nob Hill Road, Cheshire, CT 06410
Phone: 203.272.6731
Fax: 203.272.8550
Email: ahgoffice@earthlink.net
http://www.americanherbalistsguild.com/

Naturopathic Physicians

Naturopathic physicians are trained in clinical nutrition, acupuncture, homeopathic medicine, botanical medicine, psychology, and counseling. They are fully trained to be primary care providers and are a licensed profession in 13 states. Naturopatic physicians are identified by the initials "ND" after their name.

http://naturopathic.org/

Chinese Herbalists

If you are looking for a practitioner of Chinese herbal medicine, a good place to start is the National Certification Commission for Acupuncture and Oriental Medicine. This organization ensures a minimum level of training and compliance with ethical practices.

http://www.nccaom.org/

In the United Kingdom

In the United Kingdom, look for members of the National Institute of Medical Herbalists. Professional members have graduated from reputable medical herbalist training programs, must meet strict professional requirements, and must follow the NIMH's code of ethics. The U.K. has some of the best-trained Western herbalists in the world, and the NIMH has some of the most rigorous criteria for membership in the U.K. Professional herbalist members of the Institute are identified by the acronym "M.N.I.M.H." after their name.

NIHM Head Office
Elm House
54 Mary Arches Street
Exeter EX4 3BA
Tel: +44 (0) 1392 426022
Fax: +44 (0) 1392 498963
E-mail: nimh@ukexeter.freeserve.co.uk
http://www.nimh.org.uk/

In Australia

Australia has the National Herbalists Association of Australia, which promotes education, and professional and ethical standards. Membership in the NHAA implies a certain level of education and adherence to a code of ethics.

NHAA Office PO Box 45 CONCORD WEST, NSW 2138
Ph: (02) 8765 0071 Overseas: +61 2 8765 0071
Fax: (02) 8765 0091 Overseas: +61 2 8765 0091
http://www.nhaa.org.au/

Miscellaneous Resources

Multilingual database of plant names
http://www.plantnames.unimelb.edu.au/Sorting/Frontpage.html

Matches common names to scientific name and vice versa. Includes information from sixty languages and twenty scripts.

National Institutes of Health
International Bibliographical Resources on Dietary Supplements
http://grande.nal.usda.gov/ibids/index.php

Contains abstracts of published studies about herbs and supplements.

American Herbal Products Association
http://www.ahpa.org/

Contains a list of reliable herbal resources on the Web. Also has a list of members who agree to abide by the association's code of ethics.

The Dietary Supplement Information Board
http://www.supplementinfo.org/HN_HerbalAZ.asp

Information about dosage and safety for herbs and dietary supplements.

The FDA
http://www.cfsan.fda.gov/~dms/wsearch.html

U.S. Government Nutrition Information Clearinghouse
http://www.nutrition.gov

Medline Plus Medical Encyclopedia
http://www.nlm.nih.gov/medlineplus/encyclopedia.html

U.S. Office of Dietary Supplements
http://ods.od.nih.gov/Health_Information/IBIDS.aspx

National Center for Complementary and Alternative Medicine
http://nccam.nih.gov/

Food and Nutrition Information Center
http://www.nal.usda.gov/fnic/etext/000015.html

Department of Health and Human Service Healthfinder
http://www.healthfinder.gov/

Herb Med
http://www.herbmed.org/

Glossary

adaptogen The term dates back to 1947, when a Russian scientist named Lazarev needed a word for herbs that generated a nonspecific resistance to stressors. He defined an "adaptogen" as an agent that allows an organism to counteract adverse physical, chemical, or biological stressors and respond appropriately, instead of with an overreactive stress reaction.[1798]

analgesic Relieves pain.

anodyne Something that relieves pain. Peppermint oil is an anodyne.

antibacterial Kills or limits the growth of germs (bacteria).

antiemetic Relieves vomiting or nausea.

antiexudative A substance that limits the amount of fluids seeping from a damaged blood vessel into the surrounding tissue. Horse chestnut is an antiexudative.

antiflatulent Relieves intestinal gas. Lavender is an anti-flatulent

antifungal Kills or inhibits the growth of fungi.

antihidrotic A substance that inhibits sweating. Sage is an antihidrotic.

antihistamine Drugs or herbs that protect tissue from the histamine released during an allergic reaction. In doing so antihistamines decrease the symptoms caused by allergies."

anti-inflammatory A substance that counteracts inflammation or swelling.

antimicrobial A substance that kills or limits the growth of microorganisms like bacteria (antibacterial), fungi (antimycotic), viruses (antiviral), or parasites (antiparasitic).

antimycotic Kills or limits the growth of fungus. Antimicotics include garlic.

antioxidant Slows the body's production of free radicals, compounds that can cause cell damage.

antiphlogistic Reduces inflammation and fever. Antiphlogistic herbs include goldenrod.

antipruritic Prevents or relieves itching

antipyretic Reduces fever.

antiseptic Prevents or slows the growth of microorganisms.

antispasmodic Relieves cramps or spasms, usually of muscles.

antithrombotic Slows or prevents blood clotting. Antithrombotic drugs and herbs help prevent unwanted blood clots from clogging arteries.

antiviral Kills or inhibits the growth of viruses.

aromatherapy A branch of alternative medicine that uses the smell of essential oils to affect health and mood.

astringent Tightens or increases the tone of tissues. Myrrh is an astringent.

autogenic Originating within the body.
carminative Quiets spasms in and fosters the expulsion of gas from the gastrointestinal tract. Peppermint is a carminative.
cataplasm A poultice or plaster.
catarrhs Discharge from or blockage of the nose due to excess mucus. Nasal congestion. Runny nose. Postnasal drip
cathartic Has a strong laxative effect.
cholagogue Promotes the flow of bile. Lavender is a cholagogue.
choleretic Stimulates the liver to increase output of bile.
colliquative Characterized by excessive liquid discharge, or by liquefaction of tissue
counterirritant When applied topically counterirritants produce minor skin-surface irritation that reduces decreases pain or inflammation in adjacent tissues. Mint, rosemary are counterirritants.
decoction A liquid extract. The herb is simmered or boiled to extract its active ingredients. Decoction is typically used for tough, fibrous ingredients like roots and bark.
demulcent Softens and soothes irritation of mucous membranes.
diaphoretic Promotes perspiration
digestive Aids in the digestion of food.
diuretic Helps the body get rid of water. Diuretics increase urine output.
emollient A topical preparation applied to soften and smooth the skin
esculent An edible plant, one suitable for food use. Fenugreek is an esculent as well as a medicinal herb.
essential oil The oil found naturally in herbs. It is normally extracted using some kind of distillation method. It is consequently much stronger than any other herbal byproduct.
expectorant: Promotes the elimination of mucus from the respiratory tract.
folium Latin name for the leaves of a plant.
galenic preparation Preparation by infusion, decoction, or tincture as opposed to chemical formulation. Also known as galenic pharmacy.
GRAS Generally recognized as safe.
hemostatic Stops bleeding.
hyperemic Increases blood flow to tissues.
hyperglycemic High blood sugar
hyperhidrosis Excess sweating, a medical condition in which a person sweats either unpredictably or too much.
hyperlipidemia Elevated lipids in the bloodstream. These lipids may include cholesterol, triglycerides, or estersphospholipids.
hypnotic When a drug or herb is said to be "hypnotic," it induces sleep. (It doesn't cause the user to become hypnotized).
hypotensive Lowers blood pressure.
immunosuppressant Causing a suppression of the immune system.
in vitro "Test-tube" studies that don't involve testing on animals or people.

infused oil Oil from a second plant (such as olive, sesame, grapeseed, etc.) in which herbs have been soaked. Some of the properties of the herbs transfer to the oil. Infused oil can be made by either hot or cold infusion.

infusion Also known as tea. Herbs are steeped in hot water to transfer the plant properties to the liquid. This method is typically used for the delicate parts of the plant such as leaves and flowers.

myalgia Muscle pain.

pulmonary Having to do with the lungs.

relaxant Promotes relaxation.

rubefacient Stimulates blood flow to the skin's surface.

salve A topical preparation made by combining an oil with an emulsifier such as beeswax.

sedative Decreases nervousness or agitation. Lavender is mildly sedative.

semen In a Latin botanical name, "semen" means seed. For example, *Hippocastani Semen* is the seed of a horsechestnut tree.

sensitizing When your reaction to something becomes more and more problematic with repeated use.

sialogogue Stimulates salivary gland tissues to produce saliva.

spasmolytic Antispasmodic. Peppermint has a spasmolytic effect on the smooth muscle of the digestive tract.

stimulant A substance that temporarily increases functional energy in the body.

stomachic Improves the function and tone of the stomach.

tincture Herbs are steeped in alcohol or glycerin to extract active ingredients.

topical Applied to the surface of the skin.

vascular Having to do with the veins.

vasodilatory Causes blood vessels to open and widen.

visceral Related to the internal organs of the body.

vulnerary A substance that promotes the healing of new cuts and wounds.

Notes

Chapter One: Using Herbs Safely

1. E. Ernst, "Adverse Effects of Herbal Drugs in Dermatology," *The British Journal of Dermatology* 143, no. 5 (November 2000): 923–9.

2. J. Garrard J, et al, "Variations in Product Choices of Frequently Purchased Herbs: *Caveat Emptor,*" *Archives of Internal Medicine* 163, no. 19 (October 2003): 2290–5.

3. F. Firenzuoli, et al, ["Herbs on the Internet: Risky Information,"] *Recenti Progressi in Medicina* 97, no. 4 (April 2006):189–92 (Article in Italian).

4. N. G. Bisset, ed., *Herbal Drugs and Phytopharmaceuticals* (Stuttgart: Medpharm GmbH Scientific Publishers, 1994).

5. Institute of Medicine, "Preventing Medication Errors," National Academies Press, http://www.iom.edu/Object.File/Master/35/943/medication%20errors%20new.pdf.

Chapter Two: The Herbal

6. Huron H. Smith, "Ethnobotany of the Meskwaki Indians." *Bulletin of the Public Museum of the City of Milwaukee* 4 (1928): 241.

7. According to Germany's Commission E as reported in wholehealthmd.com.

8. Andrea Pierce, *Practical Guide to Natural Medicines.* (New York: Stonesong Press, 1999): 24.

9. Michael Moore, "Herbs Best as Standard Infusion," *Materia Medica Factsheet,* http://www.swsbm.com/ManualsMM/StdInfus.txt.

10. Pierce, *Practical Guide to Natural Medicines,* 25.

11. Lane P. Johnson, *Pocket Guide to Herbal Remedies,* (Malden, MA: Blackwell Science, 2002): 4.

12. Pierce, *Practical Guide to Natural Medicines,* 25.

13. Herbalgram.org, "Aloe," *American Botanical Council,* http://www.herbalgram.org/default.asp?c'aloe.

14. Herbalgram.org, "Aloe."

15. Herbasin, "Aloe (*Lu Hui*)," *Herbasin Chinese Herb Database.* http://www.herbasin.com/database/luhui.htm.

16. Kathi J. Kemper, "Aloe Vera," *The Longwood Herbal Task Force,* http://www.mcp.edu/herbal/default.htm .

17. M. Rodriguez-Bigas, N. I. Cruz, and A. Suarez, "Comparative Evaluation of Aloe Vera in The Management of Burn Wounds in Guinea Pigs." *Plastic and Reconstructive Surgery* 81 (1988): 386–9; N. Bunyapraphatsara, S. Jirakulchaiwong, S. Thirawarapan, and J. Manonukul, "The Efficacy Of Aloe Vera Cream In The Treatment Of First, Second And Third Degree Burns In Mice." *Phytomedicine* 2 (1996): 247–51.

18. V. Visuthikosol, et al., "Effect of Aloe Vera Gel to Healing of Burn Wound a Clinical and Histologic Study." *Journal of the Medical Association of Thailand* 78, no. 8 (August 1995): 403–9.

19. Steven B. Karch, *The Consumer's Guide to Herbal Medicine* (Hauppauge, NY: Advanced Research Press, 1999): 29.

20. Karch, *The Consumer's Guide to Herbal Medicine*, 29; L. Lorenzetti, R. Salisbury, and Baldwin J. Beal, "Bacteriostatic Property Of Aloe Vera," *Journal of Pharmacological Sciences* 53 (1964): 1287.

21. B. K. Vogler and E. Ernst, "Aloe Vera: A Systematic Review of its Clinical Effectiveness," *The British Journal of General Practice* 49, no. 447 (October 1999): 823–8.

22. Kemper, "Aloe Vera."

23. J. M. Schmidt and J. S. Greenspoon, "Aloe Vera Dermal Wound Gel is Associated with a Delay in Wound Healing," *Obstetrics and Gynecology* 78, no. 1 (July 1991): 115–7.

24. Schmidt, "Aloe Vera Dermal Wound Gel is Associated with a Delay in Wound Healing."

25. D. Hunter and A. Frumkin, "Adverse Reactions to Vitamin E and Aloe Vera Preparations after Dermabrasion and Chemical Peel," *Cutis: Cutaneous Medicine For The Practitioner* 47, no. 3 (March 1991): 193–6.

26. Herbalgram.org, "Aloe."

27. Karch, *The Consumer's Guide to Herbal Medicine*, 29

28. Holly J. Bayne, "FDA Issues Final Rule Banning Use of Aloe and *Cascara sagrada* in OTC Drug Products," *HerbalGram: The Journal of the American Botanical Council* 56 (2002): 56.

29. Medline Plus, "Aloe Vera," http://www.nlm.nih.gov/medlineplus/druginfo/natural/patient–aloe.html.

30. Medline Plus, "Aloe Vera."

31. Erika Lenz, "Andrographis," *Encyclopedia of Alternative Medicine*, http://www.findarticles.com/p/articles/mi_g2603/is_0001/ai_2603000154.

32. K. Bone, "The Story of *Andrographis paniculata*, a New "Immune System" Herb," *Nutrition and Healing* (September 1998): 3–9.

33. Joanna Thompson Coon and Edzard Ernst, "Andrographis Paniculata in the Treatment of Upper Respiratory Tract Infections: A Systematic Review of Safety and Efficacy," *Planta Medica* 80 (2004): 293–298; Karen W. Martin and Edzard Ernst, "Antiviral Agents from Plants and Herbs: A Systematic Review." *Antiviral Therapy* 8 (2003):77–90.

34. E. S. Gabrielian, et al., "A Double Blind, Placebo-Controlled Study of Andrographis Paniculata Fixed Combination Kan Jang in the Treatment of Acute Upper Respiratory Tract Infections Including Sinusitis," *Phytomedicine* 9, no. 7 (October 2002): 589–97.

35. N. Poolsup, et al. "Andrographis Paniculata in the Symptomatic Treatment of Uncomplicated Upper Respiratory Tract Infection: Systematic Review of Randomized Controlled Trials," *Journal of Clinical Pharmacy and Therapeutics* 29, no. 1 (February 2004): 37–45.

36. Gabrielian, "A Double Blind, Placebo-Controlled Study Of Andrographis Paniculata," 589–97.

37. J. Limsong, et al., "Inhibitory Effect of Some Herbal Extracts on Adherence of *Streptococcus mutans*," *Journal of Ethnopharmacology* 92, no. 2–3 (June 2004): 281–9.

38. A. Puri, et al., "Immunostimulant Agents from Andrographis Paniculata," *Journal of Natural Products* 56, no. 7 (July 1993): 995–9.

39. Y. C. Shen, et al., "Andrographolide Prevents Oxygen Radical Production by Human Neutrophils: Possible Mechanism(s) Involved in its Anti-Inflammatory Effect," *British Journal of Pharmacology* 135, no. 2 (January 2002): 399–406.

40. D. D. Caceres, J. L. Hancke, and R. A. Burgos, et al., "Prevention of Common Colds with Andrographis Paniculata Dried Extract: A Pilot Double Blind Trial," *Phytomedicine* 4 (1997): 101–104.

41. Bone, "The Story of Andrographis Paniculata," 101–104.

42. Bone, "The Story Of Andrographis Paniculata," 101–104.

43. Paul B. Hamel and Mary U. Chiltoskey, *Cherokee Plants and Their Uses: A 400 Year History* (Sylva, N.C.: Herald Publishing Co., 1975): 23.

44. M. H. Boskabady, et al., "Relaxant Effect of *Pimpinella anisum* on Isolated Guinea Pig Tracheal Chains and its Possible Mechanism(s)," *Journal of Ethnophamacology* 74, no. 1 (January 2001): 83–8.

45. Karch, *The Consumer's Guide to Herbal Medicine*, 34.

46. I. Kosalec, et al., "Antifungal Activity of Fluid Extract and Essential Oil from Anise Fruits (*Pimpinella Anisum L., Apiaceae*)," *Acta Pharmaceutica* 55, no. 4 (December 2005): 377–85; Soliman KM, et al., "Effect of Oil Extracted from Some Medicinal Plants on Different Mycotoxigenic Fungi," *Food and Chemical Toxicology* 40, no. 11 (November 2002):1669–75.

47. Ahmed Nm Chaudhry, et al., "Bactericidal Activity of Black Pepper, Bay Leaf, Aniseed and Coriander against Oral Isolates," *Pakistan Journal of Pharmaceutical Sciences* 19, no. 3 (July 2006): 214–218.

48 Moore, "Herbs Best as Standard Infusion."

49. David L. Hoffmann, "Herbal Materia Medica," *Health World*, http://www.healthy.net.

50. Commission E, "Star Anise Seed," *The Commission E Monographs: IHerb Health Encyclopedia*. http://www.herbalgram.org/iherb/commissione/Monographs/Monograph_0348.html.

51. Commission E, "Star Anise Seed."

52. Karch, *The Consumer's Guide to Herbal Medicine*, 35.

53. David L. Hoffmann, "Herbal Materia Medica," *Health World*. http://www.healthy.net.

54. United States Food and Drug Administration, Title 21—Food and Drugs; Chapter I—Food and Drug Administration, Department of Health and Human Services; Part 182—substances Generally Recognized as Safe. http://www.cfsan.fda.gov/~lrd/fcf182.html (June 6, 2006).

55. Karch, *The Consumer's Guide to Herbal Medicine*, 34.

56. Johnson, *Pocket Guide to Herbal Remedies*, 115.

57. S. I. Kreydiyyeh, et al., "Aniseed Oil Increases Glucose Absorption and Reduces Urine Output in the Rat," *Life Sciences* 19, no. 5 (December 2003): 663–73.

58. M. Albert-Puleo, "Fennel and Anise as Estrogenic Agents," *Journal of Ethnophamacology* 2, no. 4 (December 1980): 337–44.

59. "Japanese Star Anise," *Wikipedia*, http://en.wikipedia.org/wiki/Japanese_star_anise.

60. USDA Natural Resources Conservation Service, "*Arnica chamissonis Less.*: Chamisso arnica," *Plants Database*, http://plants.usda.gov/java/profile?symbol=ARCH3.

61. Karch, *The Consumer's Guide to Herbal Medicine*, 36.

62. University of Michigan, Dearborn, "Native American Ethnobotony," http://herb.umd.umich.edu/.

63. Pierce, *Practical Guide to Natural Medicines*, 699.

64. B. M. Seeley, et al., "Effect of Homeopathic Arnica Montana on Bruising in Face-Lifts: Results of a Randomized, Double-Blind, Placebo-Controlled Clinical Trial," *Archives of Facial Plastic Surgery* 8, no. 1 (January–February 2006): 54–9.

65. A. Totonchi and B. Guyuron, "A Randomized, Controlled Comparison Between Arnica and Steroids in the Management of Postrhinoplasty Ecchymosis and Edema," *Plastic and Reconstructive Surgery* 120, no. 1 (July 2007): 271–4.

66. D. Alonso, et al., "Effects of Topical Arnica Gel on Post-Laser Treatment Bruises," *Dermatologic Surgery* 28, no. 8 (August 2002): 686–8.

67. O. Knuesel, et al., "Arnica Montana Gel in Osteoarthritis of the Knee: An Open, Multicenter Clinical Trial," *Advances in Therapy* 19, no. 5 (September–October 2002): 209–18.

68. R. Widrig, et al., "Choosing Between NSAID and Arnica for Topical Treatment of Hand Osteoarthritis in a Randomised, Double-Blind Study," *Rheumatology International* 27, no. 6 (April 2007): 585–91.

69. G.S. Kaziro, "Metronidazole (Flagyl) and Arnica Montana in the Prevention of Post-Surgical Complications: A Comparative Placebo Controlled Clinical Trial," *British Journal of Oral Maxillofacial Surgery* 22, no. 1 (1984) 42-9.

70. Steffen Wagner, et al., "Skin Penetration Studies of Arnica Preparations and of their Sesquiterpene Lactones," *Planta Medica* 70 (2004): 897–903.

71. Hoffmann, "Arnica," *Herbal Materia Medica*.

72. Claire Kowalchik and William Hylton, eds., *Rodale's Illustrated Encyclopedia of Herbs* (Emmaus, Pennsylvania: Rodale Press, 1987).

73. Arnica, *Whole Health MD*, http://www.wholehealthmd.com/.

74. Pierce, *Practical Guide to Natural Medicines*, 45.

75. Karch, *The Consumer's Guide to Herbal Medicine*, 37.

76. Pierce, *Practical Guide to Natural Medicines*, 45.

77. Karch, *The Consumer's Guide to Herbal Medicine*, 37.

78. Karch, *The Consumer's Guide to Herbal Medicine*, 37.

79. E. Ernst and M. H. Pittler, "Efficacy of Homeopathic Arnica: A Systematic Review of Placebo-Controlled Clinical Trials," *Archives of Surgery* 133, no. 11 (November 1998): 1187–90.

80. Pierce, *Practical Guide to Natural Medicines*, 49.

81. R. Archana and A. Namasivayan, "Antistressor Effect Of *Withania somnifera*," *Journal of Ethnophamacology* 64 (1999): 91–93.

82. S. K. Bhattacharya, "Anti-stress Activity of Sitoindosides VII and VIII, New Acylsterylglucosides from *Withania somnifera*," *Phytotherapy Research* 1, no. 1 (1987): 32–37.

83. S. Sharma, S. Dahanukar, and S. M. Karandikar, "Effects of Long-Term Administration of the Roots of Ashwagandha (*Withania somnifera*) and Shatavari (*Asparagus racemosus*) in Rats," *Indian Drugs* 23 (1986): 133–139.

84. S. Venkataraghavan, C. Seshadri, T. P. Sundaresan, et al., "The Comparative Effect of Milk Fortified with Aswagandha, Aswagandha and Punarnava in Children—A Double-Blind Study," *Journal of Research in Ayurveda and Siddha* 1 (1980): 370–385.

85. Bone K., "Clinical Applications of Ayurvedic and Chinese Herbs," *Monographs for the Western Herbal Practitioner*, (Australia: Phytotherapy Press, 1996): 137–141.

86. Pierce, *Practical Guide to Natural Medicines*, 49.

87. M.K. al-Hindawi et al., "Anti-Inflammatory Activity of some Iraqi Plants Using Intact Rats," *Journal of Ethnopharmacology* 26 (1989): 163–168.

88. R. Archana and A. Namasivayan, "Antistressor Effect of *Withania Somnifera*," *Journal of Ethnophamacology* 64 (1999): 91–93.

89. C. L. Malhotra, P. K. Das, N. S. Dhalla, and K. Prasad, "Studies on *Withania ashwagandha,* Kaul. III. The Effect Of Total Alkaloids On The Cardiovascular System And Respiration," *Indian Journal of Medical Research* 49 (1981): 448–460.

90. R. Fontaine and A. Erdoes, ["On the Central Effect of Different Withania-Extracts after Oral Applications to Animals,"] *Planta Medica* 30 (1976): 242. [German]; C. L. Malhotra, V. L. Mehta, P. K. Das, and N. S. Dhalla, "Studies On Withania-Ashwagandha,"; V. Kaul, "The Effect of Total Alkaloids (Ashwagandholine) on the Central Nervous System," *Indian Journal of Physiology and Pharmacology* 9 (1965): 127–136.

91. S. K. Bhattacharya, K. S. Satyan, A. Chakrabarti, "Effect of Trasina, an Ayurvedic Herbal Formulation, on Pancreatic Islet Superoxide Dismutase Activity in Hyperglycaemic Rats," *Indian Journal of Experimental Biology* 35 (1997): 297–299.

92. S. Ghosal, J. Lal, R. Srivastava, et al., "Immunomodulatory and CNS Effects of Sitoindosides IX and X, Two New Glycowithanolides from *Withania Somnifera*," *Phytotherapy Research* 3 (1989): 201–206.

93. K. Anbalagan and J. Sadique, "Influence of an Indian Medicine (Ashwagandha) on Acute-Phase Reactants in Inflammation," *Indian Journal of Experimental Biology* 19 (1981): 245–249.

94. V. H. Begum and J. Sadique, "Long Term Effect of Herbal Drug *Withania Somnifera* on Adjuvant Induced Arthritis in Rats," *Indian Journal of Experimental Biology* 26 (1988): 877–882.

95. R. R. Kulkarni, P. S. Patki, and V. P. Jog, et al., "Treatment of Osteoarthritis with a Herbomineral Formulation: A Double-Blind, Placebo-Controlled, Cross-Over Study," *Journal of Ethnophamacology* 33 (1991): 91–95.

96. Pierce, *Practical Guide to Natural Medicines*, 49.

97. Richo Cech, *Making Plant Medicine*, (Williams, OR: Horizon Herbs, 2000): 105.

98. S. K. Bhattacharya, et al., "Adaptogenic Activity of Withania Somnifera: An Experimental Study Using a Rat Model of Chronic Stress," *Pharmacology, Biochemistry, and Behavior* 75, no. 3 (June 2003): 547–55.

99. C. S. van der Hooft, et al., ["Thyrotoxicosis Following the Use of Ashwagandha,"] *Nederlands Tijdschrift Voor Geneeskunde* 149, no. 47 (November 19, 2005): 2637–8 (Article in Dutch).

100. M. Rasool, et al., "Immunomodulatory Role of *Withania Somnifera* Root Powder on Experimental Induced Inflammation: An In Vivo and In Vitro Study," *Vascular Pharmacology* 44, no. 6 (June 2006): 406–10.

101. S. N. Arseculeratne, A. A. Gunatilaka, and R. G. Panabokk, "Studies of Medicinal Plants of Sri Lanka. Part 14: Toxicity of Some Traditional Medicinal Herbs," *Journal of Ethnophamacology* 13, no. 3 (July 1985): 323–35.

102. I. Ilayperuma, et al., "Effect of Withania Somnifera Root Extract on the Sexual Behaviour of Male Rats," *Asian Journal Of Andrology* 4, no. 4 (December 2002): 295–8.

103. A. C. Sharada, et al., "*Withania somnifera* Root Extract in Rat and Mice," *International Journal of Pharmacognosy* 31, no. 3 (1993): 205–12.

104. Karch, *The Consumer's Guide to Herbal Medicine*, 40–41.

105. Karch, *The Consumer's Guide to Herbal Medicine*, 40–41.

106. H. Yunde, et al., "Effect of Radix *Astragali Seu Hedysari* on the Interferon System," *Chinese Medical Journal* 94, no. 1 (1981): 35–40.

107. McCaleb, *The Encyclopedia of Popular Herbs*, 64.

108. H. M. Chang and P. P. H. But, *Pharmacology and Applications of Chinese Materia Medica*. Volume 2. (Hong Kong: World Scientific, 1987).

109. Astragalus (*Astragalus membranaceus*). *MedLine Plus Herbs and Supplements*, http://www.nlm.nih.gov/medlineplus/druginfo/natural/patient-astragalus.html.

110. Pierce, *Practical Guide to Natural Medicines*, 53.

111. Y. Zhang, Q. Xu, X. Liu, S. Wang, J. Shen, and L. You, "The Anti-Leukocytopenic and Anti-Stress Effects of *Astragalus saponins* (ASI, SK) on Mice," *Nanjing Yixueyuan Xuebao* 12, no. 3 (1992): 244–8.

112. Y. Z. Yang, et al., ["Observation on Collaborative Treatment of Dilated Cardiomyopathy,"] *Zhongguo Zhong Xi Yi Jie He Za Zhi*. 21, no. 4 (April 2001): 254–6. (Article in Chinese); Z. Y. Lei, et al., ["Action of *Astragalus Membranaceus* on Left Ventricular Function of Angina Pectoris,"] *Chung Kuo Chung Hsi I Chieh Ho Tsa Chih* 14, no. 4 (April 1994): 195, 199–202 (Article in Chinese).

113. H. Wang, et al., ["The Effect of Herbal Medicine Including *Astragalus Membranaceus (Fisch) Bge, Codonpsis Pilosula* and *Glycyrrhiza uralensis Fisch* on Airway Responsiveness,"] *Zhonghua Jie He He Hu Xi Za Zhi*, 21, no. 5 (May 1998): 287–8 (Article in Chinese).

114. Hoffmann, "Astragalus," *Herbal Materia Medica*.

115. Cech, *Making Plant Medicine*, 106.

116. Pierce, *Practical Guide to Natural Medicines*, 53.

117. Johnson, *Pocket Guide to Herbal Remedies*, 21.

118. McCaleb, *The Encyclopedia of Popular Herbs*, 66.

119. "Astragalus," *Web MD*.

120. "Astragalus," *Web MD*.

121. Karch, *The Consumer's Guide to Herbal Medicine*, 40.

122. Johnson, *Pocket Guide to Herbal Remedies*, 21.

123. Johnson, *Pocket Guide to Herbal Remedies*, 21.

124. Johnson, *Pocket Guide to Herbal Remedies*, 21.

125. K. Panter, W. Hartley, L. James, H. Mayland, B. Stegelmeier, and P. Kechele, "Comparative Toxicity of Selenium from Selno-DL-Methionine, Sodium Selenate and *Astragalus Bisulcatus* in Pigs," *Fundamentals of Applied Toxicology* 32 (1996): 217–23.

126. Johnson, *Pocket Guide to Herbal Remedies*, 21.

127. Johnson, *Pocket Guide to Herbal Remedies*, 21.

128. MedLine Plus Herbs and Supplements. "Astragalus (Astragalus membranaceus)."

129. MedLine Plus Herbs and Supplements. "Astragalus (Astragalus membranaceus)."

130. MedLine Plus Herbs and Supplements. "Astragalus (Astragalus membranaceus)."

131. MedLine Plus Herbs and Supplements. "Astragalus (Astragalus membranaceus)."

132. MedLine Plus Herbs and Supplements. "Astragalus (Astragalus membranaceus)."

133. MedLine Plus Herbs and Supplements. "Astragalus (Astragalus membranaceus)."

134. W. Kalt and J. E. McDonald, "Chemical Composition Of Lowbush Blueberry Cultivars," *Journal of the American Society of Horticultural Science* 121 (1996): 142–146.

135. O. Polunin, *Flowers of Europe: A Field Guide*, (New York: Oxford University Press, 1969).

136. McCaleb, *The Encyclopedia of Popular Herbs*, 70–71.

137. E. R. Muth, J. M. Laurent, and P. Jasper, "The Effect of Bilberry Nutritional Supplementation on Night Visual Acuity and Contrast Sensitivity," *Alternative Medicine Review* 5, no. 2 (April 2000): 164–73.

138. K. A. Head. "Natural Therapies for Ocular Disorders, Part Two: Cataracts and Glaucoma," *Alternative Medicine Review* 6, no. 2 (April 2001): 141–66.

139. V. Bettini, R. Aragno, M. Bettini, G. Braggion, L. Calore, and G. Penada, "Anoxia and Coronary Vasodilation by *Vaccinium myrtillus* Anthocyanosides," *Cuore* 9 (1992): 343–53.

140. Steven Foster, "Bilberry: Food and Medicine," *The Herb Companion* (1997): 68–69.

141. L. Sauebin, et al., "Effect of Anthocyanins Contained in a Blackberry Extract on the Circulatory Failure and Multiple Organ Dysfunction Caused by Endotoxin in the Rat," *Planta Medica* 70, no. 8 (August 2004): 745–52.

142. I. Erlund, et al., "Consumption of Black Currants, Lingonberries and Bilberries Increases Serum Quercetin Concentrations," *European Journal of Clinical Nutrition* 57, no. 1 (January 2003): 37–42.

143. P. M. Laplaud, A. Lelubre, and M. J. Chapman, "Antioxidant Action of *Vaccinium myrtillus* Extract on Human Low Density Lipoproteins In Vitro: Initial Observations," *Fundamental and Clinical Pharmacology* 11, no. 1 (1997): 35–40.

144. R. Puupponen-Pimia, L. Nohynek, H. L. Alakomi, and K. M. Oksman-Caldentey, "Bioactive Berry Compounds: Novel Tools Against Human Pathogens," *Applied Microbiology and Biotechnology* 67, no. 1 (April 2005): 8–18.

145. "Bilberry," *Whole Health MD*, http://www.wholehealthmd.com/.

146. McCaleb, *The Encyclopedia of Popular Herbs*, 74.

147. Richard Harkness and Steven Bratman, *Handbook of Drug–Herb and Drug-Supplement Interactions* (St. Louis, MO: Mosby, 2003): 134.

148. Johnson, *Pocket Guide to Herbal Remedies*, 178.

149. Karch, *The Consumer's Guide to Herbal Medicine*, 42.

150. Penelope Ody, *The Complete Medicinal Herbal* (London: Dorling Kindersley, 1993): 41.

151. Maud Grieve, "Borage," *Botanical.com: A Modern Herbal*, http://www.botanical.com/botanical/mgmh/b/borage66.html.

152. Grieve, *Botanical.com: A Modern Herbal.*

153. "Borage Oil," *Whole Health MD*, http://www.wholehealthmd.com.

154. "Borage Oil," *Whole Health MD.*

155. L. J. Leventhal, et al., "Treatment of Rheumatoid Arthritis with Gammalinolenic Acid," *Annals of Internal Medicine* 119, no. 9 (1993): 867–73.

156. "Borage Oil," *Whole Health MD.*

157. Pierce, *Practical Guide to Natural Medicines*, 111.

158. D. E. Mills, et al., "Dietary Fatty Acid Supplementation Alters Stress Reactivity and Performance in Man," *Journal Of Human Hypertension* 3, no. 2 (April 1989): 111–6.

159. D. F. Horrobin, "Essential Fatty Acid Metabolism and its Modification in Atopic Eczema," *American Journal of Clinical Nutrition* 71, no. 1 Supplemental (January 2000): 367–372.

160. "Borage Oil," *Whole Health MD.*

161. Pierce, *Practical Guide to Natural Medicines*, 110.

162. "Borage Oil," *Whole Health MD.*

163. "Borage Oil," *Whole Health MD.*

164. Karch, *The Consumer's Guide to Herbal Medicine*, 47

165. Karch, *The Consumer's Guide to Herbal Medicine*, 47

166. "Borage Oil," *Whole Health MD.*

167. "Borage Oil," *Whole Health MD.*

168. U.S. Food and Drug Administration. "Pyrrolizidine Alkaloids," *Foodborne Pathogenic Microorganisms and Natural Toxins Handbook*, http://www.cfsan.fda.gov/~mow/chap42.html.

169. "Borage Oil," *Whole Health MD.*

170. Thomson Healthcare, "Borage Oil," *PDR Health*, http://www.pdrhealth.com/drug_info/nmdrugprofiles/nutsupdrugs/bor_0039.shtml.

171. Thomson Healthcare. "Borage Oil."

172. Johnson, *Pocket Guide to Herbal Remedies*, 26.

173. Karch, *The Consumer's Guide to Herbal Medicine*, 47

174. "Bromelain," *Whole Health MD* http://www.wholehealthmd.com.

175. C. Neumayer, et al., "Combined Enzymatic and Antioxidative Treatment Reduces Ischemia-Reperfusion Injury in Rabbit Skeletal Muscle," *Journal of Surgical Research*, 133, no. 2 (June 15, 2006): 150–8.

176. M. Masson, ["Bromelain in Blunt Injuries of the Locomotor System: A Study of Observed Applications in General Practice,"] *Fortschritte der Medizin* 113, no. 19 (July 10, 1995): 303–6 (Article in German).

177. J. L. Blonstein, "Control of Swelling in Boxing Injuries," *Practitioner* 185 (1960): 78.

178. H. R. Maurer, "Bromelain: Biochemistry, Pharmacology and Medical Use," *Cellular and Molecular Life Sciences* 58 (2001): 1234–45.

179. A. F. Walkee, et al., "Bromelain Reduces Mild Acute Knee Pain and Improves Well-Being in a Dose-Dependent Fashion in an Open Study of Otherwise Healthy Adults," *Phytomedicine* 9, no. 8 (December 2002): 681–6.

180. Sarah Brien et al., "Bromelain as a Treatment for Osteoarthritis: A Review of Clinical Studies," *Evidence-based Complementary and Alternative Medicine* 1, no. 3 (December 2004): 251–257.

181. "Bromelain," *Whole Health MD.*

182. E. R. Secor, Jr., et al., "Bromelain Exerts Anti-Inflammatory Effects in an Ovalbumin-Induced Murine Model of Allergic Airway Disease," *Cellular Immunology* 237, no. 1 (September 2005): 68–75.

183. M. B. Stone, et al., "Preliminary Comparison of Bromelain and Ibuprofen for Delayed Onset Muscle Soreness Management," *Clinical Journal of Sport Medicine* 12 (November 2002): 373–8.

184. P. C. Miller, et al., "The Effects of Protease Supplementation on Skeletal Muscle Function and DOMS Following Downhill Running," *Journal of Sports Science* 22, no. 4 (April 2004): 365–72.

185. "Bromelain," *Whole Health MD.*

186. "Bromelain," *Health Notes.* http://www.drugstore.com/templates/hnotes/default.asp?catid=42744&trx=SRCH-0-HN-BB&trxp1=bromelain&trxp2=42744.

187. A. R. Gaby, "The Story Of Bromelain," *Nutrition and Healing* (May 1995): 3, 4, 11.

188. Gaby, "The Story Of Bromelain," 4, 11.

189. Gregory S. Kelly, "Bromelain: A Literature Review and Discussion of its Therapeutic Applications," *Alternative Medicine Review* 1, no. 4 (1996): 253.

190. Kelly, "Bromelain: A Literature Review and Discussion of its Therapeutic Applications," 243–257.

191. R. Heinicke, L. van der Wal, and M. Yokoyama, "Effect of Bromelain (Ananase) on Human Platelet Aggregation," *Experientia* 28 (1972): 844–5.

192. "Bromelain," *Whole Health MD.*

193. "Bromelain," *Whole Health MD.*

194. Kelly, "Bromelain: A Literature Review and Discussion of its Therapeutic Applications," 243–257.

195. "Bromelain," *Whole Health MD.*

196. E. Nettis, G. Napoli, A. Ferrannini, and A. Tursi, "IgE–Mediated Allergy to Bromelain," *Allergy* 56 (2001): 257–8.

197. E. Batanero, M. Villalba, R. I. Monsalve, et al., "Cross-Reactivity Between the Major Allergen from Olive Pollen and Unrelated Glycoproteins: Evidence of an Epitope in the Glycan Moiety of the Allergen," *Journal of Clinical Immunology* 97 (1996): 1264–1271.

198. "*Calendula officinalis*," *Wikipedia* http://en.wikipedia.org/wiki/Calendula_officinalis.

199. Kathi J. Kemper, "Calendula (*Calendula officinalis*)," *The Longwood Herbal Task Force*, http://www.mcp.edu/herbal/default.htm.

200. G. Dumenil, R. Chemli, C. Balansard, H. Guiraud, and M. Lallemand, ["Evaluation of Antibacterial Properties of Marigold Flowers (*Calendula Officinalis L.*) and Mother Homeopathic Tinctures of *C. Officinalis L.* and *C. Arvensis L.*,"] *Annales Pharmaceutiques Françaises* 38, no. 6 (1980): 493–9 (Article in French).

201. Z. Kalvatchev, "Anti-HIV Activity of Extracts from Calendula Officinalis Flowers," *Biomedicine and Pharmacotherapy* 51, no. 4 (1997): 176–80.

202. R. Della Loggia, et al., "The Role of Triterpenoids in the Topical Anti-Inflammatory Activity of Calendula Officinalis Flowers," *Planta Medica* 60, no. 6 (December 1994): 516–20.

203. E. Klouchek-Popova, A. Popov, N. Pavlova, and S. Krusteva, "Influence of the Physiological Regeneration and Epithelialization Using Fractions Isolated from *Calendula Officinalis*," *Acta Physiologica et Pharmacologica Bulgarica* 8, no. 4 (1982): 63–7.

204. P. Pommier, F. Gomez, M. P. Sunyach, et al., "Phase III Randomized Trial of *Calendula officinalis* Compared with Trolamine for the Prevention of Acute Dermatitis During Irradiation for Breast Cancer," *Journal of Clinical Oncology* 22, no. 8 (2004): 1447–1453.

205. A. M. Fleischner, "Plant Extracts: To Accelerate Healing and Reduce Inflammation," *Cosmetics And Toiletries* 100, no. 1010 (1985): 45–58 (Article in French).

206. V. Duran, et al., "Results of the Clinical Examination of an Ointment with Marigold (*Calendula officinalis*) Extract in the Treatment of Venous Leg Ulcers," *International Journal of Tissue Reactions* 27, no. 3 (2005): 101–6.

207. Karch, *The Consumer's Guide to Herbal Medicine*, 183.

208. Kemper, "Calendula."

209. "Calendula," *Whole Health MD.* http://www.wholehealthmd.com.

210. E. Barrie Kavasch, and Karen Baar, *American Indian Healing Arts* (New York: Bantam, 1999): 179.

211. U.S. National Library of Medicine. "Calendula (*Calendula officinalis L.*)," http://www.nlm.nih.gov/medlineplus/druginfo/natural/patient-calendula.html.

212. Kemper, "Calendula."

213. U.S. National Library of Medicine. "Calendula (*Calendula officinalis L.*)."

214. American Botanical Council, "Calendula flower," *Herbal Information: Commission E Monographs.* http://www.herbalgram.org/default.asp?c=comm_e_calendula.

215. Pierce, *Practical Guide to Natural Medicines*, 130.

216. Johnson, *Pocket Guide to Herbal Remedies*, 27.

217. U.S. National Library of Medicine. "Calendula (*Calendula officinalis L.*)."

218. Hoffmann, "Calendula," *Herbal Materia Medica.*

219. U.S. National Library of Medicine. "Calendula (*Calendula officinalis L.*)."

220. N. Reider, et al., "The Seamy Side of Natural Medicines: Contact Sensitization to Arnica (*Arnica Montana L.*) and Marigold (*Calendula Officinalis L.*)," *Contact Dermatitis* 45, no. 5 (November 2001): 269–72.

221. U.S. National Library of Medicine. "Calendula (*Calendula officinalis L.*)."

222. Pierce, *Practical Guide to Natural Medicines*, 130.

223. U.S. National Library of Medicine. "Calendula (*Calendula officinalis L.*)."

224. "Cayenne," *Whole Health MD*, http://www.wholehealthmd.com.

225. "Capsaicin," *Wikipedia.* http://en.wikipedia.org/wiki/Capsaicin; A. Dray, "Mechanism of Action of Capsaicin-like Molecules on Sensory Neurons" *Life Sciences* 51, no. 23 (1992): 1759–65.

226. W. Keitel, et al., "Capsicum Pain Plaster in Chronic Non-Specific Low Back Pain," *Arzneimittelforschung* 51, no. 11 (November 2001): 896–903.

227. H. Frerick, et al., "Topical Treatment of Chronic Low Back Pain with a Capsicum Plaster," *Pain* 106, no. 1–2 (November 2003): 59–64.

228. The Associated Press. "Chile 'Sauce' in Wounds may Deaden Surgery Pain," *Arizona Daily Star*, October 30, 2007.

229. The Associated Press. "Chile 'Sauce' in Wounds may Deaden Surgery Pain."

230. S. C. Cruwys, et al., "Sensory Denervation with Capsaicin Attenuates Inflammation and Nociception in Arthritic Rats," *Neuroscience Letters* 193, no. 3 (July 7, 1995): 205–7; F. C. Colpaert, "Effects of Capsaicin on Inflammation and an the Substance P Content of Nervous Tissues in Rats with Adjuvant Arthritis," *Life Sciences* 32, no. 16 (April 18, 1983): 1827–34; F. Y. Lam, et al., "Capsaicin Suppresses Substance P–Induced Joint Inflammation in the Rat," *Neuroscience Letters* 105, no. 1-2 (October 23, 1989): 155–8.

231. E. Winocur, et al., "Topical Application of Capsaicin for the Treatment of Localized Pain in the Temporomandibular Joint Area," *Journal of Orofacial Pain* 14, no. 1 (Winter 2000): 31–6.

232. G. M. McCarthy, et al., "Effect of Topical Capsaicin in the Therapy of Painful Osteoarthritis of the Hands." *Journal of Rheumatology* 19 (1992): 604–7.

233. C. L. Deal, et al., "Treatment Of Arthritis with Topical Capsaicin: A Double-Blind Trial." *Clinical Therapeutics* 13 (1991): 383–95.

234. R. H. Cichewicz and P.A. Thorpe, "The Antimicrobial Properties of Chile Peppers (Capsicum Species) and Their Uses in Mayan Medicine," *Journal of Ethnopharmacology* 52, no. 2 (1996): 62–70.

235. Hamel and Chiltoskey, *Cherokee Plants and Their Uses*, 48.

236. Kowalchik and Hylton, *Rodale's Illustrated Encyclopedia of Herbs.*

237. S. Marabini, et al., "Beneficial Effects of Intranasal Applications of Capsaicin in Patients with Vasomotor Rhinitis," *European Archives Of Oto-Rhino-Laryngology* 248, no. 4 (1991): 191–4.

238. E. Rau, "Treatment of Acute Tonsillitis with a Fixed-Combination Herbal Preparation," *Advances in Therapy* 17, no. 4 (July–August 2000): 197–203.

239. M. Yoshioka, et al., "Effects of Red–Pepper Diet on the Energy Metabolism in Men," *Journal of Nutritional Science and Vitaminology (Tokyo)* 41, no. 6 (December 1995): 647–56.

240. K. Lim, et al., "Dietary Red Pepper Ingestion Increases Carbohydrate Oxidation at Rest and During Exercise in Runners," *Medicine and Science in Sports and Exercise* 29, no. 3 (March 1997): 355–61.

241. Ody, *The Complete Medicinal Herbal*, 46.

242. Kowalchik and Hylton, *Rodale's Illustrated Encyclopedia of Herbs.*

243. Moore, "Dry Plant Percolation Preferences," *Materia Medica.*

244. "*Capsicum annuum*," *PDR for Herbal Medicine* (Montvale, NJ: Medical Economics Company, 1998): 715.

245. Kowalchik and Hylton, *Rodale's Illustrated Encyclopedia of Herbs.*

246. Kowalchik and Hylton, *Rodale's Illustrated Encyclopedia of Herbs.*

247. "Scoville Scale," *Wikipedia* http://en.wikipedia.org/wiki/Scoville_scale.

248. Karch, *The Consumer's Guide to Herbal Medicine*, 58.

249. Commission E, "Paprika (Cayenne)," *The Commission E Monographs: IHerb Health Encyclopedia.* http://www.herbalgram.org/iherb/commissione/Monographs/Monograph_0282.html.

250. "Cayenne," *Whole Health MD.*

251. "Cayenne," *Whole Health MD.*

252. Karch, *The Consumer's Guide to Herbal Medicine*, 58.

253. "Cayenne Pepper Fruit, *Capsicum annuum*," *Herbalgram.* http://www.herbalgram.org/default.asp?c=reference_guide.

254. "Capsicum Annuum," *PDR for Herbal Medicine*, 715.

255. Commission E. "Paprika (Cayenne)," *The Commission E Monographs: IHerb Health Encyclopedia.* http://www.herbalgram.org/iherb/commissione/Monographs/Monograph_0282.html.

256. "Cayenne," *Whole Health MD.*

257. "Cayenne," *Whole Health MD.*

258. "Capsicum Annuum," *PDR for Herbal Medicine*, 715.

259. International College of Herbal Medicine. "Chilli, *Capsicum Minimum*, *C. Fructescens*," *Herb of the Month*, January/February 2004. http://www.herbcollege.com/herbofthemonth.asp?id=61.

260. Kowalchik and Hylton, *Rodale's Illustrated Encyclopedia of Herbs.*

261. P. Milke, et al., "Gastroesophageal Reflux in Healthy Subjects Induced by Two Different Species of Chilli (*Capsicum Annum*)," *Digestive Diseases* 24, no. 1–2 (2006): 184–8.

262. D. F. Altomare, et al., "Red Hot Chili Pepper and Hemorrhoids: The Explosion of a Myth: Results of a Prospective, Randomized, Placebo-Controlled, Crossover Trial," *Diseases of the Colon and Rectum* 49, no. 7 (July 2006): 1018–23.

263. K. G. Yeoh, et al., "Chili Protects Against Aspirin–Induced Gastroduodenal Mucosal Injury in Humans." *Digestive Diseases and Sciences*, 40, no. 3 (March 1995): 580–3.

264. Cayenne Pepper Fruit, Capsicum annuum. Herbalgram. http://www.herbalgram.org/default.asp?c=reference_guide.

265. S. Tuntipopipat, et al., "Chili, But Not Turmeric, Inhibits Iron Absorption in Young Women from an Iron-Fortified Composite Meal," *Journal of Nutrition* 136, no. 12 (December 2006): 2970–4.

266. Pierce, *Practical Guide to Natural Medicines*, 134.

267. J. Thompson Coon and E. Ernst, "Systematic Review: Herbal Medicinal Products For Non-Ulcer Dyspepsia," *Alimentary Pharmacology & Therapeutics* 18, no. 10 (October 2002): 1689–99.

268. A. Madisch, C. J. Heydenreich, V. Wieland, R. Hufnagel, and J. Hotz, "Treatment of Functional Dyspepsia with a Fixed Peppermint Oil and Caraway Oil Combination Preparation as Compared to Cisapride: A Multicenter, Reference-Controlled Double-Blind Equivalence Study," *Arzneimittelforschung* 49, no. 11 (November 1999): 925–32.

269. N. S. Lacobellis, P. Lo Cantore, F. Capasso, and F. Senatore, "Antibacterial Activity Of *Cuminum cyminum L.* and *Carum carvi L.* Essential Oils," *Journal of Agricultural and Food Chemistry* 12, no. 1 (January 2005): 57–61.

270. Grieve, "Caraway," *Botanical.com: A Modern Herbal.*

271. International College of Herbal Medicine, "Caraway *Carum carvi*," *Herb of the Month*, (September/October 2006) http://www.herbcollege.com/herbofthemonth.asp?id=96.

272. "Carum Carvi," *PDR for Herbal Medicine*, 722.

273. Food and Drug Administration, Department of Health and Human Services, Title 21—Food and Drugs, Chapter I, Part 182—Substances Generally Recognized as Safe, http://www.cfsan.fda.gov/~lrd/fcf182.html.

274. "Carum Carvi," *PDR for Herbal Medicine*, 722.

275. Pierce, *Practical Guide to Natural Medicines*, 135.

276. Pierce, *Practical Guide to Natural Medicines*, 147.

277. George R. Swank, *The Ethnobotany of the Acoma and Laguna Indians* (University of New Mexico, M.A. Thesis, 1932): 55.

278. Hamel and Chiltoskey, *Cherokee Plants and Their Uses*, 28

279. James William Herrick, *Iroquois Medical Botany* (Albany: State University of New York, PhD Thesis, 1977): 423.

280. Gladys Tantaquidgeon, *A Study of Delaware Indian Medicine Practice and Folk Beliefs* (Harrisburg: Pennsylvania Historical Commission, 1942): 67.

281. Pierce, *Practical Guide to Natural Medicines*, 148.

282. Pierce, *Practical Guide to Natural Medicines*, 138.

283. Kowalchik and Hylton, *Rodale's Illustrated Encyclopedia of Herbs*, 284.

284. Michael Moore, *Herbal Formulas for Clinic and Home* (Bisbee, AZ: Southwest School of Botanical Medicine, 1995).

285. Pierce, *Practical Guide to Natural Medicines*, 147.

286. Kowalchik and Hylton, *Rodale's Illustrated Encyclopedia of Herbs*, 284.

287. K.C. Osterhoudt, et al., "Catnip and the Alteration of Human Consciousness," *Veterinary and Human Toxicology* 30, no. 6 (December 1997): 373–5.

288. Johnson, *Pocket Guide to Herbal Remedies*, 104.

289. "*Nepeta cataria*," *PDR for Herbal Medicine*, 991.

290. C. O. Massoco, et al., "Behavioral Effects of Acute and Long-Term Administration of Catnip (*Nepeta cataria*) in Mice," *Veterinary and Human Toxicology* 37, no. 6 (December 1995): 530–3.

291. "Nepeta Cataria," *PDR for Herbal Medicine*, 991.

292. Raintree Nutrition, "Cat's Claw," *Tropical Plant Database*, http://www.rain-tree.com/catclaw.htm.

293. Raintree Nutrition, "Cat's Claw."

294. R. Aquino, V. De Feo, F. De Simone, C. Pizza, and G. Cirino, "Plant Metabolites. New Compounds and Anti-Inflammatory Activity of *Uncaria tomentosa*," *Journal of Natural Products* 54 (1991): 54:453–9.

295. E. Mur, et al., "Randomized Double Blind Trial of an Extract from The Pentacyclic Alkaloid-Chemotype of Uncaria Tomentosa for the Treatment of Rheumatoid Arthritis," *Journal of Rheumatology* 29, no. 4 (April 2002): 678–81.

296. J. Piscoya, et al., "Efficacy and Safety of Freeze-Dried Cat's Claw in Osteoarthritis of the Knee: Mechanisms of Action of the Species *Uncaria Guianensis*" *Inflammation Research* 50, no. 9 (September 2001): 442–8.

297. "Cat Claw," *Whole Health MD*, http://www.wholehealthmd.com.

298. Kathi J. Kemper, "Cat's Claw (*Uncaria tomentosa*)," *The Longwood Herbal Task Force*, http://www.mcp.edu/herbal/default.htm.

299. Raintree Nutrition, "Cat's Claw."

300. "Cat Claw," *Whole Health MD*.

301. Raintree Nutrition, "Cat's Claw."

302. Karch, *The Consumer's Guide to Herbal Medicine*, 55.

303. Raintree Nutrition, "Cat's Claw."

304. Piscoya, "Efficacy and Safety of Freeze-Dried Cat's Claw in Osteoarthritis of the Knee," 442–8.

305. Karch, *The Consumer's Guide to Herbal Medicine*, 55.

306. Memorial Sloan Kettering Cancer Center, "Cat's Claw," *About Herbs*. http://www.mskcc.org/mskcc/html/11571.cfm?recordid=390.

307. Memorial Sloan Kettering Cancer Center, "Cat's Claw."

308. Raintree Nutrition. "Cat's Claw."

309. Karch, *The Consumer's Guide to Herbal Medicine*, 56.

310. Raintree Nutrition, "Cat's Claw."

311. "Cat Claw," *Whole Health MD*.

312. "Cat Claw," *Whole Health MD*.

313. *PDR for Herbal Medicine*, 735, 962

314. Robert S. McCaleb, Evelyn Leigh, and Krista Morien, *The Encyclopedia of Popular Herbs* (Roseville, CA: Prima Health, 2000): 107.

315. McCaleb, *The Encyclopedia of Popular Herbs*, 105.

316. Hoffmann, *Herbal Materia Medica*.

317. H. Viola, et al., "Apigenin, a Component of *Matricaria recutita* Flowers, is a Central Benzodiazepine Receptors-Ligand with Anxiolytic Effects," *Planta Medica* 61 (1995): 213–216.

318. Viola, "Apigenin, a component of *Matricaria recutita* flowers," 213–216; Della Loggia, R. et al., "Depressive Effects of *Chamomilla recutita* (L.), Raisch, Tubular Flowers on Central Nervous System in Mice," *Pharmacological Research Communications* 14, no. 2 (1982): 153–162.

319. R. Carle, and O. Isaac, "Effect And Effectiveness: A Commentary on the Monograph of *Matricaria Flos* (Chamomile Blossoms)." *Zeitschrift für Phytotherapie* 8 (1987): 67–77.

320. Paula Gardiner, "Chamomile (*Matricaria recutita, Anthemis nobilis*), *The Longwood Herbal Task Force* http://www.mcp.edu/herbal/default.htm.

321. Gardiner, "Chamomile."

322. Leung and Foster, *Encyclopedia of Common Natural Ingredients Used in Food, Drugs, and Cosmetics*.

323. Hoffmann, "Herbal Materia Medica."

324. Y. Kobayashi, et al., "Dietary Intake of the Flower Extracts of German Chamomile (*Matricaria Recutita* L.) Inhibited Compound 48/80-Induced Itch-Scratch Responses in Mice," *Phytomedicine* 10, no. 8 (November 2003): 657–64.

325. H. J. Glowania, et al., "The Effect of Chamomile in Healing Wounds: A Clinical, Double-Blind Study." *Zeitschrift für Hautkrankheiten* 17, no. 62 (1987): 1262–1271.

326. R. Saller, et al., "Dose-Dependency of Symptomatic Relief of Complaints by Chamomile Steam Inhalation in Patients with Common Cold." *European Journal of Pharmacology* 183 (1990):728–729.

327. N.R. Farnsworth and B.M. Morgan, "Herb Drinks: Chamomile Tea," *Journal of the American Medical Association* 221 (1972): 410.

328. "Chamomile," *Whole Health MD* http://www.wholehealthmd.com.

329. "Chamomile," *Whole Health MD.*

330. "Chamomile," *Whole Health MD.*

331. Saller, "Dose-Dependency Of Symptomatic Relief Of Complaints By Chamomile," 728–729.

332. "Chamomile," *Whole Health MD.*

333. Hoffmann, "Arnica."

334. "Chamomile," *Medline Plus Herb and Supplement.* http://www.nlm.nih.gov/medlineplus/druginfo/natural/patient-chamomile.html.

335. "Chamomile," *Whole Health MD.*

336. "*Chamaemelum nobile*," *PDR for Herbal Medicine*, 735.

337. "Chamomile," *Medline Plus Herb and Supplement.*

338. R. Segal and L. Pilote, "Warfarin Interaction with *Matricaria chamomilla*," *Canadian Medical Association Journal.* 174, no. 9 (April 2006): 1281–2.

339. McCaleb, *The Encyclopedia of Popular Herbs*, 111.

340. "Chamomile," *Medline Plus Herb and Supplement.*

341. Grieve, "Chamomiles," *Botanical.com: A Modern Herbal.*

342. Judy McBride, "Cinnamon Extracts Boost Insulin Sensitivity," *Agricultural Research Magazine* 48, no. 7 (July 2000): 21.

343. E. J. Verspohl, et al., "Antidiabetic Effect of *Cinnamomum cassia* and *Cinnamomum zeylanicum* In Vivo and In Vitro," *Phytotherapy Research* 19, no. 3 (March 2005): 203–6.

344. H. B. Singh, et al., "Cinnamon Bark Oil, a Potent Fungitoxicant against Fungi Causing Respiratory Tract Mycoses," *Allergy* 50, no. 12 (December 1995): 995–9.

345. M. P. Tampieri, et al., "The Inhibition of *Candida albicans* by Selected Essential Oils and their Major Components," *Mycopathologia* 159, no. 3 (April 2005): 339–45.

346. J. Mau, et al., "Antimicrobial Effect of Extracts from Chinese Chive, Cinnamon, and Corni Fructus," *Journal of Agricultural and Food Chemistry* 49, no. 1 (January 2001): 183–8.

347. A. Smith-Palmer, et al., "Inhibition of Listeriolysin O and Phosphatidylcholine-Specific Production in Listeria Monocytogenes by Subinhibitory Concentrations of Plant Essential Oils," *Journal of Medical Microbiology* 51, no. 7 (July 2002): 567–74.

348. P. Hersch-Martinez, et al., "Antibacterial Effects of Commercial Essential Oils over Locally Prevalent Pathogenic Strains in Mexico," *Fitoterapia* 76, no. 5 (July 2005): 453–7; N. Matan, et al., "Antimicrobial Activity of Cinnamon and Clove Oils under Modified Atmosphere Conditions," *International Journal of Food Microbiology* 107, no. 2 (March 15, 2006): 180–5; L. S. Ooi,

et al., "Antimicrobial Activities of Cinnamon Oil and Cinnamaldehyde from the Chinese Medicinal Herb *Cinnamomum cassia Blume*," *American Journal of Chinese Medicine* 34, no. 3 (2006): 511–22.

349. B. Shan, et al., "Antioxidant Capacity of 26 Spice Extracts and Characterization of their Phenolic Constituents," *Journal of Agricultural and Food Chemistry* 53, no. 20 (October 5, 2005): 7749–59; Mancini-Filho J, et al. "Antioxidant Activity of Cinnamon (*Cinnamomum zeylanicum, Breyne*) Extracts," *Bollettino Chimico Farmaceutico* 137, no. 11 (December 1998): 443–7.

350. Judy McBride, "Cinnamon Extracts Boost Insulin Sensitivity," *Agricultural Research Magazine* 48, no. 7 (July 2000).

351. A. Khan, et al., "Cinnamon Improves Glucose and Lipids of People with Type 2 Diabetes," *Diabetes Care* 26, no. 12 (December 2003): 3215–8.

352. Kristof Vanschoonbeek, et al., "Cinnamon Supplementation Does Not Improve Glycemic Control in Postmenopausal Type 2 Diabetes Patients," *Journal of Nutrition* 136 (April 2006): 977–980.

353. E. J. Verspohl, et al., "Antidiabetic Effect of *Cinnamomum cassia* and *Cinnamomum zeylanicum* In Vivo and In Vitro," *Phytotherapy Research* 19, no. 3 (March 2005): 203–6.

354. Harry G. Preuss, et al., "Whole Cinnamon and Aqueous Extracts Ameliorate Sucrose-Induced Blood Pressure Elevations in Spontaneously Hypertensive Rats," *Journal of the American College of Nutrition* 25, no. 2 (2006): 144–150.

355. "Oligomeric Proanthocyanidin," *Wikipedia*, http://en.wikipedia.org/wiki/Oligomeric_proanthocyanidin.

356. A. Khan, et al., "Cinnamon Improves Glucose and Lipids of People with Type 2 Diabetes," *Diabetes Care* 26, no. 12 (December 2003): 3215–8.

357. "Study Finds That Peppermint and Cinnamon Lower Drivers' Frustration And Increase Alertness," *Wheeling Jesuit University News and Info*, http://www.wju.edu/about/adm_news_story.asp?iNewsID=1882&strBack=%2FDefault.asp.

358. Michael Moore, "Herbs Best Used as a Strong Decoction," *Materia Medica Factsheet*, http://www.swsbm.com/ManualsMM/DecoctPrf.txt.

359. Judy Foreman, "Cinnamon Joins Cholesterol Battle," *My Health Sense*. http://www.myhealthsense.com/F040824_cinnamon.html.

360. International College of Herbal Medicine. "Cinnamon—*Cinnamomum zeylanicum, Cinnamomum cassia. Herb of the Month, June/July 2003*, http://www.herbcollege.com/herbofthemonth.asp?id=51.

361. Johnson, *Pocket Guide to Herbal Remedies*, 40.

362. "*Cinnamomum verum*," *PDR for Herbal Medicine*, 752.

363. Khan, "Cinnamon Improves Glucose And Lipids," 3215–8.

364. "Cinnamomum Verum," *PDR for Herbal Medicine*, 752.

365. United States Food and Drug Administration, Title 21—Food and Drugs; Chapter I—Food and Drug Administration, Department of Health and Human Services; Part 182—substances Generally Recognized as Safe, http://www.cfsan.fda.gov/~lrd/fcf182.html.

366. H. Endo and T. D. Rees, "Clinical Features of Cinnamon-Induced Contact Stomatitis," *The Compendium of Continuing Education in Dentistry* 27, no. 7 (July 2006): 403–9.

367. P. A. Perry, et al., "Cinnamon Oil Abuse by Adolescents," *Veterinary and Human Toxicology* 32, no. 2 (April 1990): 162–4.

368. Joseph P. Remington and Horatio C. Woods, et al., eds., *The Dispensatory of the United States of America,* Twentieth Edition. www.swsbm.com/Dispensatory/USD-1918-complete.pdf (1918).

369. Judy Foreman, "Cinnamon Joins Cholesterol Battle," *My Health Sense,* http://www.myhealthsense.com/F040824_cinnamon.html.

370. D. M. Cohen, et al. "Cinnamon-induced Oral Erythema Multiformelike Sensitivity Reaction," *Journal of the American Dental Association* 131, no. 7 (July 2000): 929–34.

371. L. Kanerva, et al., "Occupational Allergic Contact Dermatitis from Spices," *Contact Dermatitis* 35, no. 3 (September 1996): 157–62; J. L. Garcia-Abujeta, et al., "Mud Bath Dermatitis Due to Cinnamon Oil," *Contact Dermatitis* 52, no. 4 (April 2005): 234.

372. E. Tatrai, et al., "The Pulmonary Toxicity of Cinnamon Dust in Rats," *Indian Journal of Medical Research* 102 (December 1995): 287–92.

373. M. Domaracky, et al., "Effects of Selected Plant Essential Oils on the Growth and Development of Mouse Preimplantation Embryos In Vivo," *Physiological Research* 56 (2006): 97-104.

374. B. Roffey, et al., "Cinnamon Water Extracts Increase Glucose Uptake but Inhibit Adiponectin Secretion in 3T3–L1 Adipose Cells," *Molecular Nutrition and Food Research* 50, no. 8 (August 2006): 739–45; B. Mang, et al., "Effects of a Cinnamon Extract on Plasma Glucose, Hba, and Serum Lipids in Diabetes Mellitus Type 2" *European Journal Of Clinical Investigation* 36, no. 5 (May 2006): 340–4.

375. E. Barrie Kavasch and Karen Baar. *American Indian Healing Arts.* (New York: Bantam, 1999): 223.

376. Pierce, *Practical Guide to Natural Medicines,* 181.

377. Pierce, *Practical Guide to Natural Medicines,* 181.

378. Ahmad S. Tajuddin, et. al, "Aphrodisiac Activity of 50% Ethanolic Extracts of *Myristica fragrans Houtt.* (Nutmeg) and *Syzygium aromaticum (L) Merr. & Perry.* (Clove) in Male Mice: A Comparative Study," *BMC Complementary and Alternative Medicine* 3 (October 20, 2003): 6.

379. Remington and Woods, *The Dispensatory of the United States of America.*

380. History & Special Collections of UCLA Louise M. Darling Biomedical Library, "Clove," *Spices: Exotic Flavors and Medicines,* http://unitproj1.library.ucla.edu/biomed/spice/index.cfm?displayID=7.

381. "Cloves," *Wikipedia,* http://en.wikipedia.org/wiki/Clove.

382. H. J. Dorman, et al. "Antimicrobial Agents from Plants: Antibacterial Activity of Plant Volatile Oils," *Journal of Applied Microbiology* 88, no. 2 (February 2000): 308–16.

383. Pierce, *Practical Guide to Natural Medicines,* 181.

384. C. Ghelardini, et al. "Local Anaesthetic Activity of Beta-Caryophyllene," *Farmaco* 56, no. 5–7 (May–July 2001): 387–9.

385. History and Special Collections of UCLA, Louise M. Darling Biomedical Library, "Clove," *Spices: Exotic Flavors and Medicines,* http://unitproj1.library.ucla.edu/biomed/spice/index.cfm?displayID=7.

386. A. Alqareer, et al., "The Effect of Clove and Benzocaine Versus Placebo as Topical Anesthetics," *Journal of Dentistry* 34, no. 10 (November) 2006: 747–50.

387. "Cloves," *Wikipedia.*

388. "*Syzgium aromaticum,*" *PDR for Herbal Medicine,* 752.

389. Kowalchik and Hylton, *Rodale's Illustrated Encyclopedia of Herbs.*

390. Kowalchik and Hylton, *Rodale's Illustrated Encyclopedia of Herbs.*

391. Johnson, *Pocket Guide to Herbal Remedies*, 159.

392. "Clove (*Eugenia aromatica*) and Clove Oil (Eugenol)," *MedlinePlus Herb and Supplement*, http://www.nlm.nih.gov/medlineplus/druginfo/natural/patient-clove.html.

393. Pierce, *Practical Guide to Natural Medicines*, 182.

394. Pierce, *Practical Guide to Natural Medicines*, 181.

395. Pierce, *Practical Guide to Natural Medicines*, 181.

396. A. Prashar, et al., "Cytotoxicity of Clove (*Syzygium aromaticum*) Oil and its Major Components to Human Skin Cells," *Cell Proliferation* 39, no. 4 (August 2006): 241–8.

397. Pierce, *Practical Guide to Natural Medicines*, 182.

398. "Clove (*Eugenia aromatica*) and Clove Oil (Eugenol)," *MedlinePlus Herb and Supplement.*

399. Johnson, *Pocket Guide to Herbal Remedies*, 159.

400. Herrick, *Iroquois Medical Botany*, 473.

401. Pierce, *Practical Guide to Natural Medicines*, 195.

402. Pierce, *Practical Guide to Natural Medicines*, 195.

403. M. R. Kim, et al., "Antioxidative Effects of Quercetin-Glycosides Isolated from the Flower Buds of *Tussilago farfara L.* Food and Chemical Toxicology," *Food and Chemical Toxicology* 44, no. 6 (August 2006): 1299–307.

404. J. Cho, et al., "Neuroprotective and Antioxidant Effects of the Ethyl Acetate Fraction Prepared from *Tussilago farfara L.*," *Biological and Pharmaceutical Bulletin* 28, no. 3 (March 2005): 455–60.

405. L. Kokoska, et al. "Screening of Some Siberian Medicinal Plants for Antimicrobial Activity," *Journal of Ethnophamacology* 82, no. 1 (September 2002): 51–3.

406. "*Staphylococcus aureus*," *Wikipedia*, http://en.wikipedia.org/wiki/Staphylococcus_aureus.

407. Pierce, *Practical Guide to Natural Medicines*, 195.

408. Cho, "Neuroprotective and antioxidant effects of the ethyl acetate fraction," 455–60.

409. Henriette Kress, "Absorption," *Henriette's Herbal Blog*, http://www.henriettesherbal.com/blog/?cat=6&paged=5.

410. "Coltsfoot," *Whole Health MD*, http://www.wholehealthmd.com.

411. Commission E, "Coltsfoot," *The Commission E Monographs: IHerb Health Encyclopedia*, http://www.herbalgram.org/iherb/commissione/Monographs/Monograph_0071.html.

412. I. Hirono, et al., "Carcinogenic Activity of Coltsfoot, *Tussilago farfara l.*," *Gann* 67, no. 1 (February 1976): 125–9.

413. "Tussilago Farfara," *PDR for Herbal Medicine*, 1194.

414. Pierce, *Practical Guide to Natural Medicines*, 197.

415. Johnson, *Pocket Guide to Herbal Remedies*, 172; Coltsfoot. Whole Health MD.

416. "Echinacea (*E. angustifolia DC, E. pallida, E. purpurea*)," *MedlinePlus Herb And Supplements*, http://www.nlm.nih.gov/medlineplus/druginfo/natural/patient-echinacea.html.

417. Johnson, *Pocket Guide to Herbal Remedies*, 172.

418. Johnson, *Pocket Guide to Herbal Remedies*, 172.

419. M. Roulet, R. Laurini, L. Rivier, and A. Calame, "Hepatic Veno-Occlusive Disease in Newborn Infant of a Woman Drinking Herbal Tea," *Journal of Pediatrics* 112 (1988): 433–6.

420. Johnson, *Pocket Guide to Herbal Remedies*, 172.

421. Johnson, *Pocket Guide to Herbal Remedies*,172.

422. Ody, *The Complete Medicinal Herbal*, 101.

423. T. M. Teynor1, et al., "Comfrey," *Alternative Field Crops Manual* (University of Wisconsin Extension) http://www.hort.purdue.edu/newcrop/afcm/comfrey.html.

424. "Comfrey," *National Non-Food Crops Centre*, http://www.nnfcc.co.uk/crops/info/comfrey.pdf.

425. Top Cultures, "Rosmarinic Acid," *Phytochemicals*, http://www.phytochemicals.info/phytochemicals/rosmarinic-acid.php.

426. R. Koll, et al., "Efficacy and Tolerance of a Comfrey Root Extract (*Extr. Rad. Symphyti*) in the Treatment of Ankle Distorsions: Results of a Multicenter, Randomized, Placebo-Controlled, Double-Blind Study," *Phytomedicine* 11, no. 6 (September 2004): 470–7.

427. M. Kucera, et al., "Efficacy and Safety of Topically Applied Symphytum Herb Extract Cream in the Treatment of Ankle Distortion: Results of a Randomized Controlled Clinical Double Blind Study," *Wiener Medizinische Wochenschrift* 154, no. 21–22 (November 2004): 498–507.

428. R. Koll and S. Klingenburg, ["Therapeutic Characteristance and Tolerance of Topical Comfrey Preparations: Results of an Observational Study of Patients,"] *Fortschritte der Medizin Originalien* 120, no. 1 (2002): 1–9 (Article in German).

429. H. G. Predel, et al., "Efficacy of a Comfrey Root Extract Ointment in Comparison to a Diclofenac Gel in the Treatment of Ankle Distortions: Results of an Observer-Blind, Randomized, Multicenter Study," *Phytomedicine* 12, no. 10 (November 2005): 707–14.

430. Pierce, *Practical Guide to Natural Medicines*, 198.

431. Pierce, *Practical Guide to Natural Medicines*, 198.

432. M. Kucera, et al., "Efficacy and Safety of Topically Applied Symphytum Herb Extract Cream in the Treatment of Ankle Distortion: Results of a Randomized Controlled Clinical Double Blind Study," *Wiener Medizinische Wochenschrift* 154, no. 21–22 (November 2004): 498–507.

433. Johnson, *Pocket Guide to Herbal Remedies*, 158.

434. Cech, *Making Plant Medicine*, 128.

435. Hoffmann, "Comfrey."

436. F. Stickel and H. K. Seitz, "The Efficacy and Safety of Comfrey," *Public Health Nutrition* 3, no. 4A (December 2000): 501–8.

437. International Programme on Chemical Safety, "Environmental Health Criteria 80: Pyrrolizidine Alkaloids," *Chemical Safety Information from Intergovernmental Organizations*, http://www.inchem.org/documents/ehc/ehc/ehc080.htm.

438. Cech, *Making Plant Medicine*, 128

439. International Programme on Chemical Safety, "Environmental Health Criteria 80: Pyrrolizidine Alkaloids."

440. "Echinacea," *Medlineplus Herb and Supplement*.

441. International Programme on Chemical Safety, "Environmental Health Criteria 80: Pyrrolizidine Alkaloids."

442. Johnson, *Pocket Guide to Herbal Remedies*, 158.

443. Pierce, *Practical Guide to Natural Medicines*, 198.

444. Pierce, *Practical Guide to Natural Medicines*, 224.

445. Pierce, *Practical Guide to Natural Medicines*, 224.

446. S. Chrubasik, et al., "The Quality of Clinical Trials with *Harpagophytum procumbens*," *Phytomedicine* 10, no. 6–7 (2003): 613–23.

447. Devil's Claw (*Harpagophytum procumbens DC*), *MedlinePlus Herb and Supplement*, http://www.nlm.nih.gov/medlineplus/druginfo/natural/patient-devils_claw.html.

448. I. M. Mahomed and J. A. Ojewole, "Analgesic, Anti-Inflammatory and Antidiabetic Properties of *Harpagophytum procumbens DC* (*Pedaliaceae*) Secondary Root Aqueous Extract," *Phytotherapy Research* 18, no. 12 (December 2004): 982–9.

449. J. J. Gagnier, et al., "Herbal Medicine for Low Back Pain," *Cochrane Database of Systematic Reviews* 19, no. 2 (April 2006): CD004504.

450. H. Gobel, et al., ["Effects of *Harpagophytum procumbens* LI 174 (Devil's Claw) on Sensory, Motor and Vascular Muscle Reagibility in the Treatment of Unspecific Back Pain,"] *Schmerz* 15, no. 1 (February 2001): 10–8 (Article in German).

451. M. L. Andersen, et al., "Evaluation of Acute and Chronic Treatments with Harpagophytum Procumbens on Freund's Adjuvant-Induced Arthritis in Rats," *Journal of Ethnophamacology* 91, no. 2–3 (April 2004): 325–30.

452. L. W. Whitehouse, et al., "Devil's Claw (*Harpagophytum procumbens*): No Evidence for Anti-Inflammatory Activity in the Treatment of Arthritic Disease," *Canadian Medical Association Journal* 129, no. 3 (August 1,1983): 249–51.

453. T. Wegener and N. P. Lupke, "Treatment of Patients with Arthrosis of Hip or Knee with an Aqueous Extract of Devil's Claw (*Harpagophytum procumbens* DC.)," *Phytotherapy Research* 17, no. 10 (December 2003): 1165–72.

454. "Harpagophytum Procumbens," *PDR for Herbal Medicine*, 889.

455. S. Chrubasik, ["Devil's Claw Extract as an Example of the Effectiveness of Herbal Analgesics,"] *Orthopade* 33, no. 7 (July 2004): 804–8 (Article in German).

456. Johnson, *Pocket Guide to Herbal Remedies*, 73.

457. "Harpagophytum Procumbens," *PDR for Herbal Medicine*, 889.

458. Chrubasik, ["Devil's Claw Extract As An Example Of The Effectiveness Of Herbal Analgesics,"] 804–8.

459. S. Chrubasik, et al., "Effectiveness of Harpagophytum Extracts and Clinical Efficacy," *Phytotherapy Research* 18, no. 2 (February 2004): 187–9.

460. J. J. Gagnier, et al., "Herbal Medicine for Low Back Pain," *Cochrane Database of Systematic Reviews* 2 April 19, 2006): CD004504.

461. "Devil's Claw," *MedlinePlus Herb and Supplement.*

462. "Devil's Claw," *MedlinePlus Herb and Supplement.*

463. Johnson, *Pocket Guide to Herbal Remedies*, 73.

464. Johnson, *Pocket Guide to Herbal Remedies*, 73.

465. Johnson, *Pocket Guide to Herbal Remedies*, 73.

466. Johnson, *Pocket Guide to Herbal Remedies*, 73.

467. I. Mahomed, "Analgesic, Anti-Inflammatory and Antidiabetic Properties," 982–9.

468. C. Circosta, et al., "A Drug Used in Traditional Medicine: *Harpagophytum procumbens* DC. II. Cardiovascular activity," *Journal of Ethnophamacology* 11, no. 3 (August 1984): 259–74.

469. Pierce, *Practical Guide to Natural Medicines*, 236.

470. Pierce, *Practical Guide to Natural Medicines*, 236.

471. American Botanical Council, "*Echinacea angustifolia* Herb and Root/Pallida Herb." *Expanded Commission E Online* http://www.herbalgram.org/default.asp?c=he024.

472. American Botanical Council, "*Echinacea angustifolia* Herb and Root/Pallida Herb."

473. Ody, *The Complete Medicinal Herbal*, 53.

474. Cech, *Making Plant Medicine*, 135.

475. Jeffrey A. Hart, "The Ethnobotany of the Northern Cheyenne Indians of Montana," *Journal of Ethnopharmacology* 4 (1981): 20; Grinnell, George Bird, *The Cheyenne Indians: Their History and Ways of Life*, volume 2, (Lincoln: University of Nebraska Press, 1972): 188; Vestal, Paul A. and Richard Evans Schultes, *The Economic Botany of the Kiowa Indians*. (Cambridge MA: Botanical Museum of Harvard University, 1939): 57; T. N. Campbell, "Medicinal Plants Used by Choctaw, Chickasaw, and Creek Indians in the Early Nineteenth Century," *Journal of the Washington Academy of Sciences* 41, no. 9 (1951): 288. Carlson, Gustav G. and Volney H. Jones, "Some Notes on Uses of Plants by the Comanche Indians," *Papers of the Michigan Academy of Science, Arts and Letters* 25 (1940): 521.

476. A. Wacker and W. Hilbig, ["Virus-inhibition by *Echinacea purpurea*,"] *Planta Medica* 33, no. 1 (February 1978): 89–102 (Article in German).

477. B. Barrett, "Medicinal Properties of Echinacea: a Critical Review," *Phytomedicine* 10, no. 1 (January 2003): 66–86.

478. S. Mishima, et al., "Antioxidant and Immuno-Enhancing Effects of *Echinacea purpurea*," *Biological and Pharmaceutical Bulletin* 27, no. 7 (July 2004): 1004–9.

479. J. Reichling, et al., "Echinacea Powder: Treatment of Canine Chronic and Seasonal Upper Respiratory Tract Infections," *Schweizer Archiv für Tierheilkunde* 145, no. 5 (May 2003): 223–31.

480. J. Brush, et al., "The Effect of *Echinacea purpurea*, *Astragalus membranaceus* and *Glycyrrhiza glabra* on CD69 Expression and Immune Cell Activation in Humans," *Phytotherapy Research* 20, no. 8 (June 28, 2006): 687–695.

481. V. Goel, et al., "A Proprietary Extract from the Echinacea Plant (*Echinacea purpurea*) Enhances Systemic Immune Response during a Common Cold," *Phytotherapy Research* 19, no. 8 (August 2005): 689–94.

482. E. Schwarz, et al., "Oral Administration of Freshly Expressed Juice of *Echinacea purpurea* Herbs Fail to Stimulate the Nonspecific Immune Response in Healthy Young Men: Results of a Double-Blind, Placebo-Controlled Crossover Study," *Journal of Immunotherapy* 25, no. 5 (September–October 2002): 413–20.

483. Ronald B. Turner, et al., "An Evaluation of *Echinacea angustifolia* in Experimental Rhinovirus Infections," *New England Journal of Medicine* 353, no. 4 (July 28, 2005): 341–348; B. P. Barrett, et al., "Treatment of the Common Cold with Unrefined Echinacea: A Randomized, Double-Blind, Placebo-Controlled Trial," *Annals of Internal Medicine* 137, no. 12 (December 17, 2002): 939–46.

484. V. Goel, et al., "Efficacy of a Standardized Echinacea Preparation (Echinilin) for the Treatment of the Common Cold: a Randomized, Double-Blind, Placebo-Controlled Trial," *Journal of Clinical Pharmacy and Therapeutics* 29, no. 1 (February 2004): 75–83.

485. W. Weber, et al., "*Echinacea purpurea* for Prevention of Upper Respiratory Tract Infections in Children," *Journal of Alternative and Complementary Medicine* 11, no. 6 (December 2005): 1021–6.

486. J. A. Taylor, et al., "Efficacy and Safety of Echinacea in Treating Upper Respiratory Tract Infections in Children: a Randomized Controlled Trial," *Journal Of The American Medical Association* 290, no. 21 (December 3, 2003): 2824–30.

487. S. J. Sperber, et al., "*Echinacea purpurea* for Prevention of Experimental Rhinovirus Colds," *Clinical Infectious Diseases* 38, no. 10 (May 15, 2004): 1367–71.

488. E. L. Gillespie and C. I. Coleman, "The Effect of Echinacea on Upper Respiratory Infection Symptom Severity and Quality of Life," *Connecticut Medicine* 70, no. 2 (February 2006): 93–7.

489. J. Islam and R. Carter, "Use of Echinacea in Upper Respiratory Tract Infection," *The Southern Medical Journal*98, no. 3 (March 2005): 311–8.

490. Christine M. Gilroy, et al., "Echinacea and Truth in Labeling," *Archives of Internal Medicine* 163 (2003): 699–704.

491. S. A. Shah, et al., "Evaluation of Echinacea for the Prevention and Treatment of the Common Cold: a Meta-analysis," *Lancet Infectious Diseases* 7, no. 7 (July 2007): 473–80.

492. R. Schoop, et al., "Echinacea in the Prevention of Induced Rhinovirus Colds: a Meta-analysis," *Clinical Therapeutics* 28, no. 2 (February 2006): 174–83.

493. Shah, "Evaluation Of Echinacea For The Prevention And Treatment Of The Common Cold," 473–80.

494. Pierce, *Practical Guide to Natural Medicines*, 236.

495. Shelly Katheren Kraft, *Recent Changes in the Ethnobotany of Standing Rock Indian Reservation*, (University of North Dakota, M.A. Thesis, 1990): 47; George Bird Grinnell, *The Cheyenne Indians: Their History and Ways of Life*, volume 2, (Lincoln: University of Nebraska Press, 1972): 188; Melvin R. Gilmore, *Uses of Plants by the Indians of the Missouri River Region*. (SI-BAE Annual Report #33, 1919): 131.

496. Pierce, *Practical Guide to Natural Medicines*, 238.

497. Kowalchik and Hylton, *Rodale's Illustrated Encyclopedia of Herbs*.

498. Hoffmann, "Echinacea," *Herbal Materia Medica*.

499. B. Rousseau, et al., "Investigation of Anti-Hyaluronidase Treatment on Vocal Fold Wound Healing," *Journal of Voice* (Oct 20, 2005).

500. D. L. Stuart and R. B. Wills, "Effect of Drying Temperature on Alkylamide and Cichoric Acid Concentrations of *Echinacea purpurea*," *Journal of Agricultural and Food Chemistry* 51, no. 6 (March 12, 2003): 1608–10.

501. J. Garrard, et al., "Variations in Product Choices of Frequently Purchased Herbs: Caveat Emptor," *Archives of Internal Medicine* 163, no. 19 (October 27, 2003): 2290–5.

502. R. M. Brinkeborn, et al., "Echinaforce and Other Echinacea Fresh Plant Preparations in the Treatment of the Common Cold: A Randomized, Placebo Controlled, Double-Blind Clinical Trial," *Phytomedicine* 6, no. 1 (March 1999): 1–6.

503. P.C. Bradley, ed., *British Herbal Compendium: A Handbook of Scientific Information on Widely Used Plant Drugs*, volume 1, (Bournemouth, England: British Herbal Medicine Association, 1992).

504. Pierce, *Practical Guide to Natural Medicines*, 236.

505. Cech, *Making Plant Medicine*, 135

506. Pierce, *Practical Guide to Natural Medicines*, 236.

507. K. Linde, B. Barrett, K. Wolkart, R. Bauer, and D. Melchart, "Echinacea for Preventing and Treating the Common Cold," *Cochrane Database of Systematic Reviews* 25, no. 1 (January 25, 2006): CD000530.

508. D. S. Senchina, et al., "Changes in Immunomodulatory Properties of *Echinacea spp.* Root Infusions and Tinctures Stored at 4 Degrees C for Four Days," *Clinica Chimica Acta* 355, no. 1–2 (May 2005): 67–82.

509. A. Baranauskas, et al., ["Technology of Extract Improving the Immune System,"] *Medicina (Kaunas, Lithuania)* 41, no. 8 (2005): 693–7 (Article in Lithuanian).

510. K. Woelkart, et al., "Bioavailability and Pharmacokinetics of Alkamides from the Roots of *Echinacea angustifolia* in Humans," *Journal of Clinical Pharmacology* 45, no. 6 (June 2005): 683–9.

511. Johnson, *Pocket Guide to Herbal Remedies*, 54.

512. Johnson, *Pocket Guide to Herbal Remedies*, 54.

513. "Echinacea (*E. angustifolia DC, E. pallida, E. purpurea*)," *Medlineplus Herb and Supplement*, http://www.nlm.nih.gov/medlineplus/druginfo/natural/patient-echinacea.html.

514. Johnson, *Pocket Guide to Herbal Remedies*, 54.

515. "Echinacea," *Whole Health MD*, http://www.wholehealthmd.com.

516. B. Kligler, "Echinacea," *American Family Physician* 67, no. 1 (January 1, 2003): 77–80.

517. Commission E, "Echinacea purpurea Herb," *The Commission E Monographs. IHerb Health Encyclopedia*, http://www.herbalgram.org/iherb/commissione/Monographs/Monograph_0088.html.

518. Harkness and Bratman, *Handbook of Drug-Herb and Drug-Supplement Interactions*, 70–1; L. G. Miller, "Herbal Medicines: Selected Clinical Considerations Focusing on Known or Potential Drug-Herb Interactions," *Archives of Internal Medicine* 158 (1998): 2200–11.

519. W. Abebe, "Herbal Medication: Potential for Adverse Interactions with Analgesic Drugs," *Journal of Clinical Pharmacy and Therapeutics* 27 (2002): 391–401; Benjamin Kligler "Reply to: Chronic Use of Echinacea Should Be Discouraged," *American Family Physician* 68, no. 4 (August 15, 2003): 618.

520. "Echinacea," *Medlineplus Herb and Supplement*.

521. Hamel and Chiltoskey, *Cherokee Plants and Their Uses*, 33; Jennie Goodrich and Claudia Lawson, *Kashaya Pomo Plants*, (Los Angeles: American Indian Studies Center, 1980): 42; Arthur Caswell Parker, *Iroquois Uses of Maize and Other Food Plants* (Albany, NY: University of the State of New York, 1910): 96; L. S. M. Curtin, *By the Prophet of the Earth*, (Sante Fe: San Vicente Foundation, 1949): 75; L. S. M. Curtin, "Some Plants Used by the Yuki Indians: II. Food Plants," *The Masterkey* 31 (1957): 46.

522. Albert B. Reagan, "Plants Used by the Hoh and Quileute Indians," *Kansas Academy of Science* 37 (1936): 69; Lowell John Bean and Katherine Siva Saubel, *Temalpakh (From the Earth): Cahuilla Indian Knowledge and Usage of Plants* (Banning, CA: Malki Museum Press, 1972): 138; Maurice L. Zigmond, *Kawaiisu Ethnobotany* (Salt Lake City: University of Utah Press, 1981): 62; Barbara R.Bocek, "Ethnobotany of Costanoan Indians, California, Based on Collections by John P. Harrington," *Economic Botany* 38, no. 2 (1984): 240.

523. "*Sambuscus nigra*," *PDR for Herbal Medicine*, 1116.

524. R. E. Uncini Manganelli, et al., "Antiviral Activity In Vitro of *Urtica dioica L.*, *Parietaria diffusa M. et K.* and *Sambucus nigra* L.," *Journal of Ethnophamacology* 98, no. 3 (April 26, 2005): 323–7.

525. Z. Zakay-Rones, et al., "Randomized Study of the Efficacy and Safety of Oral Elderberry Extract in the Treatment of Influenza A and B Virus Infections," *The Journal of International Medical Research* 32, no. 2 (March–April 2004): 132–40.

526. V. Barak, et al. "The Effect of Sambucol, a Black Elderberry-Based, Natural Product, on the Production of Human Cytokines: I. Inflammatory Cytokines," *European Cytokine Network*. 12, no. 2 (April–June 2001): 290–6.

527. Tantaquidgeon, *Folk Medicine of the Delaware and Related Algonkian Indians*, 31. Frank G. Speck, "A List of Plant Curatives Obtained From the Houma Indians of Louisiana," *Primitive Man* 14 (1941): 60; Linda Averill Taylor, *Plants Used As Curatives by Certain Southeastern Tribes*. (Cambridge, MA: Botanical Museum of Harvard University, 1940): 59; Frank G. Speck, R. B. Hassrick and E. S. Carpenter, "Rappahannock Herbals, Folk-Lore and Science of Cures," *Proceedings of the Delaware County Institute of Science* 10 (1942): 34; Herrick, *Iroquois Medical Botany*, 448.

528. Hamel and Chiltoskey, *Cherokee Plants and Their Uses*, 33, Brian Douglas Compton, *Upper North Wakashan and Southern Tsimshian Ethnobotany: The Knowledge and Usage of Plants*, (University of British Columbia, Ph.D. Dissertation, 1993): 229.

529. V. K. Chestnut, "Plants Used by the Indians of Mendocino County, California," *Contributions from the U.S. National Herbarium* 7 (1902): 388.

530. M. A. Ebrahimzadeh, et al., "Anti-Inflammatory Activity of Sambucus Ebulus Hexane Extracts," *Fitoterapia* 77, no. 2 (February 2006): 146–8.

531. E. Harokopakis, et al., "Inhibition of Proinflammatory Activities of Major Periodontal Pathogens by Aqueous Extracts from Elder Flower (*Sambucus nigra*)," *Journal of Periodontology* 77, no. 2 (February 2006): 271–9.

532. Z. Zakay-Rones, et al., "Inhibition of Several Strains of Influenza Virus In Vitro and Reduction of Symptoms by an Elderberry Extract (*Sambucus nigra* L.) During an Outbreak of Influenza B Panama," *Journal of Alternative and Complementary Medicine* 1, no. 4 (Winter 1995): 361–9; Barak, "The Effect of Sambucol, a Black Elderberry-based, Natural Product," 290–6.

533. "*Sambuscus nigra*," *PDR for Herbal Medicine*, 1116.

534. Pierce, *Practical Guide to Natural Medicines*, 241.

535. United States Food and Drug Administration, Title 21—Food and Drugs; Chapter I—Food and Drug Administration, Department of Health and Human Services; Part 182—substances Generally Recognized as Safe. http://www.cfsan.fda.gov/~lrd/fcf182.html.

536. Pierce, *Practical Guide to Natural Medicines*, 302.

537. K. Asano, et al., "Effect of *Eleutherococcus senticosus* Extract on Human Physical Working Capacity," *Planta Medica* 52 (1986): 175–76.

538. Hartz AJ, et al., "Randomized Controlled Trial of Siberian Ginseng for Chronic Fatigue," *Psychological Medicine* 34, no. 1 (January 2004): 51–61.

539. Pierce, *Practical Guide to Natural Medicines*, 302.

540. Johnson, *Pocket Guide to Herbal Remedies*, 56.

541. Pierce, *Practical Guide to Natural Medicines*, 302.

542. Commission E. "Eleuthero (Siberian Ginseng) Root," *The Commission E Monographs: IHerb Health Encyclopedia*, http://www.herbalgram.org/iherb/commissione/Monographs/Monograph_0092.html.

543. Pierce, *Practical Guide to Natural Medicines*, 302.

544. Johnson, *Pocket Guide to Herbal Remedies*, 56.

545. Johnson, *Pocket Guide to Herbal Remedies*, 56.

546. Johnson, *Pocket Guide to Herbal Remedies*, 56.

547. Woodbridge Metcalf, "Eucalyptus Trees Around the World," *Journal of the California Horticultural Society* (April–June 1958): 31.

548. "Eucalyptol," *Wikipedia*, http://en.wikipedia.org/wiki/Eucalyptol.

549. Akaiko Akana, *Hawaiian Herbs of Medicinal Value* (Honolulu: Pacific Book House, 1922): 73.

550. S. Pattnaik, et al., "Antibacterial and Antifungal Activity of Ten Essential Oils In Vitro," *Microbios* 86, no. 349 (1996): 237–46.

551. K. Takarada, et al., "A Comparison of the Antibacterial Efficacies of Essential Oils Against Oral Pathogens," *Oral Microbiology and Immunology* 19, no. 1 (February 2004): 61–4.

552. C. H. Charles, et al., "Effect of an Essential Oil-Containing Dentifrice on Dental Plaque Microbial Composition," *American Journal of Dentistry* 13 (September 2000): 26C–30C.

553. T. Takahashi, et al., "Antimicrobial Activities of Eucalyptus Leaf Extracts and Flavonoids from *Eucalyptus maculate*," *Letters in Applied Microbiology* 39, no. 1 (2004): 60–4.

554. Akana, *Hawaiian Herbs of Medicinal Value*, 73.

555. Remington and Woods, *The Dispensatory of the United States of America*.

556. P. H. Warnke, et al. "Antibacterial Essential Oils in Malodorous Cancer Patients: Clinical Observations in 30 Patients," *Phytomedicine* 13, no. 7 (July 2006): 463–7.

557. Bean and Saubel, *Temalpakh (From the Earth)*, 73.

558. Remington and Woods, *The Dispensatory of the United States of America*.

559. P. Schnitzler, et al., "Antiviral Activity of Australian Tea Tree Oil and Eucalyptus Oil against Herpes Simplex Virus in Cell Culture," *Pharmazie* 56, no. 4 (April 2001): 343–7.

560. L. N. Coelho-de-Souza, et al., "Relaxant Effects of the Essential Oil of *Eucalyptus tereticornis* and its Main Constituent 1,8–cineole on Guinea-Pig Tracheal Smooth Muscle, *Planta Medica* 71, no. 12 (December 2005): 1173–5.

561. U. R. Juergens, et al., "Anti-inflammatory Activity of 1.8–cineol (Eucalyptol) in Bronchial Asthma: a Double-Blind Placebo-Controlled Trial," *Respiratory Medicine* 97, no. 3 (March 2003): 250–6.

562. S. Pattnaik, et al., "Antibacterial and Antifungal Activity of Ten Essential Oils In Vitro," *Microbios* 86, no. 349 (1996): 237–46.

563. T. Takahashi, Antimicrobial Activities of Eucalyptus Leaf Extracts, 60–4.

564. S. K. Shahi, et al., "Broad Spectrum Herbal Therapy Against Superficial Fungal Infections," *Skin Pharmacology and Applied Skin Physiology* 13, no. 1 (January–February 2000): 60–4.

565. R. S. Ramsewak, et al., "In Vitro Antagonistic Activity of Monoterpenes and their Mixtures Against 'Toe Nail Fungus' Pathogens," *Phytotherapy Research* 14, no. 4 (April 2003): 376–9.

566. J. Silva, et al., "Analgesic and Anti-Inflammatory Effects of Essential Oils of Eucalyptus," *Journal of Ethnophamacology* 89, no. 2–3 (December 2003): 277–83.

567. Pierce, *Practical Guide to Natural Medicines*, 250.

568. W. Weyers and R. Brodbeck. ["Skin Absorption of Volatile Oils: Pharmacokinetics,"] *Pharmazie in Unserer Zeit* 18, no. 3 (May 1989): 82–6 (Article in German).

569. J. Ilmberger, et al., The Influence of Essential Oils on Human Attention," *Chemical Senses* 26, no. 3 (March 2001): 239–45.

570. Pierce, *Practical Guide to Natural Medicines*, 249.

571. "Eucalyptol," *Wikipedia*, http://en.wikipedia.org/wiki/Eucalyptol.

572. "Eucalyptol," *Wikipedia*.

573. Weyers and Brodbeck, ["Skin Absorption Of Volatile Oils."] 82–6.

574. "*Eucalyptus globulus*," *PDR for Herbal Medicine*, 838.

575. "Eucalyptus oil," *MedlinePlus herb and supplement*, http://www.nlm.nih.gov/medlineplus/druginfo/natural/patient-eucalyptus.html.

576. Commission E, "Eucalyptus leaf," *The Commission E Monographs: IHerb Health Encyclopedia* http://www.herbalgram.org/iherb/commissione/Monographs/Monograph_0095.html.

577. Commission E, "Eucalyptus leaf."

578. Cech, *Making Plant Medicine*,140.

579. Cech, *Making Plant Medicine*, 140.

580. Commission E, "Eucalyptus leaf."

581. E. Galdi, et al. "Exacerbation of Asthma Related to Eucalyptus Pollens and to Herb Infusion Containing Eucalyptus," *Monaldi Archives for Chest Disease* 59, no. 3 (July–September 2003): 220–1.

582. Cech, *Making Plant Medicine*, 140.

583. P. R. Burkhard, et al., "Plant-Induced Seizures: Reappearance of an Old Problem," *Journal of Neurology* 246, no. 8 (August 1999): 667–70; Leung and Foster, *Encyclopedia of Common Natural Ingredients Used in Food, Drugs, and Cosmetics*, 232–3.

584. Commission E, "Eucalyptus leaf."

585. Johnson, *Pocket Guide to Herbal Remedies*, 59.

586. Johnson, *Pocket Guide to Herbal Remedies*, 59.

587. Pierce, *Practical Guide to Natural Medicines*, 250.

588. N. J. Webb and W. R. Pitt, "Eucalyptus Oil Poisoning in Childhood: 41 Cases in South-East Queensland," *Journal of Paediatrics and Child Health* 29, no. 5 (October 1993): 368–71.

589. J. Tibballs, "Clinical Effects and Management of Eucalyptus Oil Ingestion in Infants and Young Children," *The Medical Journal of Australia* 21, no. 4 (August 1995): 177–80.

590. T. Darben, et al. "Topical Eucalyptus Oil Poisoning," *The Australasian Journal of Dermatology* 39, no. 4 November 1998): 265–7.

591. L. M. Day, et al. "Eucalyptus Oil Poisoning Among Young Children: Mechanisms of Access and the Potential for Prevention," *Australian and New Zealand Journal of Public Health* 21, no. 3 (June 1997): 297–302.

592. "Eucalyptus Oil," *Medlineplus Herb and Supplement.*

593. "Eucalyptus Oil," *Medlineplus Herb and Supplement.*

594. Remington and Woods, *The Dispensatory of the United States of America.*

595. K. J. Kemper, "Evening primrose (*Oenethera biennis*)," *The Longwood, Duke Herbal Taskforce and the Center for Holistic Pediatric Education and Research* http://www.mcp.edu/herbal/epo/epo.pdf.

596. Johnson, *Pocket Guide to Herbal Remedies*, 106.

597. "Borage Oil," *Whole Health MD*, http://www.wholehealthmd.com.

598. M. Fukushima, et al., "Comparative Hypocholesterolemic Effects of Six Vegetable Oils in Cholesterol-Fed Rat," *Lipids* 31, no. 4 (April 1996): 415–9.

599. Fukushima, "Comparative Hypocholesterolemic Effects Of Six Dietary Oils," 1069–74.

600. J. P. De La Cruz, et al., "Effect of Evening Primrose Oil on Platelet Aggregation in Rabbits Fed an Atherogenic Diet," *Thrombosis Research* 87, no. 1 (July 1, 1997): 141–9.

601. M. A. Villalobos, et al., Effect of Dietary Supplementation with Evening Primrose Oil on Vascular Thrombogenesis in Hyperlipemic Rabbits," *Thrombosis and Haemostasis* 80, no. 4 (October

1998): 696–701; J. P. De La Cruz, et al., "Antioxidant Potential of Evening Primrose Oil Administration in Hyperlipemic Rabbits," *Life Sciences* 65, no. 5 (1999): 543–55.

602. R. Knorr and M. Hamburger, "Quantitative Analysis of Anti-Inflammatory and Radical Scavenging Triterpenoid Esters in Evening Primrose Oil," *Journal of Agricultural and Food Chemistry* 52, no. 11 (June 2, 2004): 3319–24.

603. J. J. Belch and A. Hill, "Evening Primrose Oil and Borage Oil in Rheumatologic Conditions," *American Journal of Clinical Nutrition* 71, no 1 supplemental (January 2000): 352S–6S.

604. M. Brzeski, et al. "Evening Primrose Oil in Patients with Rheumatoid Arthritis and Side-effects of Non-Steroidal Anti-Inflammatory Drugs," *British Journal of Rheumatology* 30, no. 5 (October 1991): 370–2; J. J. Belch, et al., "Effects of Altering Dietary Essential Fatty Acids on Requirements for Non-Steroidal Anti-Inflammatory Drugs in Patients with Rheumatoid Arthritis: a Double Blind Placebo Controlled Study," *Annals of the Rheumatic Diseases* 47, no. 2 (February 1988): 96–104; D. F. Horrobin, "Essential Fatty Acid and Prostaglandin Metabolism in Sjogren's Syndrome, Systemic Sclerosis and Rheumatoid Arthritis," *Scandinavian Journal of Rheumatology Suppl* 61 (1986): 242–5.

605. J. Jantti, et al., "Evening Primrose Oil and Olive Oil in Treatment of Rheumatoid Arthritis," *Clinical Rheumatology* 8 (June 1989): 238–44.

606. Leland C. Wyman, and Stuart K. Harris, *The Ethnobotany of the Kayenta Navaho*, (Albuquerque: The University of New Mexico Press, 1951): 33.

607. "Evening Primrose Oil," *Whole Health MD,* http://www.wholehealthmd.com.

608. Remington and Woods, *The Dispensatory of the United States of America.*

609. "Evening Primrose Oil," *MedlinePlus Herb And Supplements*, http://www.nlm.nih.gov/medlineplus/druginfo/natural/patient-primrose.html.

610. Knorr and Hamburger, "Quantitative Analysis of Anti-Inflammatory and Radical Scavenging Triterpenoid Esters," 3319–24.

611. Y. N. Shukla, et al., "Phytotoxic and Antimicrobial Constituents of *Argyreia speciosa* and *Oenothera biennis*," *Journal of Ethnophamacology* 67, no. 2 (November 1, 1999): 241–5.

612. K. A. Hammer, et al., "Antimicrobial Activity of Essential Oils and Other Plant Extracts," *Journal Of Applied Microbiology* 86, no. 6 (June 1999): 985–90.

613. "Evening Primrose Oil," *MedlinePlus Herb And Supplements.*

614. "Borage Oil," *Whole Health MD.*

615. Pierce, *Practical Guide to Natural Medicines*, 252.

616. M. Brzeski, et al., "Evening Primrose Oil in Patients with Rheumatoid Arthritis and Side-Effects Of Non-Steroidal Anti-Inflammatory Drugs," *British Journal of Rheumatology* 30, no. 5 (October 1991): 370–2; J. J. Belch, et al., "Effects of Altering Dietary Essential Fatty Acids on Requirements for Non-Steroidal Anti-Inflammatory Drugs in Patients with Rheumatoid Arthritis: a Double Blind Placebo Controlled Study," *Annals of the Rheumatic Diseases* 47, no. 2 (February 1988): 96–104.

617. "Borage Oil," *Whole Health MD.*

618. "Evening Primrose Oil," *MedlinePlus Herb And Supplements.*

619. "Borage Oil," *Whole Health MD.*

620. "Evening Primrose Oil (*Oenothera biennis L.*)," *MayoClinic.com*, http://www.mayoclinic.com/health/evening-primrose-oil/NS_patient-Primrose.

621. Johnson, *Pocket Guide to Herbal Remedies*, 106.

622. "Evening Primrose Oil," *MayoClinic.com.*

623. "Evening Primrose Oil," *MayoClinic.com.*

624. "Evening Primrose Oil," *MayoClinic.com.*

625. "Ginseng (American ginseng, Asian ginseng, Chinese ginseng, Korean red ginseng, *Panax ginseng*: *Panax spp*. including *P. ginseng* C.C. Meyer and *P. quincefolium* L., excluding *Eleutherococcus senticosus*)," *MedlinePlus Herb And Supplement*, http://www.nlm.nih.gov/medlineplus/druginfo/natural/patient-ginseng.html.

626. Johnson, *Pocket Guide to Herbal Remedies*, 106.

627. West TCM, "Xiao Hui Xiang," *Traditional Chinese Medicine and Acupuncture Health Information Organization*, http://tcm.health-info.org/Herbology.Materia.Medica/xiaohuixiang-properties.htm.

628. M. Blumenthal, et al, *The Complete German Commission E Manuscripts*, (Boston: Integrative Medicine Communications, 1998).

629. M. H. Boskabady, et al., "Possible Mechanism(s) for Relaxant Effects of *Foeniculum vulgare* on Guinea Pig Tracheal Chains," *Pharmazie* 59, no. 7 (July 2004): 561–4.

630. Hamel and Chiltoskey, *Cherokee Plants and Their Uses*, 33.

631. Remington and Woods, *The Dispensatory of the United States of America.*

632. A. O. Khaldun, ["Antibacterial Action of Ether Oils of Some Plants,"] *Zhurnal mikrobiologii, epidemiologii, i immunobiologii* 3 (May–June 2006): 92–3 (Article in Russian).

633. I. Dadalioglu and G. A. Evrendilek, "Chemical Compositions and Antibacterial Effects of Essential Oils of Turkish Oregano (*Origanum minutiflorum*), Bay Laurel (*Laurus nobilis*), Spanish Lavender (*Lavandula stoechas* L.), and Fennel (*Foeniculum vulgare*) on Common Foodborne Pathogens," *Journal of Agricultural and Food Chemistry* 52, no. 26 (December 29, 2004): 8255–60.

634. E. M. Choi and J. K. Hwang, "Anti-inflammatory, Analgesic and Antioxidant Activities of the Fruit of *Foeniculum vulgare*," *Fitoterapia*, 75, no. 6 (September 2004): 557–65.

635. Pierce, *Practical Guide to Natural Medicines*, 260.

636. Cech, *Making Plant Medicine*, 141

637. Commission E, "Fennel Oil," *The Commission E Monographs: IHerb Health Encyclopedia*, http://www.herbalgram.org/iherb/commissione/Monographs/Monograph_0098.html.

638. Pierce, *Practical Guide to Natural Medicines*, 262.

639. Commission E, "Fennel Seed," *The Commission E Monographs. IHerb Health Encyclopedia*. http://www.herbalgram.org/iherb/commissione/Monographs/Monograph_0099.html.

640. Pierce, *Practical Guide to Natural Medicines*, 260.

641. Kowalchik and Hylton, *Rodale's Illustrated Encyclopedia of Herbs*, 286.

642. Blumenthal, *The Complete German Commission E Manuscripts.*

643. Johnson, *Pocket Guide to Herbal Remedies*, 63.

644. "Foeniculum Vulgare," *PDR for Herbal Medicine*, 851.

645. F. Iten and R. Saller, ["Fennel Tea: Risk Assessment of the Phytogenic Monosubstance Estragole in Comparison to the Natural Multicomponent Mixture,] *Forsch Komplementarmed Klass Naturheilkd* 11, no. 2 (April 2004): 104–8 (Article in German).

646. Johnson, *Pocket Guide to Herbal Remedies*, 63.

647. Johnson, *Pocket Guide to Herbal Remedies*, 63.

648. Johnson, *Pocket Guide to Herbal Remedies*, 63.

649. Johnson, *Pocket Guide to Herbal Remedies*, 63.

650. D. Bown, *Encyclopedia of Herbs and Their Uses* (New York: DK Publishing, Inc., 1995).

651. Ody, *The Complete Medicinal Herbal*, 106.

652. M. Z. Gad, et al., "Biochemical Study of the Anti-Diabetic Action of the Egyptian Plants Fenugreek and Balanites," *Molecular and Cellular Biochemistry* 281, no. 1–2 (January 2006): 173–83; G. S. Kumar, et al., "Modulatory Effect of Fenugreek Seed Mucilage and Spent Turmeric on Intestinal and Renal Disaccharidases in Streptozotocin Induced Diabetic Rats," *Plant Foods for Human Nutrition* 60, no. 2 (June 2005): 87–91; B. Annida, et al., "Supplementation of Fenugreek Leaves Reduces Oxidative Stress in Streptozotocin-Induced Diabetic Rats," *Journal of Medicinal Food* 8, no. 3 (Fall 2005): 382–5; C. V. Anuradha and P. Ravikumar, "Restoration on Tissue Antioxidants by Fenugreek Seeds (*Trigonella foenum graecum*) in Alloxan-Diabetic Rats, *Indian Journal of Physiology and Pharmacology* 45, no. 4 (October 2001): 408–20.

653. A. Gupta, R. Gupta, and B. Lal, "Effect of *Trigonella foenum-graecum* (Fenugreek) Seeds on Glycaemic Control and Insulin Resistance in Type 2 Diabetes Mellitus: a Double Blind Placebo Controlled Study," *The Journal of the Association of Physicians of India* 49 (November 2001): 1057–61.

654. A. Bordia, et al., "Effect of Ginger (*Zingiber officinale Rosc.*) and Fenugreek (*Trigonella foenumgraecum* L.) on Blood Lipids, Blood Sugar and Platelet Aggregation in Patients with Coronary Artery Disease," *Prostaglandins, Leukotrienes, and Essential Fatty Acids* 56, no. 5 (May 1997): 379–84.

655. R. D. Sharma, et al., "Effect of Fenugreek Seeds on Blood Glucose and Serum Lipids in Type I Diabetes," *European Journal of Clinical Nutrition* 44, no. 4 (April 1990): 301–6.

656. J. Raju, et al., "Alleviation of Hepatic Steatosis Accompanied by Modulation of Plasma and Liver TNF-Alpha Levels by *Trigonella foenum graecum* (Fenugreek) Seeds in Zucker Obese (fa/fa) Rats," *International Journal of Obesity*. 30, no. 8 (August 2006): 1298–307.

657. Bordia, "Effect of Ginger and Fenugreek," 379–84.

658. P. Sowmya and P. Rajyalakshmi, "Hypocholesterolemic Effect of Germinated Fenugreek Seeds in Human Subjects," *Plant Foods for Human Nutrition* 53, no. 4 (1999): 359–65.

659. J. S. Thompson Coon, and E. Ernst, "Herbs for Serum Cholesterol Reduction: a Systematic View," *Journal of Family Practice* 52, no. 6 (June 2003): 468–78.

660. Blumenthal, *The Complete German Commission E Manuscripts*.

661. B. C. Ruby, S. E. Gaskill, D. Slivka, and S. G. Harger, "The Addition of Fenugreek Extract (*Trigonella foenum-graecum*) to Glucose Feeding Increases Muscle Glycogen Resynthesis After Exercise," *Amino Acids* 28, no. 1 (February 2005): 71–6.

662. T. Handa, et al., "Effects of Fenugreek Seed Extract in Obese Mice Fed a High-Fat Diet," *Bioscience, Biotechnology, and Biochemistry* 69, no. 6 (June 2005): 1186–8.

663. International College of Herbal Medicine, "Fenugreek (*Trigonella Foenum-graecum*): Herb of the Month, September/October 2005," http://www.herbcollege.com/herbofthemonth.asp?id=78.

664. A. A. Abdel-Nabey and A. A. Damir, "Changes in Some Nutrients of Fenugreek (*Trigonella Foenum graecum* L.) Seeds During Water Boiling," *Plant Foods for Human Nutrition*. 40, no. 4 (October 1990): 267–74.

665. Sowmya and Rajyalakshmi, "Hypocholesterolemic Effect of Germinated Fenugreek," 359–65.

666. P. Dixit, et al. "Antioxidant Properties of Germinated Fenugreek Seeds," *Phytotherapy Research* 19, no. 11 (November 2005): 977–83.

667. Pierce, *Practical Guide to Natural Medicines*, 263.

668. Johnson, *Pocket Guide to Herbal Remedies*, 169.

669. Bordia, "Effect of Ginger and Fenugreek," 379–84.

670. Pierce, *Practical Guide to Natural Medicines*, 263.

671. A. M. Flammang, et al., "Genotoxicity Testing of a Fenugreek Extract," *Food and Chemical Toxicology* 42, no. 11 (November 2004): 1769–75.

672. D. G. Ebo, et al., "Coriander Anaphylaxis in a Spice Grinder with Undetected Occupational Allergy," *Acta Clinic Belgica* 61, no. 3 (May–June 2006): 152–6.

673. S. P. Patil, et al., "Allergy to Fenugreek (*Trigonella foenum graecum*)," *Annals of Allergy, Asthma & Immunology* 78, no. 3 (March 1997): 297–300.

674. Pierce, *Practical Guide to Natural Medicines*, 264.

675. Ginseng. MedlinePlus herb and supplement.

676. A. Kassem, et al., "Evaluation of the Potential Antifertility Effect of Fenugreek Seeds in Male and Female Rabbits," *Contraception* 73, no. 3 (March 2006): 301–6; Adhikary P, et al., Anti-Implantation Activity of Some Indigenous Plants in Adult Female Rats, *Indian Journal of Pharmacology* 22, no. 1 (March 1990): 24–5.

677. Johnson, *Pocket Guide to Herbal Remedies*,169.

678. J. P. Lambert and J. Cormier, "Potential Interaction Between Warfarin and Boldo-Fenugreek," *Pharmacotherapy* 21, no. 4 (April 2001): 509–12.

679. G. B. Bartley, et al., "'Maple-syrup' Urine Odor Due to Fenugreek Ingestion, *New England Journal of Medicine* 305, no. 8 (August 20, 1981): 467.

680. Pierce, *Practical Guide to Natural Medicines*, 265.

681. Pierce, *Practical Guide to Natural Medicines*, 266.

682. Ody, *The Complete Medicinal Herbal*.

683. Pierce, *Practical Guide to Natural Medicines*, 267.

684. J. J. Murphy, et al., "Randomised Double-Blind Placebo-Controlled Trial of Feverfew in Migraine Prevention," *Lancet* 2, no. 8604 (July 23, 1988): 189–92; B. K. Vogler, et al., "Feverfew as a Preventive Treatment for Migraine: a Systematic Review," *Cephalalgia* 18, no. 10 (1998): 704–708.

685. Pierce, *Practical Guide to Natural Medicines*, 266.

686. John Bruno Romero, *The Botanical Lore of the California Indians* (New York: Vantage Press, Inc., 1954): 60.

687. M. Pattrick, "Feverfew in Rheumatoid Arthritis: a Double Blind, Placebo Controlled Study," *Annals of the Rheumatic Diseases* 48(1989): 547–49.

688. Hamel and Chiltoskey, *Cherokee Plants and Their Uses*, 34

689. Alexa T Smolinski, et al., "Comparative Effects of the Herbal Constituent Parthenolide (Feverfew) on Lipopolysaccharide-Induced Inflammatory Gene Expression in Murine Spleen and Liver," *Journal of Inflammation* 2 (June 29, 2005): 6.

690. Michael Moore, "Herbs Best as Cold Infusion."

691. Pierce, *Practical Guide to Natural Medicines*, 266.

692. Pierce, *Practical Guide to Natural Medicines*, 266.

693. Johnson, *Pocket Guide to Herbal Remedies*, 161.

694. Pierce, *Practical Guide to Natural Medicines*, 266.

695. Johnson, *Pocket Guide to Herbal Remedies*, 161.

696. Pierce, *Practical Guide to Natural Medicines*, 267.

697. D. V. C. Awang, *Canadian Pharmaceutical Journal* 122, no. 5 (1989): 266–70. Kavasch, E. Barrie and Karen Baar, *American Indian Healing Arts* (New York: Bantam, 1999): 245.

698. Johnson, *Pocket Guide to Herbal Remedies*,161.

699. Pierce, *Practical Guide to Natural Medicines*, 267.

700. Hoffmann, "Feverfew," *Herbal Materia Medica*.

701. Harkness and Bratman, *Handbook of Drug-Herb and Drug-Supplement Interactions*, 102

702. "Fish Oil More Useful for Treating Inflammation Than Flax Seed Oil," *Journal American College Nutrition* 21, no. 6 (December 2002): 495–505.

703. B. Walser, et al., "Supplementation With Omega–3 Polyunsaturated Fatty Acids Augments Brachial Artery Dilation and Blood Flow During Forearm Contraction," *European Journal Of Applied Physiology* 97, no. 3 (June 2006): 347–54.

704. "Omega–3 Fatty Acids, Fish Oil, Alpha–Linolenic Acid," *Mayo Clinic Website*. http://www.mayoclinic.com/health/fish-oil/NS_patient-fishoil. December 6, 2007.

705. "Omega–3 Fatty Acids, Fish Oil, Alpha–Linolenic Acid," *Mayo Clinic Website*.

706. U.S. Food and Drug Administration, "FDA Announces Qualified Health Claims for Omega–3 Fatty Acids," *FDA News*, http://www.fda.gov/bbs/topics/news/2004/NEW01115.html.

707. Ingeborg A. Brouwer, et al., "Effect of Fish Oil on Ventricular Tachyarrhythmia and Death in Patients With Implantable Cardioverter Defibrillators: The Study on Omega–3 Fatty Acids and Ventricular Arrhythmia (SOFA) Randomized Trial," *Journal of the American Medical Association* 295, no. 22 (June 14, 2006).

708. C. I. O'Connor, et al., "The Effect of Dietary Fish Oil Supplementation on Exercising Horses," Journal of Animal Science82, no. 10 (October 2004): 2978–84.

709. J. H. O'Keefe, Jr, et al., "Effects of Omega–3 Fatty Acids on Resting Heart Rate, Heart Rate Recovery After Exercise, and Heart Rate Variability in Men with Healed Myocardial Infarctions and Depressed Ejection Fractions," *American Journal of Cardiology* 97, no. 8 (April 15, 2006): 1127–30.

710. T. Phillips, et al., "A Dietary Supplement Attenuates IL–6 and CRP After Eccentric Exercise in Untrained Males," *Medicine and Science in Sports and Exercise* 35, no. 12 (December 2003): 2032–7.

711. J. Lenn, et al., "The Effects of Fish Oil and Isoflavones on Delayed Onset Muscle Soreness," *Medicine and Science in Sports and Exercise* 34, no. 10 (October 2002): 1605–13.

712. T. D. Mickleborough, et al., "Protective Effect of Fish Oil Supplementation on Exercise-Induced Bronchoconstriction in Asthma," *Chest* 129, no. 1 (January 2006): 39–49.

713. T. D. Mickleborough, et al., "Fish Oil Supplementation Reduces Severity of Exercise-Induced Bronchoconstriction in Elite Athletes," *American Journal of Respiratory and Critical Care Medicine* 168, no. 10 (November 15, 2003): 1181–9.

714. J. R. Hibbeln, et al., "A Replication Study of Violent and Nonviolent Subjects: Cerebrospinal Fluid Metabolites Of Serotonin and Dopamine are Predicted by Plasma Essential Fatty Acids," *Biological Psychiatry* 44, no. 4 (August 1998): 243–9; J. R. Hibbeln, et al., "Omega–3 Status and Cerebrospinal Fluid Corticotrophin Releasing Hormone in Perpetrators of Domestic Violence," *Biological Psychiatry* 56, no. 11 (December 1, 2004): 895–7.

715. E. A. Mitchell, et al., "Clinical Characteristics and Serum Essential Fatty Acid Levels in Hyperactive Children," *Clinical Pediatrics* 26, no. 8 (August 1987): 406–11; J. R. Chen, et al., "Dietary Patterns and Blood Fatty Acid Composition in Children with Attention-Deficit Hyperactivity Disorder in Taiwan," *Journal of Clinical Biochemistry and Nutrition* 15, no. 8 (August 2004): 467–72.

716. J. R. Hibbeln, et al., "Omega–3 Fatty Acid Deficiencies in Neurodevelopment, Aggression and Autonomic Dysregulation: Opportunities for Intervention," *International Review of Psychiatry* 18, no. 2 (April 2006): 107–18.

717. Hibbeln, "Omega–3 Status and cerebrospinal fluid corticotrophin releasing hormone," 895–7.

718. R. G. Voigt, et al., "A Randomized, Double-Blind, Placebo-Controlled Trial of Docosahexaenoic Acid Supplementation in Children with Attention-Deficit/Hyperactivity Disorder," *Journal of Pediatrics* 139, no. 2 (August 2001): 189–96; M. Haag "Essential Fatty Acids and the Brain," *Canadian Journal of Psychiatry* 48, no. 3 (April 2003): 195–203.

719. C. Bernard Gesch, et al., "Influence of Supplementary Vitamins, Minerals and Essential Fatty Acids on the Antisocial Behaviour of Young Adult Prisoners: Randomised, Placebo-Controlled Trial," *The British Journal of Psychiatry* 181 (2002): 22–28.

720. R. K. McNamara and S. E. Carlson, "Role of Omega–3 Fatty Acids in Brain Development and Function: Potential Implications for the Pathogenesis and Prevention of Psychopathology," *Prostaglandins, Leukotrienes, and Essential Fatty Acids* 75, no. 4–5. (October–November 2006): 329–49; M. Itomura, et al., "The Effect of Fish Oil on Physical Aggression in Schoolchildren—a Randomized, Double-Blind, Placebo-Controlled Trial," *Journal of Clinical Biochemistry and Nutrition* 16, no. 3 (March 2005): 163–71; L. Buydens-Branchey, et al., "Polyunsaturated Fatty Acid Status and Aggression in Cocaine Addicts," *Drug Alcohol Dependence* 71, no. 3 (September 10, 2003): 319–23; T. Hamazaki, et al., "The Effect of Docosahexaenoic Acid on Aggression in Elderly Thai Subjects—a Placebo-Controlled Double-Blind Study," *Nutritional Neuroscience* 5, no. 1 (February 2002): 37–41.

721. Hamazaki, "The Effect Of Docosahexaenoic Acid On Aggression In Young Adults," 1129–33.

722. T. Hamazaki, et al. "Docosahexaenoic Acid does not Affect Aggression of Normal Volunteers under Nonstressful Conditions. A Randomized, Placebo-Controlled, Double-Blind Study," *Lipids* 33, no. 7 (July 1998): 663–7.

723. A. J. Richardson, "Omega–3 Fatty Acids in ADHD and Related Neurodevelopmental Disorders," *International Review of Psychiatry* 18, no. 2 (April 2006): 155–72.

724. R. G. Voigt, et al, "A Randomized, Double-Blind, Placebo-Controlled Trial of Docosahexaenoic Acid Supplementation in Children with Attention-Deficit/Hyperactivity Disorder," *Journal of Pediatrics* 139, no. 2 (August 2001): 189–96.

725. K. Joshi, et al., "Supplementation with Flax Oil and Vitamin C Improves the Outcome of Attention Deficit Hyperactivity Disorder (ADHD)," *Prostaglandins, Leukotrienes, and Essential Fatty Acids* 74, no. 1 (January 2006): 17–21.

726. A. J. Richardson and P. Montgomery, "The Oxford-Durham study: a Randomized, Controlled Trial of Dietary Supplementation with Fatty Acids in Children with Developmental Coordination Disorder," *Pediatrics* 115, no. 5 (May 2005): 1360–6.

727. Pao-Yen Lin, and Kuan-Pin Su, "A Meta-Analytic Review of Double-Blind, Placebo-Controlled Trials of Antidepressant Efficacy of Omega–3 Fatty Acids," *Journal of Clinical Psychiatry* 68 (2007): 1056–1061.

728. S. Sliwinski, et al., "Poly Unsaturated Fatty Acids: Do they have a role in the Pathophysiology of Autism?" *Neuro Endocrinology Letters* 27, no. 4 (August 5, 2006); G. P. Amminger, et al., Omega–3 Fatty Acids Supplementation in Children with Autism: A Double-blind Randomized, Placebo-controlled Pilot Study," Biological Psychiatry (Aug 22, 2006).

729. P. C. Calder, "Dietary Modification of Inflammation with Lipids," *The Proceedings of the Nutrition Society* 61, no. 3 (August 2002): 345–58.

730. "Fish Oil More Useful for Treating Inflammation Than Flax Seed Oil," *Journal American College Nutrition* 21, no. 6 (December 2002): 495–505.

731. "Fish Oil More Useful for Treating Inflammation," 495–505.

732. R. Oh, "Practical Applications of Fish Oil (Omega–3 Fatty Acids) in Primary Care," *The Journal of the American Board of Family Practice* 18, no. 1 (January–February 2005): 28–36; A. A. Berbert, C. R. Kondo, C. L. Almendra, T. Matsuo, and I. Dichi, "Supplementation of Fish Oil and Olive Oil in Patients with Rheumatoid Arthritis, *Nutrition* 21, no. 2 (February 2005): 131–6.

733. Alison M Hill, et al., "Combining Fish-Oil Supplements with Regular Aerobic Exercise Improves Body Composition and Cardiovascular Disease Risk Factors," *American Journal of Clinical Nutrition* 85, no. 5, (May 2007): 1267–1274.

734. "Fish Oil," *Whole Health MD*, http://www.wholehealthmd.com.

735. American Heart Association, "New Guidelines Focus on Fish, Fish Oil, Omega–3 Fatty Acids," http://www.americanheart.org/presenter.jhtml?identifier=3006624.

736. American Heart Association, "New Guidelines Focus on Fish, Fish Oil, Omega–3 Fatty Acids."

737. American Heart Association, "New Guidelines Focus on Fish, Fish Oil, Omega–3 Fatty Acids."

738. "Fish Oil," *Whole Health MD*.

739. "Fish Oil," *Whole Health MD*.

740. Christine J. Lewis, "Letter Regarding Dietary Supplement: Health Claim for Omega–3 Fatty Acids and Coronary Heart Disease (Docket No. 91N–0103)," U. S. Food and Drug Administration; Center for Food Safety and Applied Nutrition, Office of Nutritional Products, Labeling, and Dietary Supplements. http://www.cfsan.fda.gov/~dms/ds-ltr11.html.

741. American Heart Association, "New Guidelines Focus on Fish, Fish Oil, Omega–3 Fatty Acids."

742. "Fish Oil," *Whole Health MD*.

743. "Fish Oil," *Whole Health MD*.

744. Natural Standard Patient Monographs, "Omega–3 Fatty Acids, Fish Oil, Alpha-Linolenic Acid," *Mayo Clinic* http://www.mayoclinic.com/health/fish-oil/NS_patient-fishoil.

745. Paul J Nestel, "Fish oil and Cardiovascular Disease: Lipids And Arterial Function," *American Journal of Clinical Nutrition* 71, no. 1, (January 2000) 228S–231S.

746. Micromedex, "Omega–3–acid Ethyl Esters (Systemic)," *MayoClinic.com* http://www.mayoclinic.com/health/drug-information/DR500573.

747. Remington and Woods, *The Dispensatory of the United States of America*.

748. Artemis P. Simopoulos, "Omega–3 Fatty Acids in Inflammation and Autoimmune Diseases," *Journal of the American College of Nutrition* 21, no. 6, (2002) 495–505.

749. Remington and Woods, *The Dispensatory of the United States of America*.

750. Grieve, "Flax," *Botanical.com: A Modern Herbal.*

751. "Flaxseed," *The Commission E Monographs* http://www.herbalgram.org/iherb/commissione/Monographs/Monograph_0176.html.

752. K. Prasad, "Hypocholesterolemic and Antiatherosclerotic Effect of Flax Lignan Complex Isolated from Flaxseed," *Atherosclerosis* 178, no. 2 (April 2005): 269–75.

753. P. J. Nestel, "Arterial Compliance in Obese Subjects is Improved with Dietary Plant n–3 Fatty Acid from Flaxseed Oil Despite Increased LDL Oxidizability," *Arteriosclerosis, Thrombosis, and Vascular Biology* 17, no. 6 (June 1997): 1163–70.

754. Pierce, *Practical Guide to Natural Medicines,* 269; S. Mandasescu, et al., "Flaxseed Supplementation in Hyperlipidemic Patients," *Revista Medico-Chirurgicală a Societății de Medici și Naturaliști din Iași* 109, no. 3 (July–September 2005): 502–6.

755. Pierce, *Practical Guide to Natural Medicines,* 269.

756. Blumenthal, *The Complete German Commission E Manuscripts.*

757. Remington and Woods, *The Dispensatory of the United States of America.*

758. R. S. Mueller, et al., "Effect of Omega–3 Fatty Acids on Canine Atopic Dermatitis," *The Journal of Small Animal Practice* 45, no. 6 (June 2004): 293–7.

759. A. Bjørneboe, E. Søyland, and G. E. Bjørneboe, et al., "Effect of Dietary Supplementation with Eicosapentaenoic Acid in the Treatment of Atopic Dermatitis," *The British Journal of Dermatology* 117 (1987): 463–9; A. Bjørnboe, E. Søyland, G. E. Bjørnboe, et al., "Effect of n–3 Fatty Acid Supplement to Patients with Atopic Dermatitis," *Journal of Internal Medicine Supplement* 225 (1989): 233–6; E. Søyland, G. Rajka, A. Bjørneboe, et al., "The Effect of Eicosapentaenoic Acid in the Treatment Of Atopic Dermatitis: A Clinical Study," *Acta Dermato-Venereologica* 144 (1989): 139; J. Berth-Jones, R. A. C. Graham-Brown, "Placebo-Controlled Trial of Essential Fatty Acid Supplementation in Atopic Dermatitis," *Lancet* 341 (1993): 1557–60.

760. J. D. Spence, et al., "The Effect of Flax Seed Cultivars with Differing Content of Alpha–Linolenic Acid and Lignans on Responses to Mental Stress, *Journal of the American College of Nutrition* 22, no 6 (December 2003): 494–501.

761. K. Joshi, et al., "Supplementation with Flax Oil and Vitamin C Improves The Outcome Of Attention Deficit Hyperactivity Disorder (ADHD)," *Prostaglandins, Leukotrienes, and Essential Fatty Acids* 74, no. 1 (January 2006): 17–21.

762. G. S. Young, J. A. Conquer, and R. Thomas, "Effect of Randomized Supplementation with High Dose Olive, Flax or Fish Oil on Serum Phospholipid Fatty Acid Levels in Adults with Attention Deficit Hyperactivity Disorder," *Reproduction, Nutrition, Development* 45, no. 5 (September–October 2005): 549–58.

763. T. Shipochliev, et al., ["Anti-Inflammatory Action of a Group of Plant Extracts,"] *Veterinarno-meditsinski Nauki* 18, no. 6 (1981): 87–94 (Article in Bulgarian).

764. D.E. Nordstrom, et al., "Alpha–Linolenic Acid in the Treatment of Rheumatoid Arthritis: A Double-Blind, Placebo-Controlled and Randomized Study: Flaxseed vs. Safflower Seed," *Rheumatology International* 14 no. 6 (1995): 231–34.

765. "Flaxseed Oil," *Whole Health MD,* http://www.wholehealthmd.com.

766. L. U. Thompson, "Experimental Studies on Lignans and Cancer," *Baillière's Clinical Endocrinology and Metabolism* 12 (1998): 691–705.

767. Michael S Donaldson, "Nutrition and Cancer: A Review of the Evidence for an Anti-Cancer Diet," Nutrition *Journal* 3 (2004): 19.

768. EBSCO CAM Review Board, "Flaxseed Oil," *Health Library* http://healthlibrary.epnet.com/GetContent.aspx?token=e0498803-7f62-4563-8d47-5fe33da65dd4&chunkiid=21715.

769. "Flaxseed," *The Commission E Monographs* http://www.herbalgram.org/iherb/commissione/Monographs/Monograph_0176.html.

770. "Flaxseed," *The Commission E Monographs.*

771. Henriette Kress, "Absorption," *Henriette's Herbal Blog* http://www.henriettesherbal.com/blog/?cat=6&paged=5.

772. Johnson, *Pocket Guide to Herbal Remedies*, 89.

773. Pierce, *Practical Guide to Natural Medicines*, 269.

774. NCCAM, "Flaxseed and Flaxseed Oil," *Herbs at a Glance*, http://nccam.nih.gov/health/flaxseed.

775. Kowalchik and Hylton, *Rodale's Illustrated Encyclopedia of Herbs.*

776. Michael S Donaldson, "Nutrition and Cancer: A Review of the Evidence for an Anti-Cancer Diet," *Nutrition Journal* 3 (2004): 19.

777. Eunyoung Cho, et al, "Polyunsaturated fatty acids are potent neuroprotectors" *American Journal of Clinical Nutrition* 73, no. 2(2001): 209–218.

778. J. Waldschlager, et al., "Flax-Seed Extracts with Phytoestrogenic Effects on a Hormone Receptor-Positive Tumour Cell Line," *Anticancer Research* 25, no. 3A (May–June 2005): 1817–22.

779. U.S. National Institute of Health, "Flaxseed and Flaxseed Oil (*Linum usitatissimum*)," *MedlinePlus Herb and Supplements*, http://www.nlm.nih.gov/medlineplus/druginfo/natural/patient-flaxseed.html.

780. Johnson, *Pocket Guide to Herbal Remedies*, 89.

781. Pierce, *Practical Guide to Natural Medicines*, 269.

782. Pierce, *Practical Guide to Natural Medicines*, 269.

783. M. T. Murray, *The Healing Properties Of Herbs* (Rocklin, CA: Prima Publishing, 1995).

784. D. Heber, "Vegetables, Fruits and Phytoestrogens in the Prevention of Diseases," *Journal of Postgraduate Medicine* 50, no. 2 (April–June 2004): 145–9.

785. American Botanical Council, "Garlic," *Expanded Commission E Online* http://www.herbalgram.org/default.asp?c=he037.

786. Grieve, "Garlic," *Botanical.com: A Modern Herbal.*

787. M. Castleman, *The Healing Herbs* (New York: Bantam Books, 1995).

788. Y. L. Lee, et al., "Antibacterial Activity of Vegetables and Juices," *Nutrition* 19, no. 11–12 (November–December 2003): 994–6.

789. I. M. Bakri and C. W. Douglas, "Inhibitory Effect of Garlic Extract on Oral Bacteria," *Archives of Oral Biology* 50, no. 7 (July 2005): 645–51; B. A. Iwalokun, et al., "In Vitro Antimicrobial Properties of Aqueous Garlic Extract against Multidrug-Resistant Bacteria and Candida Species from Nigeria," *Journal of Medicinal Food* 7, no. 3 (Fall 2004): 327–33; I. A. Adeleye and L. Opiah, "Antimicrobial Activity of Extracts of Local Cough Mixtures on Upper Respiratory Tract Bacterial Pathogens," *The West Indian Medical Journal* 52, no. 3 (September 2003): 188–90.

790. K. Van-Kessel, et al., "Common Complementary and Alternative Therapies for Yeast Vaginitis and Bacterial Vaginosis: A Systematic Review," *Obstetrical & Gynecological Survey* 58, no. 5 (May 2003): 351–8; Michael R. Tansey and Judith A. Appleton, "Inhibition of Fungal Growth by Garlic Extract," *Mycologia* 67, no. 2 (March–April 1975): 409–413.

791. Y. Tsai, et al. "Antiviral Properties of Garlic: In Vitro Effects on Influenza B, Herpes Simplex and Coxsackie Viruses," *Planta Medica* 5 (October 1985): 460–1.

792. B. Turner, C. Molgaard, and P. Marckmann, "Effect of Garlic (*Allium sativum*) Powder Tablets on Serum Lipids, Blood Pressure and Arterial Stiffness in Normo-Lipidaemic Volunteers: A Randomised, Double-Blind, Placebo-Controlled Trial," *The British Journal of Nutrition* 92, no. 4 (October 2004): 701–6.

793. I. Durak, et al, "Effects of Garlic Extract Consumption on Blood Lipid and Oxidant/Antioxidant Parameters in Humans with High Blood Cholesterol," *The Journal of Nutritional Biochemistry* 15, no. 6 (June 2004): 373–7.

794. A. Peleg, et al., "Effect of Garlic on Lipid Profile and Psychopathologic Parameters in People with Mild to Moderate Hypercholesterolemia," *The Israel Medical Association Journal* (September 2003): 637–40.

795. P. Satitvipawee, et al., "No Effect of Garlic Extract Supplement on Serum Lipid Levels in Hypercholesterolemic Subjects," *Journal of the Medical Association of Thailand* (August 2003): 750–7.

796. R. Bakhsh and M. I. Chughtai, "Influence of Garlic on Serum Cholesterol, Serum Triglycerides, Serum Total Lipids and Serum Glucose in Human Subjects," *Nahrung* 28, no. 2 (1984): 159–63.

797. A. Bordia, "Effect Of Garlic On Blood Lipids In Patients With Coronary Heart Disease," *American Journal of Clinical Nutrition* 34, no. 10 (October 1981): 2100–3.

798. Tieraona Low Dog and David Riley, "Management of Hyperlipidemia," *Alternative Therapies* 9, no. 3 (May–June 2003): 28–41.

799. Hamel and Chiltoskey, *Cherokee Plants and Their Uses*, 35.

800. Grieve, "Garlic," *Botanical.com: A Modern Herbal.*

801. P. Josling, "Preventing the Common Cold with a Garlic Supplement: A Double-Blind, Placebo-Controlled Survey," *Advances in Therapy* 18, no. 4 (July–August 2001): 189–93.

802. K. C. Srivastava, "Evidence for the Mechanism by which Garlic Inhibits Platelet Aggregation," *Prostaglandins, Leukotrienes, and Medicine* 22, no. 3 (June 1986): 313–21; K. Rahman and D. Billington, Dietary Supplementation with Aged Garlic Extract Inhibits ADP-Induced Platelet Aggregation in Humans," *Journal of Nutrition* 130, no. 11 (November 2000): 2662–5.

803. Low Dog and Riley, "Management of Hyperlipidemia," 28–41; A. Gonen, et al., The Antiatherogenic Effect of Allicin: Possible Mode of Action," *Pathobiology* 72, no. 6 (2005): 325–34; Pierce, *Practical Guide to Natural Medicines*, 283.

804. N. Morihara, et al., "Aged Garlic Extract Maintains Cardiovascular Homeostasis in Mice and Rats,"*Journal of Nutrition* 136, no. 3 suppl (March 2006): 777S–781S.

805. A. Harauma and T. Moriguchi, "Aged Garlic Extract Improves Blood Pressure in Spontaneously Hypertensive Rats More Safely Than Raw Garlic," *Journal of Nutrition* 136, no. 3 suppl (March 2006): 769S–773S; I. Durak, et al., "Effects of Garlic Extract Consumption on Blood Lipid and Oxidant/Antioxidant Parameters in Humans with High Blood Cholesterol," *Journal of Clinical Biochemistry and Nutrition* 15, no. 6 (June 2004): 373–7.

806. N. Morihara, "Aged Garlic Extract Ameliorates Physical Fatigue," *Biological & Pharmaceutical Bulletin* 29, no. 5 (May 2006): 962–6.

807. N. Morihara, et al., "Aged Garlic Extract Enhances Production of Nitric Oxide," *Life Science* 71, no. 5 (June 21, 2002): 509–17.

808. S. K. Verma, et al., "Effect of Garlic (*Allium sativum*) Oil on Exercise Tolerance in Patients with Coronary Artery Disease," *Indian Journal of Physiology and Pharmacology* 49, no. 1 (January 2005): 115–8.

809. K. M. Lemar, et al., "Garlic (*Allium sativum*) as an Anti-Candida Agent: A Comparison of the Efficacy of Fresh Garlic and Freeze-Dried Extracts," *Journal of Applied Microbiology* 93, no. 3 (2002): 398–405.

810. Pierce, *Practical Guide to Natural Medicines*, 283.

811. Joyce A. Wardwell, *The Herbal Home Remedy Book* (Pownal: Storey Publishing, 1998): 111.

812. M. L. Motsei, et al., "Screening of Traditionally Used South African Plants for Antifungal Activity Against *Candida albicans*," *Journal of Ethnophamacology* 86, no. 2–3 (June 2003): 235–41.

813. Wardwell, *The Herbal Home Remedy Book*, 111.

814. S. Gorinstein, et al., "Raw and Boiled Garlic Enhances Plasma Antioxidant Activity and Improves Plasma Lipid Metabolism in Cholesterol-Fed Rats," *Life Science* 78, no. 6 (January 2, 2006): 655–63.

815. S. K. Chutani and A. Bordia, "The Effect of Fried Versus Raw Garlic on Fibrinolytic Activity in Man," *Atherosclerosis* 38, no. 3–4 (February–March 1981): 417–21.

816 .H. K. Berthold, T. Sudhop, and K. von Bergmann, "Effect of a Garlic Oil Preparation on Serum Lipoproteins and Cholesterol Metabolism: A Randomized Controlled Trial," *Journal of the American Medical Association* 279, no. 23 (1998): 1900–1902.

817. Low Dog and Riley, "Management of Hyperlipidemia," 28–41.

818. Tieraona Low Dog, "Some Clinically Tested Products Sold in the United States," *DrLowDog.com* http://www.drlowdog.com/DrLowDog.com/Publications_files/Clinically%20Tested%20Herbs.pdf.

819. "Garlic," *Whole Health MD* http://www.wholehealthmd.com.

820. Pierce, *Practical Guide to Natural Medicines*, 283.

821. "Garlic (*Allium sativum L.*)," *Medlineplus Herb and Supplements* http://www.nlm.nih.gov/medlineplus/druginfo/natural/patient-garlic.html.

822. "Garlic," *Whole Health MD*.

823. "Garlic," *Whole Health MD*.

824. Johnson, *Pocket Guide to Herbal Remedies*, 6; Pierce, *Practical Guide to Natural Medicines*, 283.

825. "Garlic," *Whole Health MD*.

826. "Garlic," *Whole Health MD*.

827. "Garlic (*Allium sativum L.*)," *Medlineplus Herb and Supplements*.

828. "Garlic (*Allium sativum L.*)," *Medlineplus Herb and Supplements*.

829. Pierce, *Practical Guide to Natural Medicines*, 283.

830. "Garlic (*Allium sativum L.*)," *Medlineplus Herb and Supplements*.

831. R. K. Yadav and N. S. Verma, "Effects of Garlic (*Allium sativum*) Extract on the Heart Rate, Rhythm and Force of Contraction in Frog: A Dose-Dependent Study," *Indian Journal of Experimental Biology* 42, no. 6 (June 2004): 628–31.

832. Harkness and Bratman, *Handbook of Drug-Herb and Drug-Supplement Interactions*, 134.

833. "Garlic (*Allium sativum L.*)," *Medlineplus Herb and Supplements*.

834. Pierce, *Practical Guide to Natural Medicines*, 283.

835. American Botanical Council, "Garlic," *Expanded Commission E Online* http://www.herbalgram.org/default.asp?c=he037.

836. "Garlic (*Allium sativum L.*)," *Medlineplus Herb and Supplements.*

837. Harkness and Bratman, *Handbook of Drug-Herb and Drug-Supplement Interactions*, 134.

838. Harkness and Bratman, *Handbook of Drug-Herb and Drug-Supplement Interactions*, 319; Low Dog and Riley, "Management of Hyperlipidemia," 28–41.

839. E. Sussman, "Garlic Supplements can Impede HIV Medication," *AIDS* 16, no. 9 (June 14, 2002): N5.

840. V. E. Tyler, *Herbs of Choice* (Binghampton, NY: Haworth Press, 1994).

841. West TCM, "Sheng Jiang," *Traditional Chinese Medicine and Acupuncture Health Information Organization* http://tcm.health-info.org/Herbology.Materia.Medica/shengjiang-properties.htm.

842. "Ginger," *Whole Health MD* http://www.wholehealthmd.com.

843. "Ginger," *Whole Health MD.*

844. S. Sontakke, V. Thawani, and M. S. Naik, "Ginger as an Antiemetic in Nausea and Vomiting Induced by Chemotherapy: A Randomized, Crossover, Double Blind Study," *Indian Journal of Pharmacology* 35 (2003): 32–36.

845. D. S. Qian and Z. S. Liu, Pharmacologic Studies of Antimotion Sickness Actions of Ginger, *Zhongguo Zhong Xi Yi Jie He Za Zhi* 12, no. 2 (1992): 95–98.

846. J. J. Stewart, et al., "Effects of Ginger on Motion Sickness Susceptibility and Gastric Function," *Pharmacology* 42, no. 2 (1991): 111–20.

847. S. Visalyaputra, N. Petchpaisit, and K. Somcharoen, et al., "The Efficacy of Ginger Root in the Prevention of Postoperative Nausea and Vomiting After Outpatient Gynaecological Laparoscopy," *Anaesthesia* 53, no. 5 (1998): 506–510; Z. Arfeen, H. Owen, and J. L Plummer, et al., A Double-Blind Randomized Controlled Trial of Ginger for the Prevention of Postoperative Nausea and Vomiting," *Anaesthesia and Intensive Care* 23, no. 4 (1995): 449–452.

848. "Ginger," *Whole Health MD.*

849. D.B. Mowrey and D.E. Clayson, "Motion Sickness, Ginger, and Psychophysics," *Lancet.* 1 (1982): 655–57.

850. R. Schmid, T. Schick, R. Steffen, et al., "Comparison of Seven Commonly Used Agents for Prophylaxis of Seasickness," *Journal of Travel Medicine* 1, no. 4 (1994): 203–206.

851. Maryland Medical Center Programs Center for Integrative Medicine, "Ginger Research," http://www.umm.edu/altmed/ConsHerbs/Gingerch.html.

852. Sontakke, "Ginger as an Antiemetic," 32–36.

853. R. Grzanna, L. Lindmark, and C. G. Frondoza, "Ginger—an Herbal Medicinal Product with Broad Anti-Inflammatory Actions," *Journal of Medicinal Food* 8, no. 2 (Summer 2005): 125–32.

854. C. L. Shen, K. J. Hong, and S. W. Kim, Effects of Ginger (*Zingiber officinale Rosc.*) on Decreasing the Production of Inflammatory Mediators in Sow Osteoarthrotic Cartilage Explants," *Journal of Medicinal Food* 6, no. 4 (Winter 2003): 323–8.

855. J. N. Sharma, K. C. Srivastava, and E. K. Gan, "Suppressive Effects of Eugenol and Ginger Oil on Arthritic Rats," *Pharmacology* 49, no. 5 (1994): 314–318; H. Y. Young, et al., "Analgesic and Anti-Inflammatory Activities of [6]-gingerol," *Journal of Ethnopharmacology* 96, no. 1–2 (January 4, 2005): 207–10.

856. K. Srivastava, et al., "Ginger (*Zingiber officinale*) and Rheumatic Disorders," *Medical Hypotheses* 29 (1989): 25–28.

857. I. Wigler, et al., "The Effects of Zintona EC (a ginger extract) on Symptomatic Gonarthritis," *Osteoarthritis-Cartilage* 11, no. 11 (November 2003): 783–9; R. D. Altman and K. C. Marcussen, "Effects of a Ginger Extract on Knee Pain in Patients with Osteoarthritis," *Arthritis and Rheumatism* 44, no. 11 (November 2001): 2531–8.

858. H. Bliddal, A. Rosetzsky, and P. Schlichting, et al., "A Randomized, Placebo-Controlled, Cross-Over Study Of Ginger Extracts And Ibuprofen In Osteoarthritis," *Osteoarthritis Cartilage* 8, no. 1 (2000): 9–12.

859. West TCM "Sheng Jiang," *Traditional Chinese Medicine and Acupuncture Health Information Organization* http://tcm.health-info.org/Herbology.Materia.Medica/shengjiang-properties.htm.

860. "Ginger," *Whole Health MD.*

861. S. Inouye et al., *Microbial Biochemistry* 100 (1984): 232; J. F. Akoachere, et al. "Antibacterial Effect of *Zingiber officinale* and *Garcinia kola* on Respiratory Tract Pathogens," *East African Medical Journal* 79, no. 11 (November 2002): 588–92.

862. C. Thongson, P. M. Davidson, W. Mahakarnchanakul, and P. Vibulsresth, "Antimicrobial Effect of Thai Spices Against *Listeria monocytogenes* and *Salmonella typhimurium* DT104," *Journal of Food Protection* 68, no. 10 (2005): 2054–8.

863. Remington and Woods, *The Dispensatory of the United States of America.*

864. Grieve, "Ginger," *Botanical.com: A Modern Herbal.*

865. M. N. Ghayur and A. H. Gilani, "Pharmacological Basis for The Medicinal Use of Ginger in Gastrointestinal Disorders, *Digestive Diseases and Sciences* 50, no. 10 (October 2005): 1889–97.

866. "Ginger," *Whole Health MD.*

867. B. Fuhrman, M. Rosenblat, and T. Hayek, et al., "Ginger Extract Consumption Reduces Plasma Cholesterol, Inhibits LDL Oxidation and Attenuates Development of Atherosclerosis in Atherosclerotic, Apolipoprotein E-Deficient Mice," *Journal of Nutrition* 130, no. 5 (2000): 1124–1131.

868. Low Dog and Riley, "Management of Hyperlipidemia," 28–41

869. M. Thomson, et al., "The use of Ginger (*Zingiber officinale* Rosc.) as a Potential Anti-Inflammatory and Antithrombotic Agent," *Prostaglandins, Leukotrienes, and Essential Fatty Acids* 67, no. 6 (December 2002): 475–8.

870. U. Bhandari, et al., "The Protective Action of Ethanolic Ginger (*Zingiber officinale*) Extract in Cholesterol Fed Rabbits," *Journal of Ethnopharmacology* 61, no. 2 (June 1998): 167–71.

871. P. L. Janssen, et al., "Consumption of Ginger (*Zingiber officinale roscoe*) does not Affect Ex Vivo Platelet Thromboxane Production in Humans," *European Journal of Clinical Nutrition* 50, no. 11 (November 1996): 772–4.

872. A. Bordia, et al., "Effect of Ginger (*Zingiber officinale* Rosc.) and Fenugreek (*Trigonella foenumgraecum* L.) on Blood Lipids, Blood Sugar and Platelet Aggregation in Patients with Coronary Artery Disease," *Prostaglandins, Leukotrienes, and Essential Fatty Acids* 56, no. 5 (May 1997): 379–84.

873. Low Dog and Riley, "Management of Hyperlipidemia," 28–41.

874. West TCM, "Sheng Jiang."

875. Akana, *Hawaiian Herbs of Medicinal Value*, 19.

876. S. C. Penna, et al., "Anti-inflammatory Effect of the Hydralcoholic Extract of *Zingiber officinale* Rhizomes on Rat Paw and Skin Edema," *Phytomedicine* 10, no. 5 (2003): 381–5.

877. "Ginger," *Whole Health MD.*

878. "Ginger," *Whole Health MD.*

879. "Ginger," *Whole Health MD.*

880. H. A. Schwertner, D. C. Rios, and J. E. Pascoe, "Variation in Concentration and Labeling of Ginger Root Dietary Supplements," *Obstetrics and Gynecology* 107, no. 6 (June 2006): 1337–43.

881. "Ginger," *Whole Health MD.*

882. "Ginger," *Whole Health MD.*

883. "Ginger," *Whole Health MD.*

884. Remington and Woods, *The Dispensatory of the United States of America.*

885. "Ginger," *Whole Health MD.*

886. "Ginger," *Whole Health MD.*

887. "Ginger," *Whole Health MD.*; Antoine Al-Achi, "A Current Look at Ginger Use," *The U.S. Pharmacist* http://www.uspharmacist.com/oldformat.asp?url=newlook/files/Comp/ginger2.htm&pub%20id=8&article%20id=772.

888. Commission E, "Ginger Root," *The Commission E Monographs: IHerb Health Encyclopedia* http://www.herbalgram.org/iherb/commissione/Monographs/Monograph_0181.html.

889. "Ginger," *Whole Health MD.*

890. Commission E, "Ginger Root."

891. Low Dog and Riley, "Management of Hyperlipidemia," 28–41.

892. X. Jiang, et al., "Effect of Ginkgo and Ginger on the Pharmacokinetics and Pharmacodynamics of Warfarin in Healthy Subjects," *British Journal of Clinical Pharmacology* 59, no. 4 (April 2005): 425–32; D. J. Brown, "Ginkgo and Ginger do not Affect the Pharmacokinetics and Pharmacodynamics of Warfarin or Coagulation in Healthy Adults," *HerbalGram* 68 (Fall 2005): 30–31.

893. W. Abebe, "Herbal Medication: Potential for Adverse Interactions with Analgesic Drugs," *Journal of Clinical Pharmacy and Therapeutics* 27, no. 6 (December 2002): 391–401; Harkness and Bratman, *Handbook of Drug-Herb and Drug-Supplement Interactions*, 322.

894. M. N. Ghayur and A. H. Gilani, "Ginger Lowers Blood Pressure through Blockade of Voltage-Dependent Calcium Channels," *Journal of Cardiovascular Pharmacology* 45, no. 1 (January 2005): 74–80; M. S. Weidner, and K. Sigwart, "The Safety of a Ginger Extract in the Rat," *Journal of Ethnopharmacology* 73, no. 3 (December 2000): 513–20.

895. K. Sekiya, A. Ohtani, and S. Kusano, "Enhancement of Insulin Sensitivity in Adipocytes by Ginger," *Biofactors* 22, no. 1–4 (2004): 153–6.

896. N. R. Farnsworth, A. S. Bingel, and G. A Cordell, et al., "Potential Value of Plants as Sources of New Antifertility Agents I," *Journal of Pharmaceutical Sciences* 64 (1975): 535–598.

897. J. M. Wilkinson, "Effect of Ginger Tea on the Fetal Development of Sprague-Dawley Rats," *Reproductive Toxicology (Elmsford, N.Y.)* 14, no. 5 (November–December 2000): 507–12.

898. Antoine Al-Achi, "A Current Look at Ginger Use," *The US Pharmacist* http://www.uspharmacist.com/oldformat.asp?url=newlook/files/Comp/ginger2.htm&pub%20id=8&article%20id=772.

899. Al-Achi, "A Current Look at Ginger Use."

900. Maryland Medical Center Programs Center for Integrative Medicine, "Ginger Research,"

901. Johnson, *Pocket Guide to Herbal Remedies*, 190.

902. Pierce, *Practical Guide to Natural Medicines*, 292.

903. Cor Kwant, "Ginkgo Biloba: History," *The Ginkgo Pages*, http://www.xs4all.nl/~kwanten/history.htm.

904. American Botanical Council, "Ginkgo Biloba Leaf Extract," *herbalgram.com* http://www.herbalgram.org/default.asp?c=he040.

905. Pierce, *Practical Guide to Natural Medicines*, 293.

906. A. Walesiuk, E. Trofimiuk, and J. J. Braszko, "Ginkgo Biloba Normalizes Stress and Corticosterone–Induced Impairment of Recall in Rats," *Pharmacological Research* 53, no. 2 (February 2006): 123–8; A. Walesiuk, et al., Gingko Biloba Extract Diminishes Stress–Induced Memory Deficits In Rats," *Pharmacological Reports* 57, no. 2 (March–April 2005): 176–87; M. Zhang and J. Cai, "Extract of Ginkgo Biloba Leaves Reverses Yohimbine-Induced Spatial Working Memory Deficit in Rats," *Behavioural Pharmacology* 16, no. 8 (December 2005): 651–6.

907. J. Reichling, et al., "Reduction of Behavioral Disturbances in Elderly Dogs Supplemented with a Standardised Ginkgo Leaf Extract," *Schweizer Archiv für Tierheilkunde* 148, no. 5 (May 2006): 257–63.

908. G. Vorberg,. "Ginkgo Biloba Extract (GBE): a Long-Term Study of Chronic Cerebral Insufficiency in Geriatric Patients," *Clinical Trials Journal* 22 (1985):149–57.

909. K. A. Wesnes, et al., "The Memory Enhancing Effects of a Ginkgo Biloba/Panax Ginseng Combination in Healthy Middle–Aged Volunteers," *Psychopharmacology* 152, no. 4 (November 2000): 353–61.

910. C. Stough, J. Clarke, J. Lloyd, and P. J. Nathan, "Neuropsychological Changes After 30-Day Ginkgo Biloba Administration In Healthy Participants," *The International Journal of Neuropsychopharmacology* 4, no. 2 (June 2001): 131–4.

911. S. Mills and K. Bone, "Principles and practice of phytotherapy," *Modern Herbal Medicine* (Churchill Livingstone, 2000).

912. M. vanDongen, et al. "Ginkgo for Elderly People with Dementia and Age-Associated Memory Impairment: A Randomized Clinical Trial," *Journal of Clinical Epidemiology* 56, no. 4 (April 2003): 367–76; Paul R. Solomon, et al., "Ginkgo for Memory Enhancement: A Randomized Controlled Trial," *Journal of the American Medical Association* 288, no. 7 (August 21, 2002): 835–40; N. R. Burns, J. Bryan, and T. Nettelbeck, "Ginkgo Biloba: No Robust Effect on Cognitive Abilities or Mood in Healthy Young or Older Adults," *Human Psychopharmacology* 21, no. 1 (January 2006): 27–37.

913. R. Ihl, "The Impact of Drugs against Dementia on Cognition in Aging and Mild Cognitive Impairment," *Pharmacopsychiatry* 36, Supplement 1 (June 2003): S38–43.

914. S. Elsabagh, et al., Limited Cognitive Benefits in Stage +2 Postmenopausal Women after 6 Weeks of Treatment with Ginkgo Biloba," *Journal of Psychopharmacology* 19, no. 2 (March 2005): 173–81.

915. S. Nishida and H. Satoh, "Age-Related Changes in the Vasodilating Actions of Ginkgo Biloba Extract and its Main Constituent, Bilobalide, in Rat Aorta," *Clinica Chimica Acta* 354, no. 1–2 (April 2005): 141–6.

916. Z. Subhan and I. Hindmarsh, "The Psychopharmacological effects of Ginkgo Biloba extract in Normal Healthy Volunteers," *International Journal of Clinical and Phamacologic Research* 4 (1984): 89–93.

917. J. Persson, et al., "The Memory–Enhancing Effects of Ginseng and Ginkgo Biloba in Healthy Volunteers," *Psychopharmacology* 172, no. 4 (April 2004): 430–4; P. L. Moulton, et al., "The Effect of Ginkgo Biloba on Memory in Healthy Male Volunteers," Physiology & Behavior 73, no. 4 (July 2001): 659–65.

918. S. Elsabagh, et al., "Differential Cognitive Effects of Ginkgo Biloba after Acute and Chronic Treatment in Healthy Young Volunteers," *Psychopharmacology*. 179, no. 2 (May 2005): 437–46.

919. M. Shen, et al., ["Effects of an Extract of Ginkgo Biloba on the Blood Flow of Brains and Back Legs of Dogs,"] *Zhong Yao Cai* 23, no. 12 (December 2000): 764–6.

920. American Botanical Council, "Ginkgo Biloba Leaf Extract," *Herbal Information: Expanded Commission E Online* http://www.herbalgram.org/default.asp?c=he040.

921. D. Rai, et al., "Anti–Stress Effects of Ginkgo Biloba and *Panax ginseng*: A Comparative Study," *Journal of Pharmacological Sciences* 93, no. 4 (December 2003): 458–64.

922. P. Braquet, "The Gingkolides: Potent Platelet–Activating Factor Antagonists Isolated from Gingko Biloba Extract," *Drugs of the Future* 12 (1987): 643–99.

923. G. Sener, G. Z. Omurtag, O. Sehirli, A. Tozan, M. Yuksel, F. Ercan, and N. Gedik, "Protective Effects of Ginkgo Biloba against Acetaminophen–Induced Toxicity in Mice," *Molecular and Cellular Biochemistry* 283, no. 1–2 (February 2006): 39–45.

924. K. P. Loh, et al., "A Comparison Study of Cerebral Protection Using Ginkgo Biloba Extract and Losartan on Stroked Rats," *Neuroscience Letters* 398, no. 1–2 (May 1, 2006): 28–33; Hu, B, et al. "Protective Effects of Ginkgo Biloba Extract on Rats During Cerebral Ischemia/Reperfusion," *Chinese Medical Journal* 115, no. 9 (September 2002): 1316–20.

925. G. Sener, et al. "Ginkgo Biloba Extract Protects against Ionizing Radiation–Induced Oxidative Organ Damage in Rats," *International Journal of Clinical Pharmacology Research* 53, no. 3 (March 2006): 241–52.

926. Q. H. Gong, et al., "Protective Effects Of Ginkgo Biloba Leaf Extract On Aluminum–Induced Brain Dysfunction In Rats," *Life Sciences* 77, no. 2 (May 27, 2005): 140–8.

927. Y. Yamamoto, ["Effect of Ginkgo Biloba Extract on Memory Deficits in Radial Maze Performance Induced by Some Drugs in Rats,"] *Japanese Journal of Psychopharmacology* 25, no. 2 (April 2005): 85–90.

928. S. Z. Huang, "Effect of Ginkgo Biloba Extract on Livers in Aged Rats," *World Journal of Gastroenterology* 11, no. 1 (January 7, 2005): 132–5.

929. K. Lamm and W. Arnold, "The Effect of Blood Flow Promoting Drugs on Cochlear Blood Flow, Perilymphatic Po(2) and Auditory Function in the Normal and Noise–Damaged Hypoxic and Ischemic Guinea Pig Inner Ear," *Hearing Research* 141, no. 1–2 (March 2000): 199–219.

930. N. Holstein, ["Ginkgo Special Extract EGb 761 in Tinnitus Therapy: An Overview of Results of Completed Clinical Trials,"] *Fortschritte der Medizin* 118, no. 4 (January 11, 2001): 157–64 (Review in German); Morgenstern, C : Biermann, E. "The Efficacy of Ginkgo Special Extract EGb 761 in Patients with Tinnitus," *International Journal of Clinical Pharmacology and Therapeutics* 40, no. 5 (May 2002): 188–97.

931. D. Rejali, et al., "Ginkgo Biloba does not Benefit Patients with Tinnitus: A Randomized Placebo–Controlled Double–Blind Trial and Meta–Analysis of Randomized Trials," *Clinical Otolaryngology* 29, no. 3 (June 2004): 226–31.

932. P. F. Smith, et al., "Ginkgo Biloba Extracts for Tinnitus: More Hype than Hope?" *Journal of Ethnopharmacology* 100, no. 1–2 (August 22, 2005): 95–9.

933. Pierce, *Practical Guide to Natural Medicines*, 293.

934. Pierce, *Practical Guide to Natural Medicines*, 295.

935. Pierce, *Practical Guide to Natural Medicines*, 292.

936. D. Mantle, et al., "Comparison of Antioxidant Activity in Commercial Ginkgo Biloba Preparations," *Journal of Alternative and Complementary Medicine* 9, no. 5 (October 2003): 625–9.

937. Commission E, "Ginkgo Biloba Leaf Extract," *The Commission E Monographs: Iherb Health Encyclopedia* http://www.herbalgram.org/iherb/commissione/Monographs/Monograph_0183.html.

938. Pierce, *Practical Guide to Natural Medicines*, 295.

939. P. L. Le Bars and J. Kastelan, "Efficacy and Safety of a Ginkgo Biloba Extract," *Public Health Nutrition* 3, no. 4A (December 2000): 495–9.

940. C. Cianfrocca, et al., "Ginkgo Biloba–Induced Frequent Ventricular Arrhythmia," *Italian Heart Journal* 3, no. 11 (November 2002): 689–91.

941. Y. Kubota, et al., "Effects of Ginkgo Biloba Extract Feeding on Salt–Induced Hypertensive Dahl Rats," *Biological and Pharmaceutical Bulletin* 29, no. 2 (February 2006): 266–9.

942. Y. Kubota, et al, "Effects of Ginkgo Biloba Extract on Blood Pressure and Vascular Endothelial Response by Acetylcholine in Spontaneously Hypertensive Rats," *The Journal of Pharmacy and Pharmacology* 58, no. 2 (February 2006): 243–9.

943. Z. Hu, et al., "Herb–Drug Interactions: A Literature Review," *Drugs* 65, no. 9 (2005): 1239–82.

944. Pierce, *Practical Guide to Natural Medicines*, 295.

945. O. Q. Yin, et al. "Pharmacogenetics and Herb–Drug Interactions: Experience with Ginkgo Biloba and Omeprazole," *Pharmacogenetics* 14, no. 12 (December 2004): 841–50.

946. S. Bent, H. Goldberg, A. Padula, and A. L. Avins, "Spontaneous Bleeding Associated with Ginkgo Biloba: A Case Report and Systematic Review of the Literature," *Journal of General Internal Medicine* 20, no. 7 (July 2005): 657–61.

947. S. Kohler, et al., "Influence of a 7–Day Treatment with Ginkgo Biloba Special Extract EGb 761 on Bleeding Time and Coagulation: A Randomized, Placebo–Controlled, Double–Blind Study in Healthy Volunteers," *Blood Coagulation & Fibrinolysis* 15, no. 4 (June 2004): 303–9.

948. Harkness and Bratman, *Handbook of Drug-Herb and Drug-Supplement Interactions*, 324.

949. F. W. Fraunfelder, "Ocular Side Effects from Herbal Medicines and Nutritional Supplements," *American Journal of Ophthalmology* 138, no. 4 (October 2004): 639–47.

950. H. S. Chung, et al., "Ginkgo Biloba Extract Increases Ocular Blood Flow Velocity," *Journal of Ocular Pharmacology and Therapeutics* 15, no. 3 (June 1999): 233–40.

951. C. A. Haller, K. H. Meier, and K. R. Olson, "Seizures Reported in Association with Use of Dietary Supplements," *Clinical Toxicology (Philadelphia, Pa.)* 43, no. 1 (2005): 23–30.

952. Haller, et al. "Seizures Reported In Association With Use Of Dietary Supplements," 23–30.

953. Yo Kajiyama, et al., "Ginkgo Seed Poisoning," *Pediatrics* 109, no. 2 (February 2002): 325–7.

954. "Ginseng," *Medlineplus Herb And Supplement.*

955. A. Sparreboom, et al., "Herbal Remedies in the United States: Potential Adverse Interactions with Anticancer Agents," *Journal of Clinical Oncology* 22, no. 2 (June 15, 2004): 2489–503.

956. Pierce, *Practical Guide to Natural Medicines*, 298.

957. Pierce, *Practical Guide to Natural Medicines*, 298.

958. D. Q. Dou, et al., "Studies on the Characteristic Constituents of Chinese Ginseng and American Ginseng," *Planta Medica* 64, no. 6 (1998): 585–586.

959. Pierce, *Practical Guide to Natural Medicines*, 298.

960. West TCM, "Ren Shen," *Traditional Chinese Medicine and Acupuncture Health Information Organization* http://tcm.health–info.org/Herbology.Materia.Medica/renshen–properties.htm; Hamel and Chiltoskey, *Cherokee Plants and Their Uses*, 36; Tantaquidgeon, *Folk Medicine of the*

Delaware and Related Algonkian Indians, 74, 130, 32; William Sturtevant, *The Mikasuki Seminole: Medical Beliefs and Practices* (Yale University, PhD Thesis, 1954): 318.

961. Herrick, *Iroquois Medical Botany*, 396.

962. Huron H Smith, "Ethnobotany of the Menomini Indians," *Bulletin of the Public Museum of the City of Milwaukee* 4 (1923): 24.

963. S. E. Bentler, et al., "Prospective Observational Study of Treatments for Unexplained Chronic Fatigue," *Journal of Clinical Psychiatry* 66, no. 5 (May 2005): 625–32.

964. D. O. Kennedy, et al., "Electroencephalograph Effects of Single Doses of *Ginkgo biloba* and *Panax ginseng* in Healthy Young Volunteers," *Pharmacology, Biochemistry, and Behavior* 75, no. 3 (June 2003): 701–9.

965. J. L. Reay, et al., "Effects of *Panax ginseng*, Consumed with and without Glucose, on Blood Glucose Levels and Cognitive Performance During Sustained 'Mentally Demanding' Tasks, *Journal of Psychopharmacology* 20, no. 6 (November 2006): 771–81.

966. D. O. Kennedy, et al., "Modulation of Cognition and Mood Following Administration of Single Doses of Ginkgo Biloba, Ginseng, and a Ginkgo/Ginseng Combination to Healthy Young Adults," *Physiology and Behavior*. 75, no. 5 (April 15, 2002): 739–51.

967. D. O. Kennedy, et al., "Dose Dependent Changes in Cognitive Performance and Mood Following Acute Administration of Ginseng to Healthy Young Volunteers," *Nutritional Neuroscience* 4, no. 4 (2001): 295–310.

968. K. A. Wesnes, et al., "The Memory Enhancing Effects of a Ginkgo Biloba/Panax Ginseng Combination in Healthy Middle–Aged Volunteers," *Psychopharmacology (Berlin)* 152, no. 4 (November 2000): 353–61.

969. B. J. Cardinal and H. J. Engels, "Ginseng does not Enhance Psychological Well–Being in Healthy, Young Adults: Results of a Double–Blind, Placebo–Controlled, Randomized Clinical Trial," *Journal of the American Dietetic Association* 1010, no. 6 (June 2001): 655–60.

970. S. H. Kim, et al., "Effects of Panax Ginseng Extract on Exercise–Induced Oxidative Stress," *The Journal of Sports Medicine and Physical Fitness* 45, no. 2 (June 2005): 178–82.

971. M. T. Liang, et al., "*Panax notoginseng* Supplementation Enhances Physical Performance During Endurance Exercise," *Journal of Strength and Conditioning Research* 19, no. 1 (February 2005): 108–14.

972. G. Pieralisi, P. Ripari, L. Vecchiet, "Effects of a Standardized Ginseng Extract Combined with Dimethylaminoethanol Bitartrate, Vitamins, Minerals and Trace Elements on Physical Performance During Exercise," *Clinical Therapeutics* 13 (1991): 373–82.

973. A. W. Ziemba, et al., "Ginseng Treatment Improves Psychomotor Performance at Rest and During Graded Exercise in Young Athletes," *International Journal of Sport Nutrition* 9, no. 4 (December 1999): 371–7.

974. J. D. Allen, et al., "Ginseng Supplementation does not Enhance Healthy Young Adults' Peak Aerobic Exercise Performance," *Journal of the American College of Nutrition* 17, no. 5 (October 1998): 462–6; H. J. Engels and J. C. Wirth, "No Ergogenic Effects Of Ginseng (*Panax ginseng C.A. Meyer*) During Graded Maximal Aerobic Exercise," *Journal of the American Dietetic Association* 97, no. 10 (October 1997): 1110–5; A. C. Morris, et al., "No Ergogenic Effect of Ginseng Ingestion," *International Journal of Sport Nutrition* 6, no. 3 (September 1996): 263–71; C. C. Hsu, et al., "American Ginseng Supplementation Attenuates Creatine Kinase Level Induced by Submaximal Exercise in Human Beings," *World Journal of Gastroenterology* 11, no. 34 (September 14, 2005): 5327–31;

H. J. Engels, et al., "Effects of Ginseng on Secretory IgA, Performance, and Recovery from Interval Exercise," *Medicine and Science in Sports and Exercise* 35, no. 4 (April 2003): 690–6; H. J. Engels, et al., "Effects of Ginseng Supplementation on Supramaximal Exercise Performance and Short–Term Recovery," *Journal of Strength and Conditioning Research* 15, no. 3 (August 2001): 290–5.

975. Pierce, *Practical Guide to Natural Medicines*, 298.

976. Z. Song, et al. "Gerimax Ginseng Regulates Both Humoral and Cellular Immunity During Chronic *Pseudomonas aeruginosa* Lung Infection," *Journal of Alternative and Complementary Medicine* 8, no. 4 (August 2002): 459–66.

977. Pierce, *Practical Guide to Natural Medicines*, 298.

978. Moore, "Dry Plant Percolation Preferences," *Materia Medica.*

979. Johnson, *Pocket Guide to Herbal Remedies*, 108.

980. American Botanical Council, "Ginseng Root," *Herbal Information: Expanded Commission E Online* http://www.herbalgram.org/default.asp?c=he041.

981. Herrick, *Iroquois Medical Botany*, 396.

982. Pierce, *Practical Guide to Natural Medicines*, 298.

983. Bown, *Encyclopedia of Herbs and their Uses.*

984. Pierce, *Practical Guide to Natural Medicines*, 298.

985. Ody, *The Complete Medicinal Herbal*, 84; Harkness and Bratman, *Handbook of Drug-Herb and Drug-Supplement Interactions*, 93.

986. Harkness and Bratman, *Handbook of Drug-Herb and Drug-Supplement Interactions*, 134–5; J. L. Reay, et al., "The Glycaemic effects of Single Doses of *Panax ginseng* in Young Healthy Volunteers," *British Journal of Nutrition* 96, no. 4 (October 2006): 639–42.

987. Harkness and Bratman, *Handbook of Drug-Herb and Drug-Supplement Interactions*, 327; Jiang X, et al., "Investigation of The Effects of Herbal Medicines on Warfarin Response in Healthy Subjects: A Population Pharmacokinetic–Pharmacodynamic Modeling Approach," *Journal of Clinical Pharmacology* 46, no. 11 (November 2006): 1370–8.

988. "Ginseng," *Medlineplus Herb And Supplements.*

989. P. M. Stavro, et al., "North American Ginseng Exerts a Neutral Effect on Blood Pressure in Individuals with Hypertension," *Hypertension* 46, no. 2 (August 2005): 406–11.

990. World Health Organization (WHO). "*Ginseng radix.*" *WHO Monographs On Selected Medicinal Plants* Vol. 1. (Geneva: World Health Organization, 1999): 168–182.

991. Johnson, *Pocket Guide to Herbal Remedies*, 108.

992. M. F. Melzig, ["Goldenrod—A Classical Exponent In The Urological Phytotherapy,"] *Wiener Medizinische Wochenschrift* 154, no. 21–22 (November 2004): 523–7 (Article in German).

993. "Goldenrod," *Purdue Guide to Medicinal and Aromatic Plants* http://www.hort.purdue.edu/newcrop/med–aro/factsheets/GOLDENROD.html.

994. Hamel and Chiltoskey, *Cherokee Plants and Their Uses*, 36.

995. J. Leuschner, "Anti–Inflammatory, Spasmolytic and Diuretic Effects of a Commercially Available *Solidago gigantea* Herb Extract," Arzneimittelforschung 45, no. 2 (February 1995): 165–8; S. N. Okpanyi, et al., ["Anti–Inflammatory, Analgesic and Antipyretic Effect of Various Plant Extracts and their Combinations in an Animal Model,"] *Arzneimittelforschung* 39, no. 6 (June 1989): 698–703 (Article in German).

996. Pierce, *Practical Guide to Natural Medicines*, 310.

997. Top Cultures, "Rutin," *Phytochemicals* http://www.phytochemicals.info/phytochemicals/rutin.php.

998. A. F. Morel, et al., "Antimicrobial Activity of Extractives of *Solidago microglossa*," *Fitoterapia* 77, no. 6 (September 2006): 453–5.

999. G. Bader, et al., ["The Antifungal Action of Polygalacic Acid Glycosides,"] *Pharmazie* 45, no. 8 (July 1990): 618–20 (Article in German).

1000. Hamel and Chiltoskey, *Cherokee Plants and Their Uses*, 36.

1001. S. Z. Choi, et al., "Immunobiological Activity of a New Benzyl Benzoate from the Aerial Parts of *Solidago virga–aurea var. gigantean*," *Archives of Pharmacal Research* 28, no. 1 (January 2005): 49–54.

1002. J. Leuschner, "Anti–Inflammatory, Spasmolytic and Diuretic Effects of a Commercially Available *Solidago gigantea* Herb Extract," *Arzneimittelforschung* 45, no. 2 (February 1995): 165–8.

1003. M. el–Ghazaly, et al., "Study of the Anti–Inflammatory Activity Of *Populus tremula, Solidago virgaurea* and *Fraxinus excelsior, Arzneimittelforschung* 42, no. 3 (March 1992): 333–6.

1004. Hoffmann, "Golden Rod," *Herbal Materia Medica.*

1005. Hoffmann, "Golden Rod," *Herbal Materia Medica.*

1006. Johnson, *Pocket Guide to Herbal Remedies*, 153.

1007. Johnson, *Pocket Guide to Herbal Remedies*, 153. Pierce, *Practical Guide to Natural Medicines*, 313.

1008. Johnson, *Pocket Guide to Herbal Remedies*, 153.

1009. Johnson, *Pocket Guide to Herbal Remedies*, 153.

1010. Martin Schàtzle, Monika Agathos, and Reinhard Breit, "Allergic Contact Dermatitis from Goldenrod (*Herba solidaginis*) after Systemic Administration," *Contact Dermatitis* 39, no. 5 (1998): 271–272.

1011. Remington and Woods, *The Dispensatory of the United States of America.*

1012. American Botanical Council, "Market Conditions and Regulatory Climate For Herbs in the United States," *The Complete German Commission E Monographs: Therapeutic Guide to Herbal Medicines,* 1999 http://www.herbalgram.org/default.asp?c=cemarketconditions.

1013. Hamel and Chiltoskey, *Cherokee Plants and Their Uses*, 36.

1014. R. Chandler, Lois Freeman Frank, and Shirley N. Hooper, "Herbal Remedies of the Maritime Indians," *Journal of Ethnopharmacology* 1 (1979): 57.

1015. Grieve, "Golden Seal," *Botanical.com: A Modern Herbal.*

1016. Steven Foster. "Goldenseal: *Hydrastis canadensis, American Botanical Council's Botanical Booklet Series* http://www.herbalgram.org/default.asp?c=goldenseal.

1017. Pierce, *Practical Guide to Natural Medicines*, 310–15.

1018. Herrick, *Iroquois Medical Botany*, 324.

1019. Remington and Woods, *The Dispensatory of the United States of America.*

1020. J. Rehman, et al., "Increased Production of Antigen–Specific Immunoglobulins G and M Following In Vivo Treatment with the Medicinal Plants *Echinacea angustifolia* and *Hydrastis canadensis*," *Immunology Letters*. 68, no. 2–3 (June 1, 1999): 391–5.

1021. Cech, *Making Plant Medicine*, 151

1022. Pierce, *Practical Guide to Natural Medicines*, 310–15.

1023. J. E. Simon, A. F. Chadwick and L. E. Craker, "Herbs: An Indexed Bibliography, 1971–1980," *The Scientific Literature on Selected Herbs, and Aromatic and Medicinal Plants of the Temperate Zone* (Hamden, CT: Archon Books, 1984).

1024. Pierce, *Practical Guide to Natural Medicines*, 310–15.

1025. Simon, Chadwick and Craker, *Herbs: An Indexed Bibliography.*

1026. C. A. Newall, et al., *Herbal Medicines: a Guide for Health Care Professionals* (London: The Pharmaceutical Press, 1996).

1027. Cech, *Making Plant Medicine*, 151.

1028. Johnson, *Pocket Guide to Herbal Remedies*, 76.

1029. Pierce, *Practical Guide to Natural Medicines*, 310–15.

1030. Pierce, *Practical Guide to Natural Medicines*, 316–319.

1031. D. MacKay, A. L. Miller, "Nutritional Support for Wound Healing," *Alternative Medicine Review* 8, no. 4 (November 2003): 359–77.

1032. D. Herbert, et al., "In vitro Experiments with *Centella asiatica*: Investigation to Elucidate the Effect of an Indigenously Prepared Powder of This Plant on the Acid–Fastness and Viability of *M. tuberculosis*," *Indian Journal of Leprosy* 66, no. 1 (January–March 1994): 65–8.

1033. F. X. Maquart, et al., "Triterpenes from *Centella asiatica* Stimulate Extracellular Matrix Accumulation in Rat Experimental Wounds," *European Journal of Dermatology* 9, no. 4 (June 1999): 289–96.

1034. A. Shukla, et al., "Asiaticoside–Induced Elevation of Antioxidant Levels in Healing Wounds," *Phytotherapy Research* 13, no. 1 (February 1999): 50–4.

1035. A. Shukla, et al., "In Vitro and In Vivo Wound Healing Activity of Asiaticoside Isolated from *Centella asiatica*," *Journal of Ethnophamacology* 65, no. 1 (April 1999): 1–11.

1036. P. Boiteau and A.R. Ratsimamanga, ["Asiaticoside Extracted from *Centella asiatica* and its Therapeutic Uses in Cicatrization of Experimental and Refractory Wounds (Leprosy, Cutaneous Tuberculosis and Lupus),"] *Therapie* 11 (1956): 125–49 (article in French).

1037. G. L. Young and D. Jewell, "Creams for Preventing Stretch Marks in Pregnancy," *Cochrane Database of Systematic Reviews* 2 (2000): CD000066.

1038. Pierce, *Practical Guide to Natural Medicines*, 316–319.

1039. M. R. Cesarone, et al., "Flight Microangiopathy in Medium–to Long–Distance Flights: Prevention of Edema and Microcirculation Alterations with Total Triterpenic Fraction of *Centella asiatica*," *Angiology* 52 (October 2001): Suppl 2:S33–7.

1040. M. R. Cesarone, et al., ["Activity of *Centella asiatica* in Venous Insufficiency,"] *Minerva Cardioangiologica* 40, no. 4 (April 1992): 137–43 (article in Italian); Belcaro GV, et al. "Capillary Filtration and Ankle Edema in Patients with Venous Hypertension Treated with TTFCA," *Angiology* 41, no. 1 (January 1990): 12–8.

1041. Bown, *Encyclopaedia of Herbs and their Uses.*

1042. R. N. Chopra, S. L. Nayar, and I. C. Chopra, *Glossary of Indian Medicinal Plants (Including the Supplement)*, (New Delhi: Council of Scientific and Industrial Research, 1986).

1043. J. Bradwejn, et al., "A Double–Blind, Placebo–Controlled Study on the Effects of Gotu Kola (*Centella asiatica*) on Acoustic Startle Response in Healthy Subjects," *Journal of Clinical Psychopharmacology* 20, no. 6 (December 2000): 680–4.

1044. Pierce, *Practical Guide to Natural Medicines*, 316–319.

1045. Johnson, *Pocket Guide to Herbal Remedies*, 35.

1046. B. M. Hausen, "*Centella asiatica* (Indian Pennywort), an Effective Therapeutic but a Weak Sensitizer," *Contact Dermatitis* 29, no. 4 (October 1993): 175–9.

1047. H. C. Eun and A. Y. Lee, "*Contact Dermatitis* due to Madecassol," *Contact Dermatitis* 13 no. 5 (1985): 310; Gonzalo Garijo MA, et al., "Allergic Contact Dermatitis due to *Centella asiatica*: a New Case," *Allergologia et immunopathologia* 24, no. 3 (May–June 1996): 132–4.

1048. O. D. Laerum and O. H. Iverson, "Reticuloses and Epidermal Tumors in Hairless Mice after Topical Skin Applications of Cantharidin and Asiaticoside," *Cancer Research* 32 (1972): 1463–69.

1049. Bown, *Encyclopaedia of Herbs and their Uses.*

1050. Johnson, *Pocket Guide to Herbal Remedies*, 35.

1051. Johnson, *Pocket Guide to Herbal Remedies*, 35.

1052. A. S. Ramaswamy, et al., "Pharmacological Studies on *Centella asiatica* D (Brahma Manduki) Umbelliferae," *Journal of Research in Indian Medicine* 4 (1970): 160–75.

1053. American Botanical Council, "Herbal Information: Herb Reference Guide," http://www.herbalgram.org/default.asp?c=reference_guide.

1054. Pierce, *Practical Guide to Natural Medicines*, 338–340.

1055. Hamel and Chiltoskey, *Cherokee Plants and Their Uses*, 39; Smith, "Ethnobotany of the Meskwaki Indians," 250.

1056. Grieve, "Hops," *Botanical.com: A Modern Herbal.*

1057. Blumenthal, *The Complete German Commission E Manuscripts.*

1058. V. E. Tyler, "Herbs Affecting the Central Nervous System," p. 442–449. In: J. Janick (ed.), *Perspectives on New Crops and New Uses* (Alexandria, VA: ASHS Press, 1999).

1059. J. Holzl, "Inhaltsstoffe Des Hopfens," *Zeitschrist für Phytotherapie* 13 (1992): 155–61 (article in German).

1060. R. Hansel and H. H. Wagener, "Attempts to Identify Sedative-Hypnotic Active Substance in Hops," *Arzneimittel–Forschung* 17 (1967): 79.

1061. R. Schellenberg, S. Sauer, E. A. Abourashed, U. Koetter, and A. Brattström, "The Fixed Combination of Valerian and Hops (Ze91019) Acts Via a Central Adenosine Mechanism," *Planta Medica* 70, no. 7 (July 2004): 594–597.

1062. A. Fussel, et al., "Effect of a Fixed Valerian–Hop Extract Combination (Ze 91019) on Sleep Polygraphy in Patients with Non–Organic Insomnia: A Pilot Study," *European Journal of Medical Research* 5, no. 9 (September 18, 2000): 385–90.

1063. Tantaquidgeon, *Folk Medicine of the Delaware and Related Algonkian Indians*, 31.

1064. Lloyd G. Carr and Carlos Westey, "Surviving Folktales and Herbal Lore Among the Shinnecock Indians," *Journal of American Folklore* 58 (1945): 120.

1065. Blumenthal, *The Complete German Commission E Manuscripts.*

1066. Chestnut, "Plants Used by the Indians of Mendocino County, California," 344; Melvin R. Gilmore, "Uses of Plants by the Indians of the Missouri River Region," SI–*BAE Annual Report #33* (1919): 77; Alice C. Fletcher and Francis La Flesche "The Omaha Tribe," *SI–BAE Annual Report #27* (1911): 584.

1067. Grieve, "Hops," *Botanical.com: A Modern Herbal.*

1068. T. D. Morgan, A. E. Beezer, J. C. Mitchell, and A. W. Bunch, "A Microcalorimetric Comparison of the Anti–*Streptococcus mutans* Efficacy of Plant Extracts and Antimicrobial Agents in Oral Hygiene Formulations," *Journal of Applied Microbiology* 90, no. 1 (2001): 53–58.

1069. Michael Moore. "Herbs Best as Standard Infusion."

1070. Commission E, "Hops," "*The Commission E Monographs: IHerb Health Encyclopedia,*" http://www.herbalgram.org/iherb/commissione/Monographs/Monograph_0201.html.

1071. Johnson, *Pocket Guide to Herbal Remedies*, 35.

1072. National Library of Medicine and the National Institutes of Health, "Hops (*Humulus lupulus L.*)," *MedlinePlus Health Information*, http://www.nlm.nih.gov/medlineplus/druginfo/natural/patient-hops.html.

1073. Pierce, *Practical Guide to Natural Medicines*, 338–340.

1074. National Library of Medicine and the National Institutes of Health, "Hops (*Humulus lupulus L.*)."

1075. National Library of Medicine and the National Institutes of Health, "Hops (*Humulus lupulus L.*)."

1076. Pierce, *Practical Guide to Natural Medicines*, 338–340.

1077. Johnson, *Pocket Guide to Herbal Remedies*, 35.

1078. Pierce, *Practical Guide to Natural Medicines*, 338–340.

1079. Ginseng, *Medlineplus Herb And Supplement*.

1080. National Library of Medicine and the National Institutes of Health, "Hops (*Humulus lupulus L.*)."

1081. National Library of Medicine and the National Institutes of Health, "Hops (*Humulus lupulus L.*)."

1082. National Library of Medicine and the National Institutes of Health, "Hops (*Humulus lupulus L.*)."

1083. Zigmond, *Kawaiisu Ethnobotany*, 10; Bocek, *Ethnobotany of Costanoan Indians*, 23.

1084. C. R. Sirtori, "Aescin: Pharmacology, Pharmacokinetics and Therapeutic Profile," *Pharmacological Research* 44 (2001): 183–193.

1085. A. Neiss, C. Bohm, "Demonstration of the Effectiveness of the Horse-Chestnut-Seed Extract in the Varicose Syndrome Complex," *MMW: Münchener Medizinische Wochenschrift* 118 (1976): 213–216 (translated from German).

1086. H. W. Kreysel, H. P. Nissen HP, and E. Enghoffer, "A Possible Role of Lysosomal Enzymes in the Pathogenesis of Varicosis and the Reduction in their Serum Activity by Venostatin," *VASA. Zeitschrift für Gefässkrankheiten (Journal for Vascular Diseases)* 12 (1983): 377–382.

1087. EBSCO, "Horse Chestnut," *Health Library*, http://healthlibrary.epnet.com/GetContent.aspx?token=dce59228-1023-4705-b1c7-b407be7b4fc6&chunkiid=21758#ref2.

1088. Hamel and Chiltoskey, *Cherokee Plants and Their Uses*, 27.

1089. I. Sato, et al., "Anti-Inflammatory Effect Of Japanese Horse Chestnut (*Aesculus turbinata*) Seeds," *The Journal of Veterinary Medical Science* 68, no. 5 (May 2006): 487–9.

1090. C. R. Sirtori, "Aescin: Pharmacology, Pharmacokinetics and Therapeutic Profile, *Pharmacological Research* 44, no. 3 (September 2001): 183–93.

1091. C. Calabrese and P. Preston, "Report of the Results of a Double-Blind, Randomized, Single-Dose Trial of a Topical 2% Escin Gel versus Placebo in the Acute Treatment of Experimentally-Induced Hematoma in Volunteers," *Planta Medica* 59 (1993): 394–397.

1092. Salisbury University, "Horse Chestnut," *Nurse's Guide To Herbal Remedies* http://www.salisbury.edu/nursing/herbalremedies/horse_chestnut.htm.

1093. C. Diehm, "The Role of Oedema Protective Drugs in the Treatment of Chronic Venous Insufficiency: A Review of Evidence Based on Placebo–Controlled Clinical Trials with Regard to Efficacy and Tolerance," *Phlebology* 11 (1996): 23–29.

1094. G. Hitzenberger, "The Therapeutic Effectiveness of Chestnut Extract," *Wiener Medizinische Wochenschrift* 139 (1989): 385–389 (translated from German).

1095. H. Pabst, et al., "Efficacy and Tolerability of Escin/Diethylamine Salicylate Combination Gels in Patients with Blunt Injuries of the Extremities," *International Journal of Sports Medicine* 22, no. 6 (August 2001): 430–6.

1096. Pierce, *Practical Guide to Natural Medicines*, 343–345.

1097. "Horse Chestnut," *Health Notes*, http://www.deliciouslivingmag.com/healthnotes/healthnotes.cfm?org=nh&lang=EN%2CEN&ContentID=2110008.

1098. EBSCO, "Horse Chestnut."

1099. Nova Scotia Museum of Natural History, "Horse–Chestnut," *The Poison Plant Patch* http://museum.gov.ns.ca/poison/chestnut.htm.

1100. Cooperative Extension Service, Purdue University, "Ohio Buckeye Horse Chestnut," *Indiana Toxic Plant Indices*, http://www.vet.purdue.edu/depts/addl/toxic/plant44.htm.

1101. Johnson, *Pocket Guide to Herbal Remedies*, 3.

1102. K. Takegoshi, T. Tohyama, and K. Okuda, et al., "A Case of Venoplant–Induced Hepatic Injury," *Gastroenterologia Japonica* 21 (1986): 62–65.

1103. Johnson, *Pocket Guide to Herbal Remedies*, 3; Salisbury University "Horse Chestnut."

1104. Johnson, *Pocket Guide to Herbal Remedies*, 3.

1105. Salisbury University "Horse Chestnut."

1106. "Echinacea (*E. angustifolia* DC, *E. pallida*, *E. purpurea*), *Medlineplus Herb and Supplement*, http://www.nlm.nih.gov/medlineplus/druginfo/natural/patient–echinacea.html.

1107. Salisbury University "Horse Chestnut."

1108. Johnson, *Pocket Guide to Herbal Remedies*, 3.

1109. Salisbury University "Horse Chestnut."

1110. Pierce, *Practical Guide to Natural Medicines*, 343–345.

1111. Express Scripts, "Horse Chestnut," *Drug Digest Herbs and Supplements* http://www.drugdigest.org/DD/DVH/HerbsTake/0,3927,4024%7CHorse+Chestnut,00.html.

1112. Pierce, *Practical Guide to Natural Medicines*, 346–7.

1113. Pierce, *Practical Guide to Natural Medicines*, 346–7.

1114. Hamel and Chiltoskey, *Cherokee Plants and Their Uses*, 39

1115. Grieve, "Horseradish," *Botanical.com: A Modern Herbal.*

1116. Pierce, *Practical Guide to Natural Medicines*, 346–7.

1117. Tantaquidgeon, *Folk Medicine of the Delaware and Related Algonkian Indians*, 66, 82.

1118. Hamel and Chiltoskey, *Cherokee Plants and Their Uses*, 39.

1119. Grieve, "Horseradish," *Botanical.com: A Modern Herbal.*

1120. Pierce, *Practical Guide to Natural Medicines*, 346–7; Commission E, "Horse Radish," *The Commission E Monographs: IHerb Health Encyclopedia* http://www.herbalgram.org/iherb/commissione/Monographs/Monograph_0206.html.

1121. Grieve, "Horseradish," *Botanical.com: A Modern Herbal.*

1122. Pierce, *Practical Guide to Natural Medicines*, 346–7.

1123. Pierce, *Practical Guide to Natural Medicines*, 346–7.

1124. Pierce, *Practical Guide to Natural Medicines*, 346–7.
1125. Johnson, *Pocket Guide to Herbal Remedies*, 3.
1126. Pierce, *Practical Guide to Natural Medicines*, 346–7.
1127. Pierce, *Practical Guide to Natural Medicines*, 346–7.
1128. Pierce, *Practical Guide to Natural Medicines*, 346–7.
1129. Commission E, "Horseradish," *The Commission E Monographs: IHerb Health Encyclopedia* http://www.herbalgram.org/iherb/commissione/Monographs/Monograph_0206.html.
1130. Johnson, *Pocket Guide to Herbal Remedies*, 3.
1131. Johnson, *Pocket Guide to Herbal Remedies*, 3.
1132. Johnson, *Pocket Guide to Herbal Remedies*, 3.
1133. Pierce, *Practical Guide to Natural Medicines*, 346–7.
1134. Mu Zei, "Horsetail–Scouring Rush," *Traditional Chinese Medicine and Acupuncture Health Information Organization* http://tcm.health–info.org/Herbology.Materia.Medica/muzei–properties.htm.
1135. National Library of Medicine and the National Institutes of Health, "Horsetail (*Equisetum arvense L.*)," *Medlineplus Health Information* http://www.nlm.nih.gov/medlineplus/druginfo/natural/patient–horsetail.html.
1136. Nancy Chapman Turner, and Marcus A. M. Bell, "The Ethnobotany of the Southern Kwakiutl Indians of British Columbia," *Economic Botany* 27 (1973): 263.
1137. Goodrich and Lawson, *Kashaya Pomo Plants*, 58.
1138. Mu Zei, "Traditional Chinese Medicine–Acupuncture–Herbs–Formulas," http://tcm.health–info.org/Herbology.Materia.Medica/muzei–properties.htm.
1139. Grieve, "Horsetails," *Botanical.com: A Modern Herbal.*
1140. B. E. Myagmar, et al., "Free Radical Scavenging Action of Medicinal Herbs from Mongolia," *Phytomedicine* 7, no. 3 (June 2000): 221–9.
1141. N. Radulovic, et al., "Composition and Antimicrobial Activity of *Equisetum arvense* L. Essential Oil," *Phytotherapy Research* 20, no. 1 (January 2006): 85–8.
1142. F. H. Do Monte, et al., "Antinociceptive and Anti–Inflammatory Properties of the Hydroalcoholic Extract of Stems from *Equisetum arvense* L. in Mice," *Pharmacological Research* 49, no. 3 (March 2004): 239–43.
1143. "Information for Transformation," *Tuberrose.com* http://tuberose.com/Silica.html.
1144. Pierce, *Practical Guide to Natural Medicines*, 348–50.
1145. Pierce, *Practical Guide to Natural Medicines*, 348–50.
1146. National Library of Medicine and the National Institutes of Health "Horsetail (*Equisetum arvense* L.)," *MedlinePlus Health Information.*
1147. American Botanical Council, "Horsetail Herb," Herbalgram.
1148. Commission E, "Horsetail herb," *The Commission E Monographs: IHerb Health Encyclopedia* http://www.herbalgram.org/iherb/commissione/Monographs/Monograph_0207.html.
1149. National Library of Medicine and the National Institutes of Health "Horsetail (*Equisetum arvense* L.)," *MedlinePlus Health Information.*
1150. American Botanical Council, "Horsetail Herb," Herbalgram.
1151. Pierce, *Practical Guide to Natural Medicines*, 348–50.
1152. American Botanical Council, "Horsetail Herb," Herbalgram.

1153. M. A. Weiner, *Earth Medicine, Earth Food* (New York: Ballantine Books, 1980).

1154. American Botanical Council, "Horsetail Herb," Herbalgram.

1155. Pierce, *Practical Guide to Natural Medicines*, 348–50.

1156. Johnson, *Pocket Guide to Herbal Remedies*, 3.

1157. Johnson, *Pocket Guide to Herbal Remedies*, 3.

1158. B. Fabre, B. Geay, and P. Beaufils, "Thiaminase Activity in *Equisetum arvense* and its Extracts, *Plant Med Phytother* 26 (1993): 190–197.

1159. "Redundant Reprint: Herbal Medications," *HerbalGram: The Journal of the American Botanical Council* 28 (1993): 54.

1160. Weiner, *Earth Medicine, Earth Food.*

1161. National Library of Medicine and the National Institutes of Health "Horsetail (*Equisetum arvense* L.)."

1162. Pierce, *Practical Guide to Natural Medicines*, 348–50.

1163. Johnson, *Pocket Guide to Herbal Remedies*, 3.

1164. American Botanical Council, "Horsetail Herb," Herbalgram.

1165. Pierce, *Practical Guide to Natural Medicines*, 390–92.

1166. B. F. Bradley, et al., "Anxiolytic Effects of *Lavandula angustifolia* Odour on the Mongolian Gerbil Elevated Plus Maze," *Journal of Ethnophamacology* 111, no. 3 (December 27, 2006): 517–25.

1167. G. Buchbauer, et al., "Aromatherapy: Evidence for Sedative Effects of the Essential Oil of Lavender after Inhalation," *Zeitschrift für Naturforschung: Journal of Biosciences* 46, no. 11–12 (November–December 1991): 1067–72.

1168. D. L. Wells, "Aromatherapy for Travel–Induced Excitement in Dogs," *Journal of the American Veterinary Medical Association* 229, no. 6 (September 15, 2006): 964–7.

1169. R. Sakamoto, et al., "Effectiveness of Aroma on Work Efficiency: Lavender Aroma During Recesses Prevents Deterioration of Work Performance," *Chemical Senses* 30, no. 8 (October 2005): 683–91.

1170. Sakamoto, "Effectiveness of Aroma on Work Efficiency," 683–91.

1171. N. Motomura, et al., "Reduction of Mental Stress with Lavender Odorant," *Perceptual and Motor Skills* 93, no. 3 (December 2001): 713–8.

1172. M. Moss, et al., "Aromas of Rosemary and Lavender Essential Oils Differentially Affect Cognition and Mood in Healthy Adults," *The International Journal of Neuroscience* 113, no. 1 (January 2003): 15–38.

1173. J. Lehrner, et al., "Ambient Odors of Orange and Lavender Reduce Anxiety and Improve Mood in a Dental Office," *Physiology and Behavior* 86, no. (1–2) (September 15, 2005): 8692–5.

1174. P. W. Lin, et al., "Efficacy of Aromatherapy (*Lavandula angustifolia*) as an Intervention for Agitated Behaviours in Chinese Older Persons with Dementia: A Cross–Over Randomized Trial," *International Journal of Geriatric Psychiatry* 22, no. 5 (Mar 7, 2007): 405-10.

1175. S. Y. Lee, ["The Effect of Lavender Aromatherapy on Cognitive Function, Emotion, and Aggressive Behavior of Elderly with Dementia,"] *Taehan Kanho Hakhoe Chi* 35, no. 2 (April 2005): 303–12 (Article in Korean).

1176. T. Field, et al., "Lavender Fragrance Cleansing Gel Effects on Relaxation," *The International Journal of Neuroscience* 115, no. 2 (February 2005): 207–22.

1177. S. Akhondzadeh, et al., "Comparison of *Lavandula angustifolia* Mill. Tincture and Imipramine in the Treatment of Mild to Moderate Depression: A Double–Blind, Randomized Trial," *Progress in Neuro-Psychopharmacology & Biological Psychiatry* 27, no. 1 (February 2003): 123–7.

1178. C. E. Campenni, et al., "Role of Suggestion in Odor–Induced Mood Change," *Psychological Reports* 94, no. 3, part 2 (June 2004): 1127–36.

1179. G. T. Lewith, et al., "A Single–Blinded, Randomized Pilot Study Evaluating the Aroma of *Lavandula augustifolia* as a Treatment for Mild Insomnia," *Journal of Alternative and Complementary Medicine* 11, no. 4 (August 2005): 631–7.

1180. M. Hardy, et al., "Replacement of Drug Treatment for Insomnia by Ambient Odour," *The Lancet* 346 (September 9, 1995): 701.

1181. I. S. Lee, and G. J. Lee, ["Effects of Lavender Aromatherapy on Insomnia and Depression in Women College Students,"] *Taehan Kanho Hakhoe Chi* 36, no. 1 (February 2006): 136–43 (Article in Korean).

1182. Pierce, *Practical Guide to Natural Medicines*, 390–92.

1183. Grieve, "Lavender," *Botanical.com: A Modern Herbal.*

1184. Pierce, *Practical Guide to Natural Medicines*, 390–92; P. E. Lusby, et al., "A Comparison of Wound Healing Following Treatment with *Lavandula* x *Allardii* Honey or Essential Oil," *Phytotherapy Research* 20, no. 9 (September 2006): 755–7.

1185. F. D. D'Auria, et al., "Antifungal Activity of *Lavandula angustifolia* Essential Oil Against *Candida albicans* Yeast And Mycelial Form," *Medical Mycology* 43, no. 5 (August 2005): 391–6.

1186. K. Takarada, et al., "A Comparison of the Antibacterial Efficacies of Essential Oils Against Oral Pathogens," *Oral Microbiology and Immunology* 19, no. 1 (February 2004): 61–4.

1187. T. Moon, et al., "Antiparasitic Activity of Two Lavandula Essential Oils against *Giardia duodenalis, Trichomonas vaginalis* and *Hexamita inflate*," *Parasitology Research* 99, no. 6 (November 2006): 722–8.

1188. S. Sosa, et al., "Extracts and Constituents of *Lavandula multifida* with Topical Anti–Inflammatory Activity," *Phytomedicine* 12, no. 4 (April 2005): 271–7.

1189. V. Hajhashemi, et al., "Anti–inflammatory and Analgesic Properties of the Leaf Extracts and Essential Oil of *Lavandula angustifolia* Mill," *Journal of Ethnophamacology* 89, no. 1 (November 2003): 67–71.

1190. C. Ghelardini, et al., "Local Anaesthetic Activity of the Essential Oil of *Lavandula angustifolia*," *Planta Medica* 65, no. 8 (December 1999): 700–3.

1191. M. Hur and S. H. Han, "Clinical Trial of Aromatherapy on Postpartum Mother's Perineal Healing," *Taehan Kanho Hakhoe Chi* 34, no. 1 (February 2004): 53–62.

1192. Remington and Woods, *The Dispensatory of the United States of America.*

1193. Pierce, *Practical Guide to Natural Medicines*, 390–92.

1194. Grieve, "Lavenders," *Botanical.com: A Modern Herbal.*

1195. J. J. Gedney, et al., "Sensory and Affective Pain Discrimination after Inhalation of Essential Oils," *Psychosomatic Medicine* 66, no. 4 (July–August 2004): 599–606.

1196. F. Ginsberg, J. P. Famaey, "A Double–Blind Study of Topical Massage with Rado–Salil Ointment in Mechanical Low Back Pain," *The Journal of International Medical Research* 15 (1987): 148–153.

1197. Michael Moore, "Herbs Best as Standard Infusion."

1198. Pierce, *Practical Guide to Natural Medicines*, 390–92.

1199. S. Sosa, et al. "Extracts and Constituents of *Lavandula multifida* with Topical Anti-Inflammatory Activity," *Phytomedicine* 12, no. 4 (April 2005): 271–7.

1200. Pierce, *Practical Guide to Natural Medicines*, 390–92.

1201. National Library of Medicine and the National Institutes of Health "Lavender (*Lavandula angustifolia Miller*)," *MedlinePlus Health Information* http://www.nlm.nih.gov/medlineplus/druginfo/natural/patient-lavender.html.

1202. National Library of Medicine and the National Institutes of Health. "Lavender (*Lavandula angustifolia* Miller)," *MedlinePlus Health Information.*

1203. A. Prashar, et al., "Cytotoxicity of Lavender Oil and its Major Components to Human Skin Cells," *Cell Proliferation* 37, no. 3 (June 2004): 221–9.

1204. Johnson, *Pocket Guide to Herbal Remedies*, 3.

1205. Pierce, *Practical Guide to Natural Medicines*, 390–92.

1206. National Library of Medicine and the National Institutes of Health. "Lavender (*Lavandula angustifolia Miller*)," *MedlinePlus Health Information.*

1207. Jeffrey G. Ghassemi. "Aromatherapy: Evidence for Sedative Effects of the Essential Oil of Lavender after Inhalation," *Washington Post* (July 4, 2006): HE02 http://www.washingtonpost.com/wp-dyn/content/article/2006/07/03/AR2006070300769.html.

1208. Johnson, *Pocket Guide to Herbal Remedies*, 3.

1209. American Herbal Pharmacology Delegation. "Herbal Pharmacology in the People's Republic of China," (Washington D.C.: National Academy of Sciences) http://www.swsbm.com/Ephemera/China_herbs.pdf.

1210. J. A. Duke and E. S. Ayensu, *Medicinal Plants of China* (Algonac, MI: Reference Publications, Inc, 1985).

1211. Gan Cao. "TCM Chinese Herb Pictures," http://tcm.health-info.org/Herbology.Materia.Medica/gancao-properties.htm.

1212. University of Michigan, Dearborn. "Native American Ethnobotony," http://herb.umd.umich.edu/.

1213. "Licorice," *Wikipedia* http://en.wikipedia.org/wiki/Licorice.

1214. "Licorice," *Wikipedia.*

1215. Pierce, *Practical Guide to Natural Medicines*, 399–403.

1216. R. F. Chandler, "Licorice, More than Just a Flavour," *Canadian Pharmaceutical Journal* 118 (1985): 420–24.

1217. Pierce, *Practical Guide to Natural Medicines*, 399–403.

1218. S. Shibata, "A Drug Over the Millennia: Pharmacognosy, Chemistry, and Pharmacology of Licorice," *Yakugaku Zasshi* 120, no. 10 (October 2000): 849–62.

1219. Pierce, *Practical Guide to Natural Medicines*, 399–403.

1220. E. Sugishita, et al., "Studies on the Combination of *Glycyrrhizae Radix* in Shakuyaku-kanzo-To," *Journal of Pharmacobio-Dynamics* 7, no. 7 (July 1984): 427–35.

1221. Moore, "Herbs Best Used as a Strong Decoction," *Materia Medica Factsheet* http://www.swsbm.com/ManualsMM/DecoctPrf.txt.

1222. Cech, *Making Plant Medicine*, 165.

1223. Cech, *Making Plant Medicine*, 166.

1224. Pierce, *Practical Guide to Natural Medicines*, 399–403.

1225. L. Folkersen, et al., ["Licorice. A Basis for Precautions one More Time!"] *Ugeskrift for Laeger* 158, no. 51 (December 1996): 7420–1 (Article in Danish).

1226. A. Chubachi, et al., "Acute Renal Failure Following Hypokalemic Rhabdomyolysis Due to Chronic Glycyrrhizic Acid Administration," *Internal Medicine (Tokyo, Japan)* 31, no. 5 (May 1992): 708–11.

1227. Pierce, *Practical Guide to Natural Medicines*, 399–403.

1228. Johnson, *Pocket Guide to Herbal Remedies*, 3.

1229. B. Fu, et al., "The Application of Macroporous Resins in the Separation of Licorice Flavonoids and Glycyrrhizic Acid," *Journal of Chromatography A* 1089, no. 1–2 (September 30, 2005): 18–24.

1230. S. K. Das, et al., "Deglycyrrhizinated Liquorice in Aphthous Ulcers," *The Journal of the Association of Physicians of India* 37, no. 10 (October 1989): 647.

1231. National Library of Medicine and the National Institutes of Health, "Licorice (*Glycyrrhiza glabra L.*) and DGL (deglycyrrhizinated licorice)," *MedlinePlus Health Information* http://www.nlm.nih.gov/medlineplus/druginfo/natural/patient–licorice.html.

1232. Pierce, *Practical Guide to Natural Medicines*, 399–403.

1233. Commission E "Licorice Root," *The Commission E Monographs: IHerb Health Encyclopedia* http://www.herbalgram.org/iherb/commissione/Monographs/Monograph_0227.html.

1234. Cech, *Making Plant Medicine*, 165.

1235. Johnson, *Pocket Guide to Herbal Remedies*, 3.

1236. Harkness and Bratman, *Handbook of Drug-Herb and Drug-Supplement Interactions*, 82.

1237. Harkness and Bratman, *Handbook of Drug-Herb and Drug-Supplement Interactions*, 219.

1238. Harkness and Bratman, *Handbook of Drug-Herb and Drug-Supplement Interactions*, 235.

1239. Harkness and Bratman, *Handbook of Drug-Herb and Drug-Supplement Interactions*, 190.

1240. A. M. Heck, et al., "Potential Interactions Between Alternative Therapies and Warfarin," *American Journal of Health-System Pharmacy* 57, no. 13 (July 1, 2000): 1221–7.

1241. D. Armanini, et al., "Licorice Consumption and Serum Testosterone in Healthy Man," *Experimental and Clinical Endocrinology & Diabetes* 111, no. 6 (September 2003): 341–3.

1242. T. E. Strandberg, et al., "Birth Outcome in Relation to Licorice Consumption During Pregnancy," *American Journal of Epidemiology* 153, no. 11 (June 1, 2001): 1085–8.

1243. J. Lietava, "Medicinal Plants in a Middle Paleolithic Grave Shanidar IV?" *Journal of Ethnopharmacology* 35 (1992): 263–6.

1244. Pierce, *Practical Guide to Natural Medicines*, 417–420.

1245. Grieve, "Mallows," *Botanical.com: A Modern Herbal.*

1246. Pierce, *Practical Guide to Natural Medicines*, 417–420.

1247. G. Nosal'ova, et al., "Antitussive Action of Extracts and Polysaccharides of Marshmallow (*Althaea officinalis* L., var. Robusta)," *Pharmazie* 47, no. 3 (1992): 224–26.

1248. L. Iauk, et al., "Antibacterial Activity of Medicinal Plant Extracts Against Periodontopathic Bacteria," *Phytotherapy Research* 17, no. 6 (June 2003): 599–604.

1249. Pierce, *Practical Guide to Natural Medicines*, 417–420.

1250. M. C. Recio, et al., "Antimicrobial Activity of Selected Plants Employed in the Spanish Mediterranean Area. II.," *Phytotherapy Research* 3 (1989): 77–80.

1251. A. Kardosova, et al., "Antioxidant Activity of Medicinal Plant Polysaccharides," *Fitoterapia* 77, no. 5 (July 2006): 367–73.

1252. M. Tomoda, R. Gonda, N. Shimizu, and H. Yamada, "Plant Mucilages. XLII. An Anti–Complementary Mucilage from the Leaves of *Malva sylvestris* var. mauritiana," *Chemical and Pharmaceutical Bulletin* 37 (1989): 3029–3032.

1253. D. F. Wang, et al., ["Analgesic and Anti–Inflammatory Effects of the Flower of *Althaea rosea* (L.) Cav."] *Zhongguo Zhong Yao Za Zhi* 14, no. 1 (January 1989): 46–8, 64 (Article in Chinese).

1254. Ody, *The Complete Medicinal Herbal*, 35.

1255. Michael Moore, "Herbs Best as Cold Infusion," *Materia Medica Factsheet*, http://www.swsbm.com/ManualsMM/CldInfus.txt.

1256. Remington and Woods, *The Dispensatory of the United States of America.*

1257. Pierce, *Practical Guide to Natural Medicines*, 417–420.

1258. Henriette Kress, "Absorption," *Henriette's Herbal Blog* http://www.henriettesherbal.com/blog/?cat=6&paged=5.

1259. Pierce, *Practical Guide to Natural Medicines*, 417–420.

1260. National Library of Medicine and the National Institutes of Health, "Marshmallow (*Althaea officinalis* L.), *MedlinePlus Health Information* http://www.nlm.nih.gov/medlineplus/druginfo/natural/patient–marshmallow.html.

1261. Pierce, *Practical Guide to Natural Medicines*, 417–420.

1262. Commission E, "Marshmallow Leaf," *The Commission E Monographs: IHerb Health Encyclopedia* http://www.herbalgram.org/iherb/commissione/Monographs/Monograph_0245.html.

1263. National Library of Medicine, "Marshmallow (*Althaea officinalis* L.)."

1264. Remington and Woods, *The Dispensatory of the United States of America.*

1265. Grieve, "Myrrh," *Botanical.com: A Modern Herbal.*

1266. Grieve, "Myrrh," *Botanical.com: A Modern Herbal.*

1267. Mo Yao. "TCM Herb Pictures," http://tcm.health–info.org/Herbology.Materia.Medica/moyao–properties.htm.

1268. M. Tariq, et al., "Anti–Inflammatory Activity of *Commiphora molmol*," *Agents Actions* 17, no. 3–4 (January 1986): 381–2; A. H. Atta and A. Alkofahi, "Anti–Nociceptive and Anti–Inflammatory Effects of Some Jordanian Medicinal Plant Extracts," *Journal of Ethnophamacology* 60, no. 2 (March 1998): 117–24.

1269. O. A. Olajide, "Investigation of the Effects of Selected Medicinal Plants on Experimental Thrombosis," *Phytotherapy Research* 13, no. 3 (May 1999): 231–2.

1270. Piero Dolara, et al., "Analgesic Effects of Myrrh," *Nature* 379, no. 6560 (January 4, 1996): 1–98.

1271. Commission E, "Myrrh," *The Commission E Monographs: IHerb Health Encyclopedia* http://www.herbalgram.org/iherb/commissione/Monographs/Monograph_0263.html.

1272. D. A. Tipton, et al., "In Vitro Cytotoxic and Anti–Inflammatory Effects of Myrrh Oil on Human Gingival Fibroblasts and Epithelial Cells," *Toxicology in Vitro* 17, no. 3 (June 2003): 301–10; M. M. al–Harbi, et al., "Gastric Antiulcer and Cytoprotective Effect of *Commiphora molmol* in rats," *Journal of Ethnophamacology* 55, no. 2 (January 1997): 141–50.

1273. Pierce, *Practical Guide to Natural Medicines*, 449–451.

1274. Johnson, *Pocket Guide to Herbal Remedies*, 43.

1275. Johnson, *Pocket Guide to Herbal Remedies*, 43.

1276. Cech, *Making Plant Medicine*, 178.

1277. Pierce, *Practical Guide to Natural Medicines*, 454–457.

1278. Nancy J. Turner and Barbara S. Efrat, *Ethnobotany of the Hesquiat Indians of Vancouver Island* (Victoria: British Columbia Provincial Museum, 1982): 76.

1279. Nancy J. Turner, John Thomas, Barry F. Carlson and Robert T, *Ogilvie Ethnobotany of the Nitinaht Indians of Vancouver Island* (Victoria: British Columbia Provincial Museum, 1983): 128, 140, 289; Catherine S. Fowler, *Willards Z. Park's Ethnographic Notes on the Northern Paiute of Western Nevada 1933–1940* (Salt Lake City: University of Utah Press, 1989): 126; Erna Gunther, *Ethnobotany of Western Washington* (Seattle: University of Washington Press, 1973): 28; Goodrich and Lawson, *Kashaya Pomo Plants*, 77

1280. I. Gulcin, et al., "Antioxidant, Antimicrobial, Antiulcer and Analgesic Activities of Nettle (*Urtica dioica L.*), *Journal of Ethnophamacology* 90, no. 2–3 (February 2004): 90205–15.

1281. K. Riehemann, et al., "Plant Extracts From Stinging Nettle (*Urtica dioica*), an Antirheumatic Remedy, Inhibit The Proinflammatory Transcription Factor NF–kappaB. *FEBS Letters* 442, no. 1 (January 8, 1999): 89–94; B. Obertreis, et al., ["Anti–Inflammatory Effect of *Urtica dioica folia* Extract in Comparison to Caffeic Malic Acid,"] *Arzneimittelforschung* 46, no. 1 (January 1996): 52–6 (Article in German).

1282. C. Randall, H. Randall, F. Dobbs, C. Hutton, and H. Sanders, "Randomized Controlled Trial of Nettle Sting for Treatment of Base–of–Thumb Pain," *Journal of the Royal Society of Medicine* 93, no. 6 (June 2000): 305–9.

1283. Grieve, "Nettles," *Botanical.com: A Modern Herbal.*

1284. P. Mittman, "Randomized, Double Blind Study Of Freeze Dried *Urtica dioica* in the Treatment of Allergic Rhinitis," *Planta Medica* 56 (1990): 44–47.

1285. Mittman, "Randomized, Double–Blind Study of Freeze–Dried *Urtica dioica*," 44–47.

1286. Nancy J. Turner and Barbara S. Efrat, *Ethnobotany of the Hesquiat Indians of Vancouver Island* (Victoria: British Columbia Provincial Museum, 1982): 76.

1287. Gunther, *Ethnobotany of Western Washington*, 28.

1288. Bean and Saubel, *Temalpakh (From the Earth)*, 143.

1289. Pierce, *Practical Guide to Natural Medicines*, 454–457.

1290. Remington and Woods, *The Dispensatory of the United States of America.*

1291. Gulcin, "Antioxidant, Antimicrobial, Antiulcer and Analgesic Activities of Nettle (*Urtica dioica* L.), 90205–15.

1292. Moore, "Herbs Best as Cold Infusion."

1293. Pierce, *Practical Guide to Natural Medicines*, 454–457.

1294. Johnson, *Pocket Guide to Herbal Remedies*, 175.

1295. Mittman "Randomized, Double Blind Study of Freeze Dried *Urtica dioica* in the Treatment of Allergic Rhinitis," 44–47.

1296. Pierce, *Practical Guide to Natural Medicines*, 454–457.

1297. Johnson, *Pocket Guide to Herbal Remedies*, 175.

1298. Hoffmann, *Herbal Materia Medica.*

1299. Pierce, *Practical Guide to Natural Medicines*, 454–457.

1300. Pierce, *Practical Guide to Natural Medicines*, 454–457.

1301. Pierce, *Practical Guide to Natural Medicines*, 454–457.

1302. Cech, *Making Plant Medicine*, 179.

1303. Pierce, *Practical Guide to Natural Medicines*, 454–457.

1304. Pierce, *Practical Guide to Natural Medicines*, 454–457.

1305. Johnson, *Pocket Guide to Herbal Remedies*, 175.

1306. Johnson, *Pocket Guide to Herbal Remedies*, 175.

1307. K. Dhawan, et al., "Aphrodisiac Activity of Methanol Extract of Leaves of *Passiflora incarnata* Linn in Mice," *Phytotherapy Research* 17, no. 4 (April 2003): 401–3.

1308. Pierce, *Practical Guide to Natural Medicines*, 488–91.

1309. K. Dhawan, et al., "Anti–Anxiety Studies on Extracts of *Passiflora incarnata* Linneaus," *Journal of Ethnophamacology* 78, no. 2–3 (December 2001): 165–70.

1310. S. Akhondzadeh, et al., "Passionflower in the Treatment of Generalized Anxiety: A Pilot Double–Blind Randomized Controlled Trial with Oxazepam," *Journal of Clinical Pharmacy and Therapeutics* 26, no. 5 (October 2001): 363–7.

1311. Grieve, "Passion Flower," *Botanical.com: A Modern Herbal.*

1312. Remington and Woods, *The Dispensatory of the United States of America.*

1313. Pierce, *Practical Guide to Natural Medicines*, 488–91.

1314. N. Aoyagi, et al., "Anti–Anxiety Studies on Extracts of *Passiflora incarnata* Linneaus," *Chemical and Pharmaceutical Bulletin* 22 (1974): 1008.

1315. K. Shinomiya, et al., "Hypnotic Activities of Chamomile and Passiflora Extracts in Sleep–Disturbed Rats," *Biological & Pharmaceutical Bulletin* 28, no. 5 (May 2005): 808–10.

1316. Pierce, *Practical Guide to Natural Medicines*, 488–91.

1317. Hamel and Chiltoskey, *Cherokee Plants and Their Uses*, 47.

1318. J.M. Nicolls, et al., "Passicol, an Antibacterial and Antifungal Agent Produced by Passiflora Plant Species: Qualitative and Quantitative Range of Activity," *Antimicrobial Agents and Chemotherapy* 3 (1973): 110–117.

1319. K. Dhawan and A. Sharma, "Antitussive Activity of the Methanol Extract of *Passiflora incarnata* Leaves," *Fitoterapia* 73, no. 5 (August 2002): 397–9.

1320. A. B. Montanher, et al., "Evidence of Anti–Inflammatory Effects of *Passiflora edulis* in an Inflammation Model," *Journal of Ethnophamacology* 109, no. 2 (January 19, 2007): 281–8; Filho A. Goncalves, et al., ["Effect of *Passiflora edulis* (Passion Fruit) Extract on Rats' Bladder Wound Healing: Morphological Study,"] *Journal of the Royal Society of Medicine* 21, supplement 2 (2006): 1–8 (Article in Portuguese).

1321. Garros, ["Extract from *Passiflora edulis* on the Healing of Open Wounds in Rats,"] 55–65.

1322. Cech, *Making Plant Medicine*, 182.

1323. Pierce, *Practical Guide to Natural Medicines*, 488–91.

1324. K. Dhawan, et al., "Anxiolytic Activity of Aerial and Underground Parts of *Passiflora incarnate*," *Fitoterapia* 72, no. 8 (December 2001): 922–6.

1325. Johnson, *Pocket Guide to Herbal Remedies*, 109.

1326. Johnson, *Pocket Guide to Herbal Remedies*,109; Pierce, *Practical Guide to Natural Medicines*, 488–91.

1327. Pierce, *Practical Guide to Natural Medicines*, 488–91.

1328. Johnson, *Pocket Guide to Herbal Remedies*, 109.

1329. Pierce, *Practical Guide to Natural Medicines*, 488–91.

1330. J.M. Nicolls, et al., "Passicol, an Antibacterial and Antifungal Agent Produced by Passiflora Plant Species: Qualitative and Quantitative Range of Activity," *Antimicrobial Agents and Chemotherapy* 3 (1973): 110–117.

1331. Blumenthal, *The Complete German Commission E Manuscripts.*

1332. Pierce, *Practical Guide to Natural Medicines*, 488–91.

1333. University of Maryland Medical Center, "Passionflower," *Medical Reference: Complementary Medicine* http://www.umm.edu/altmed/articles/passionflower–000267.htm.

1334. Johnson, *Pocket Guide to Herbal Remedies*, 109.

1335. C. A. Newall, et al., *Herbal Medicines: A Guide for Health–Care Professionals* (London: The Pharmaceutical Press, 1996).

1336. Pierce, *Practical Guide to Natural Medicines*, 488–91.

1337. Johnson, *Pocket Guide to Herbal Remedies*, 109.

1338. Pierce, *Practical Guide to Natural Medicines*, 488–91.

1339. K. C. Santos, et al., "*Passiflora actinia* Hooker Extracts and Fractions Induce Catalepsy in Mice," *Journal of Ethnophamacology* 100, no. 3 (Sep 14, 2005): 306–9.

1340. Steven Foster "Peppermint: Mentha x piperita," *American Botanical Council Botanical Booklet Series* http://www.herbalgram.org/default.asp?c=peppermint.

1341. Pierce, *Practical Guide to Natural Medicines*, 498–502.

1342. Pierce, *Practical Guide to Natural Medicines*, 498–502.

1343. Pierce, *Practical Guide to Natural Medicines*, 498–502.

1344. T. Inoue, et al., "Effects of Peppermint (*Mentha piperita* L.) Extracts on Experimental Allergic Rhinitis in Rats," *Biological and Pharmaceutical Bulletin* 24, no. 1 (January 2001): 92–5.

1345. D. L. Mckay and J. B. Blumberg, "A Review of the Bioactivity and Potential Health Benefits of Peppermint Tea (*Mentha piperita* L.)," *Phytotherapy Research* 20, no. 8 (2006): 619–33.

1346. Pierce, *Practical Guide to Natural Medicines*, 498–502.

1347. "Menthol," *Wikipedia* http://en.wikipedia.org/wiki/Menthol.

1348. S. J. Davies, et al., "A Novel Treatment of Postherpetic Neuralgia Using Peppermint Oil," *The Clinical Journal of Pain* 18, no. 3 (May–June 2002): 200–2.

1349. Bo He, "TCM Chinese Herb Pictures," http://tcm.health–info.org/Herbology.Materia.Medica/bohe–properties.htm.

1350. H. Gobel, et al., "Effect of Peppermint and Eucalyptus Oil Preparations on Neurophysiological and Experimental Algesimetric Headache Parameters," *Cephalalgia* 14, no. 3 (June 1994): 228–34.

1351. "Eucalyptus," *Whole Health MD.*

1352. Pierce, *Practical Guide to Natural Medicines*, 498–502.

1353. Leung and Foster, *Encyclopedia of Common Natural Ingredients Used in Food, Drugs, and Cosmetics.*

1354. J. W. Isbary and H. Zeller, ["Experiences with Sportgel in the Ambulatory Treatment of Athletic Injuries,"] *Fortschritte der Medizin* 101, no. 29 (August 4, 1983): 1351–4 (Article in German).

1355. G.D. Bell and J. Doran, "Gall Stone Dissolution in Man Using an Essential Oil Preparation," *British Medical Journal* 278 (1979): 24.

1356. National Library of Medicine and the National Institutes of Health "Peppermint Oil (*Mentha x piperita L.*)," *MedlinePlus Health Information* http://www.nlm.nih.gov/medlineplus/druginfo/natural/patient–peppermint.html.

1357. Sharon Snider, "Banning 415 Ingredients from Seven Categories of NonPrescription Drugs," *Food and Drug Administration* P92–27 (August 25,1992) http://www.fda.gov/bbs/topics/NEWS/NEW00298.html.

1358. Pierce, *Practical Guide to Natural Medicines*, 498–502.

1359. J. G. C. Kingham, "Commentary: Peppermint Oil and Colon Spasm," *The Lancet*, 346 (October 14, 1995): 986.

1360. D. Yadegarinia, et al., "Biochemical Activities of Iranian *Mentha piperita* L. and *Myrtus communis* L. Essential Oils," *Phytochemistry* 67, no. 12 (June 2006): 1249–55.

1361. N. Mimica–Dukic, et al., "Antimicrobial and Antioxidant Activities of Three *Mentha* Species Essential Oils," *Planta Medica* 68, no. 5 (May 2003): 413–9.

1362. "Benzoic–acid," Dr. Duke's Phytochemical and Ethnobotanical Databases http://www.ars–grin.gov/cgi–bin/duke/chemical.pl?BENZOICACID.

1363. S. Behnam, et al., "Composition and Antifungal Activity of Essential Oils of *Mentha piperita* and *Lavendula angustifolia* on Post–Harvest Phytopathogens," *Communications in Agricultural and Applied Biological Sciences* 71, no. 3, part B (2006): 1321–6.

1364. D. L. McKay, et al., "A Review of the Bioactivity and Potential Health Benefits of Peppermint Tea (*Mentha piperita* L.), *Phytotherapy Research* 20, no. 8 (August 2006): 619–33.

1365. A. H. Atta, et al., "Anti–Nociceptive and Anti–Inflammatory Effects of Some Jordanian Medicinal Plant Extracts," *Journal of Ethnophamacology* 60, no. 2 (March 1998): 117–24.

1366. Pierce, *Practical Guide to Natural Medicines*, 498–502.

1367. C. Ho and C. Spence, "Olfactory Facilitation of Dual–Task Performance," *Neuroscience Letters* 389, no. 1 (November 2005): 35–40.

1368. S. Barker, et al., "Improved Performance on Clerical Tasks Associated with Administration of Peppermint Odor," *Perceptual and Motor Skills* 97, no. 3, part 1 (December 2003): 1007–10.

1369. Megan Rauscher, "Peppermint, Cinnamon Pep up Drivers," *Reuters Health* http://story.news.yahoo.com/s/nm/20060201/hl_nm/peppermint_cinnamon_dc.

1370. J. Ilmberger, et al., "The Influence of Essential Oils on Human Attention. I: Alertness," *Chemical Senses* 26, no. 3 (March 2001): 239–45.

1371. Pierce, *Practical Guide to Natural Medicines*, 498–502.

1372. C. Fang, et al., "Synergistically Enhanced Transdermal Permeation and Topical Analgesia of Tetracaine Gel Containing Menthol and Ethanol in Experimental and Clinical Studies," *European Journal of Pharmaceutics and Biopharmaceutics* 68 (2008): 735-740.

1373. Pierce, *Practical Guide to Natural Medicines*, 498–502.

1374. Johnson, *Pocket Guide to Herbal Remedies*, 97.

1375. Pierce, *Practical Guide to Natural Medicines*, 498–502.

1376. Commission E, "Peppermint Oil," *The Commission E Monographs: IHerb Health Encyclopedia* http://www.herbalgram.org/iherb/commissione/Monographs/Monograph_0290.html.

1377. Commission E, "Peppermint Oil."

1378. Commission E, "Peppermint Oil."

1379. Pierce, *Practical Guide to Natural Medicines*, 498–502.

1380. Johnson, *Pocket Guide to Herbal Remedies*, 97.

1381. Johnson, *Pocket Guide to Herbal Remedies*, 97.

1382. Pierce, *Practical Guide to Natural Medicines*, 498–502.

1383. Commission E, "Peppermint Oil."

1384. Johnson, *Pocket Guide to Herbal Remedies*, 97.

1385. Commission E, "Peppermint Oil."

1386. M. Akdogan, et al., "Effect of *Mentha piperita* (Labiatae) and *Mentha spicata* (Labiatae) on Iron Absorption in Rats," *Toxicology and Industrial Health* 20, no. 6–10 (September 2004): 119–22.

1387. Commission E, "Peppermint Oil."

1388. Leung and Foster, *Encyclopedia of Common Natural Ingredients Used in Food, Drugs, and Cosmetics*.

1389. Harkness and Bratman, *Handbook of Drug-Herb and Drug-Supplement Interactions*, 178.

1390. Pierce, *Practical Guide to Natural Medicines*, 498–502.

1391. Gregory S. Kelly, "*Rhodiola rosea*: A Possible Plant Adaptogen," *Smart Nutrition* http://smart-drugs.net/Rhodiola-rosea.htm.

1392. Smith, G. Warren, "Arctic Pharmacognosia," *Arctic* 26 (1973): 325.

1393. E. K. Boon-Niermeijer, A. van den Berg, G. Wikman, and F. A. Wiegant, "Phyto-Adaptogens Protect Against Environmental Stress-Induced Death of Embryos from the Freshwater Snail *Lymnaea stagnalis*," *Phytomedicine* 7 (2000): 389–399.

1394. H. C. Goel, et al., "Radioprotection by *Rhodiola imbricata* in Mice Against Whole-Body Lethal Irradiation," *Journal of Medicinal Food* 9, no. 2 (Summer 2006): 154–60.

1395. A. P. Azizov and R. D. Seifulla, "The Effect of Elton, Leveton, Fitoton and Adapton on the Work Capacity of Experimental Animals," *Eksperimental'naia i Klinicheskaia Farmakologiia* 61 (1998): 61–63 (Article in Russian).

1396. Gregory S. Kelly, "*Rhodiola rosea*: A Possible Plant Adaptogen," *Smart Nutrition* http://smart-drugs.net/Rhodiola-rosea.htm; I. I. Brekhman, and I. V. Dardymov, "New Substances of Plant Origin which Increase Nonspecific Resistance," *Annual Review of Pharmacology* 9 (1969): 419–430.

1397. V. A. Shevtsov, et al., "A Randomized Trial of Two Different Doses of a SHR-5 *Rhodiola rosea* Extract Versus Placebo and Control of Capacity for Mental Work," *Phytomedicine* 10, no. 2–3 (2003): 95–105.

1398. K. De Bock, B. O. Eijnde, M. Ramaekers, and P. Hespel, "Acute *Rhodiola rosea* Intake can Improve Endurance Exercise Performance," *International Journal of Sport Nutrition and Exercise Metabolism* 14, no. 3 (June 2004): 298–307.

1399. S. N. Colson, et al., "*Cordyceps sinensis*- and *Rhodiola rosea*-Based Supplementation in Male Cyclists and its Effect on Muscle Tissue Oxygen Saturation," *Journal of Strength and Conditioning Research* 19, no. 2 (May 2005): 358–63.

1400. S. L. Stancheva and A. Mosharrof, "Effect of the Extract of *Rhodiola rosea* L. on the Content of the Brain Biogenic Monamines," *Med Physiol* 40 (1987): 85–87.

1401. V. Darbinyan, et al., A*Rhodiola rosea* in Stress Induced Fatigue—a Double Blind Cross-over Study of a Standardized Extract SHR-5 with a Repeated Low-Dose Regimen on the Mental Performance of Healthy Physicians during Night Duty," *Phytomedicine* 7, no. 5 (October 2000): 365–71.

1402. A. A. Spasov, et al., "A Double–Blind, Placebo–Controlled Pilot Study of the Stimulating and Adaptogenic Effect of *Rhodiola rosea* SHR–5 Extract on the Fatigue of Students Caused by Stress During an Examination Period with a Repeated Low–Dose Regimen," *Phytomedicine* 7, no. 2 (April 2000): 85–9.

1403. Kelly, "*Rhodiola rosea*: A Possible Plant Adaptogen."

1404. Heather S. Oliff, "Optimum Dosage of *Rhodiola rosea* Extract for Anti–fatigue Effects and Improved Mental Performance," *HerbalGram: The Journal of the American Botanical Council* 63 (2004): 20–21.

1405. V. A. Shevtsovl, et al., "A Randomized Trial of Two Different Doses of a SHR–5 *Rhodiola rosea* Extract Versus Placebo and Control of Capacity for Mental Work," *Phytomedicine* 10 (2003): 95–105.

1406. Shevtsov, "A Randomized Trial of Two Different Doses of a SHR–5," 95–105.

1407. Oliff, "Optimum Dosage of *Rhodiola rosea* Extract," 20–21.

1408. "*Rhodiola rosea*," *Alternative Medicine Review* 7, no. 5 (2002): 421–3.

1409. K. De Bock, B. O. Eijnde, M. Ramaekers, and P. Hespel, "Acute *Rhodiola rosea* Intake can Improve Endurance Exercise Performance," *International Journal of Sport Nutrition and Exercise Metabolism* 14, no. 3 (June 2004): 298–307.

1410. "*Rhodiola rosea*," *Alternative Medicine Review*, 421–3.

1411. Shevtsov, "A Randomized Trial of Two Different Doses of a SHR–5," 95–105.

1412. D. Franco, et al., "Processing of *Rosa rubiginosa*: Extraction of Oil and Antioxidant Substances," *Bioresource Technology* 98, no. 18 (January 2, 2007): 3506–3512; D. Hornero–Mendez, et al., "Carotenoid Pigments in *Rosa mosqueta* Hips, an Alternative Carotenoid Source for Foods," *Journal of Agricultural and Food Chemistry* 48, no. 3 (March 2000): 825–8.

1413. D. Deliorman Orhan, et al., "In Vivo Anti–Inflammatory and Antinociceptive Activity of the Crude Extract and Fractions from *Rosa canina L.* Fruits," *Journal of Ethnophamacology* 112, no 2 (March 30, 2007): 394–400.

1414. Anthony C. Dweck, "Formulating with Natural Ingredients," *Dweck Data* http://www.dweckdata.com/Published_papers/Formulating_with_Naturals.pdf.

1415. J. C. Moreno Gimenez, et al., ["Treatment of Skin Ulcer Using Oil of Mosqueta Rose,"] *Medicina Cutánea Ibero-Latino-Americana* 18, no. 1 (1990): 63–6 (Article in Spanish); F. Camacho, "Treatment of Acne Scars with Musk Rose Oil," *Medicina Cutanea Ibero–Latino–Americana* 22, no. 3 (1994): 137–142.

1416. Blumenthal, *The Complete German Commission E Manuscripts*. In Pierce, *Practical Guide to Natural Medicines*, 552–553.

1417. Pierce, *Practical Guide to Natural Medicines*, 551–554.

1418. T. Mangena, N. Y. Muyima, "Comparative Evaluation of the Antimicrobial Activities of Essential Oils of *Artemisia afra*, *Pteronia incana* and *Rosmarinus officinalis* on Selected Bacteria and Yeast Strains," *Letters in Applied Microbiology* 28, no. 4 (April 1999): 291–6.

1419. M. Moss, et al., "Aromas of Rosemary and Lavender Essential Oils Differentially Affect Cognition and Mood in Healthy Adults," *The International Journal of Neuroscience* 113, no. 1 (January 2003): 15–38.

1420. M. Moss, et al., "Aromas of Rosemary and Lavender Essential Oils," 15–38.

1421. M. R. al–Sereiti, et al., "Pharmacology of Rosemary (*Rosmarinus officinalis* Linn.) and its Therapeutic Potentials," *Indian Journal of Experimental Biology* 37, no. 2 (February 1999): 124–30.

1422. Michael Moore. "Herbs Best as Standard Infusion."

1423. Pierce, *Practical Guide to Natural Medicines*, 551–554.

1424. Ody, *The Complete Medicinal Herbal*, 92.

1425. Pierce, *Practical Guide to Natural Medicines*, 137.

1426. Johnson, *Pocket Guide to Herbal Remedies*, 137.

1427. Pierce, *Practical Guide to Natural Medicines*, 551–554.

1428. P. R. Burkhard, et al., "Plant–Induced Seizures: Reappearance of an Old Problem," *Journal of Neurology* 246, no. 8 (August 1999): 667–70.

1429. Johnson, *Pocket Guide to Herbal Remedies*, 137.

1430. Bean and Saubel, *Temalpakh (From the Earth)*, 136.

1431. V. De Leo, D. Lanzetta, R. Cazzavacca, and G. Morgante, ["Treatment of Neurovegetative Menopausal Symptoms with a Phytotherapeutic Agent,"] *Minerva Ginecologica* 50, no. 5 (May 1998): 207–11 (Article in Italian).

1432. Pierce, *Practical Guide to Natural Medicines*, 563–566.

1433. Hamel and Chiltoskey, *Cherokee Plants and Their Uses*, 53.

1434. Percy Train, James R. Henrichs, and Archer W. Andrew, *Medicinal Uses of Plants by Indian Tribes of Nevada* (Washington DC: U.S. Department of Agriculture, 1941): 136–7.

1435. Pierce, *Practical Guide to Natural Medicines*, 563–566.

1436. Pierce, *Practical Guide to Natural Medicines*, 563–566.

1437. Remington and Woods, *The Dispensatory of the United States of America*.

1438. K. Horiuchi, et al., "Potentiation of Antimicrobial Activity of Aminoglycosides by Carnosol from *Salvia officinalis*," *Biological and Pharmaceutical Bulletin* 30, no. 2 (February 2007): 287–90; R. S. Pereira, et al., ["Antibacterial Activity of Essential Oils on Microorganisms Isolated from Urinary Tract Infection,"] *Revista de Saúde Pública* 38, no. 2 (April 2004: 326–8 (Article in Portuguese).

1439. M. Ozcan, "Antioxidant Activities of Rosemary, Sage, and Sumac Extracts and their Combinations on Stability of Natural Peanut Oil," *Journal of Medicinal Food* 6, no. 3 (Fall 2003): 267–70.

1440. C. F. Lima, et al., "Water and Methanolic Extracts of *Salvia officinalis* Protect HepG2 Cells from t–BHP Induced Oxidative Damage," *Chemico-Biological Interactions* 167, no. 2 (April 25, 2007): 107–15.

1441. Pierce, *Practical Guide to Natural Medicines*, 563–566.

1442. Johnson, *Pocket Guide to Herbal Remedies*, 142.

1443. Johnson, *Pocket Guide to Herbal Remedies*, 142.

1444. Pierce, *Practical Guide to Natural Medicines*, 563–566.

1445. Pierce, *Practical Guide to Natural Medicines*, 563–566.

1446. D. L. J. Opdyke, "Monographs on Fragrance Raw Materials," *Food and Cosmetics Toxicology* 14 (1976): 857.

1447. Johnson, *Pocket Guide to Herbal Remedies*, 142.

1448. Pierce, *Practical Guide to Natural Medicines*, 563–566.

1449. Ody, *The Complete Medicinal Herbal*, 95.

1450. Johnson, *Pocket Guide to Herbal Remedies*, 142.

1451. Pierce, *Practical Guide to Natural Medicines*, 596–598.

1452. Remington and Woods, *The Dispensatory of the United States of America*.

1453. Remington and Woods, *The Dispensatory of the United States of America.*

1454. Pierce, *Practical Guide to Natural Medicines*, 596–598.

1455. Grieve, "Shepherd's Purse," *Botanical.com: A Modern Herbal.*

1456. Francis Densmore, "Menominee Music," *SI–BAE Bulletin* 102 (1932): 134.

1457. Pierce, *Practical Guide to Natural Medicines*, 596–598.

1458. S. A. Moskalenko, "Preliminary Screening of Far-Eastern Ethnomedicinal Plants for Antibacterial Activity," *Journal of Ethnopharmacology* 15 (1986): 231–59.

1459. M. S. El Abyad, et al., "Preliminary Screening of Some Egyptian Weeds for Antimicrobial Activity," *Microbios* 62, no. 250 (1990): 47–57.

1460. Pierce, *Practical Guide to Natural Medicines*, 596–598.

1461. Pierce, *Practical Guide to Natural Medicines*, 596–598.

1462. Commission E "Shepherd's Purse," *The Commission E Monographs: Iherb Health Encyclopedia* http://www.herbalgram.org/iherb/commissione/Monographs/Monograph_0338.html.

1463. Pierce, *Practical Guide to Natural Medicines*, 596–598.

1464. Johnson, *Pocket Guide to Herbal Remedies*, 29.

1465. Johnson, *Pocket Guide to Herbal Remedies*, 29.

1466. Johnson, *Pocket Guide to Herbal Remedies*, 29.

1467. Johnson, *Pocket Guide to Herbal Remedies*, 29.

1468. Pierce, *Practical Guide to Natural Medicines*, 601–602.

1469. "Illegal Stripping and Conservation of Slippery Elm Trees," *HerbalGram* 74 (2007): 54–61.

1470. Hamel and Chiltoskey, *Cherokee Plants and Their Uses*, 33.

1471. Frances Densmore, "Uses of Plants by the Chippewa Indians," *SI–BAE Annual Report* 44 (1928): 342.

1472. Herrick, *Iroquois Medical Botany*, 306.

1473. Tantaquidgeon, *Folk Medicine of the Delaware and Related Algonkian Indians*, 132.

1474. Pierce, *Practical Guide to Natural Medicines*, 601–602.

1475. Hamel and Chiltoskey, *Cherokee Plants and Their Uses*, 33.

1476. Huron H. Smith, "Ethnobotany of the Menomini Indians," *Bulletin of the Public Museum of the City of Milwaukee* 4 (1923): 56–57.

1477. Smith, "Ethnobotany of the Meskwaki Indians," 251.

1478. Albert B. Reagan, "Plants Used by the Bois Fort Chippewa (Ojibwa) Indians of Minnesota," *Wisconsin Archeologist* 7, no. 4 (1928): 231.

1479. Pierce, *Practical Guide to Natural Medicines*, 601–602.

1480. Remington and Woods, *The Dispensatory of the United States of America.*

1481. Pierce, *Practical Guide to Natural Medicines*, 601–602.

1482. Romero, *The Botanical Lore of the California Indians*, 27.

1483. Grieve, "Elm, Slippery," *Botanical.com: A Modern Herbal.*

1484. Pierce, *Practical Guide to Natural Medicines*, 601–602.

1485. Remington and Woods, *The Dispensatory of the United States of America.*

1486. Johnson, *Pocket Guide to Herbal Remedies*, 173.

1487. Johnson, *Pocket Guide to Herbal Remedies*, 173.

1488. Pierce, *Practical Guide to Natural Medicines*, 601–602.

1489. Johnson, *Pocket Guide to Herbal Remedies*, 173.

1490. Pierce, *Practical Guide to Natural Medicines*, 601–602.

1491. Johnson, *Pocket Guide to Herbal Remedies*, 173.

1492. Remington and Woods, *The Dispensatory of the United States of America.*

1493. Pierce, *Practical Guide to Natural Medicines*, 566–570.

1494. Steven Foster, "St. John's Wort: *Hypericum perforatum*," *Steven Foster Group* http://www.stevenfoster.com/education/monograph/hypericum.html.

1495. American Botanical Council "St. John's Wort," *Herbal Information: Expanded Commission E Online* http://www.herbalgram.org/default.asp?c=he094.

1496. Pierce, *Practical Guide to Natural Medicines*, 566–570.

1497. Grieve, "St. John's Wort," *Botanical.com: A Modern Herbal.*

1498. American Botanical Council "St. John's Wort."

1499. American Botanical Council "St. John's Wort"; K. Linde, et al, "St John's Wort for Depression—An Overview and Meta-Analysis of Randomised Clinical Trials," *British Medical Journal* 313 (1996): 253B258.

1500. Johnson, *Pocket Guide to Herbal Remedies*, 77.

1501. A. Szegedi, R. Kohnen, A. Dienel, and M. Kieser, "Acute Treatment of Moderate to Severe Depression with Hypericum Extract WS" 5570 (St. John's Wort): Randomized, Controlled, Double-Blind, Non-Inferiority Trial versus Peroxetine," *BMJ (Clinical Research Ed.)* (2005): 330:503.

1502. R. C. Shelton, M. B. Keller, and A. J. Gelenberg, et al. "Effectiveness of St. John's Wort in Major Depression," *Journal Of The American Medical Association* 285 (2001): 1978–86; Hypericum Depression Trial Study Group, "Effect of *Hypericum perforatum* (St John's Wort) in Major Depressive Disorder," *Journal Of The American Medical Association* 287, no. 14 (2002): 1807–1814.

1503. K. Clement, et al., "St. John's Wort and the Treatment of Mild to Moderate Depression: A Systematic Review," *Holistic Nursing Practice* 20, no. 4 (July–August 2006): 197–203.

1504. American Botanical Council, "St. John's Wort," *Herbal Information: Expanded Commission E Online.*

1505. Deutsches Grúnes Kreuz E.V., ["St. John's Wort Treatment Relieves Skin Inflammation and Pruritus in Neurodermatitis,"] *Kinderkrankenschwester* 24, no. 11 (November 2005): 479 (Article in German).

1506. Remington and Woods, *The Dispensatory of the United States of America.*

1507. Hamel and Chiltoskey, *Cherokee Plants and Their Uses*, 53.

1508. S. A. Barrett and E. W. Gifford, "Miwok Material Culture," *Bulletin of the Public Museum of the City of Milwaukee* 2, no. 4 (1933): 171.

1509. Pierce, *Practical Guide to Natural Medicines*, 566–570.

1510. Leung and Foster, *Encyclopedia of Common Natural Ingredients Used in Food, Drugs, and Cosmetics*; D. Muruelo et al. "Therapeutic Agents with Dramatic Retroviral Activity," *Proceedings of the National Academy of Science, U.S.A.* 85 (1988): 5230–34.

1511. P. K. Mukherjee and B. Suresh, "The Evaluation of Wound-Healing Potential of *Hypericum hookerianum* Leaf and Stem Extracts," *Journal of Alternative and Complementary Medicine* 6, no. 1 (February 2000): 61–9; P. K. Mukherjee, et al., "Evaluation of In-Vivo Wound Healing Activity of *Hypericum patulum* (Family: hypericaceae) Leaf Extract on Different Wound Model in Rats," *Journal of Ethnophamacology* 70, no. 3 (June 2000): 315–21.

1512. C. M. Hautarzt Schempp, ["Topical Treatment of Atopic Dermatitis with Hypericum Cream: A Randomised, Placebo–Controlled, Double–Blind Half–Side Comparison Study,"] *Der Hautarzt; Zeitschrift für Dermatologie, Venerologie, und verwandte Gebiete* 54, no. 3 (March 2003): 248–53 (Article in German).

1513. Pierce, *Practical Guide to Natural Medicines*, 566–570.

1514. American Botanical Council, "St. John's Wort," *Herbal Information: Expanded Commission E Online.*

1515. "St. John's Wort," *Wikipedia* http://en.wikipedia.org/wiki/St._John%27s_Wort.

1516. "St. John's Wort," *Wikipedia.*

1517. Johnson, *Pocket Guide to Herbal Remedies*, 77.

1518. "St. John's Wort," *Wikipedia.*

1519. Pierce, *Practical Guide to Natural Medicines*, 566–570.

1520. H. L. Kim, J. Streltzer, and D. Goebert, "St. John's Wort for Depression: A Meta–Analysis of Well–Defined Clinical Trials," *The Journal of Nervous and Mental Disease* 187, no. 9 (1999): 532–538.

1521. Harkness and Bratman, *Handbook of Drug–Herb and Drug–Supplement Interactions*, 188.

1522. "Ginseng," *Medlineplus Herb And Supplement.*

1523. Johnson, *Pocket Guide to Herbal Remedies*, 77.

1524. N. Ferko and M. A. Levine, "Evaluation of the Association Between St. John's Wort and Elevated Thyroid–Stimulating Hormone," *Pharmacotherapy* 21, no. 12 (December 2001): 1574–8.

1525. National Institute of Mental Health, "Depression," http://www.nimh.nih.gov/nimhhome/index.cfm.

1526. American Herbal Products Association, "Herb Info: FAQs," http://www.ahpa.org/Default.aspx?tabid=70.

1527. Pierce, *Practical Guide to Natural Medicines*, 628–630.

1528. Pierce, *Practical Guide to Natural Medicines*, 628–630.

1529. J. M. Concha, et al., "Antifungal Activity of *Melaleuca alternifolia* (Tea–Tree) Oil Against Various Pathogenic Organisms," *Journal of the American Podiatric Medical Association* 88, no. 10 (October 1998): 489–92.

1530. K. A. Hammer, et al., "Susceptibility of Transient and Commensal Skin Flora to the Essential Oil of *Melaleuca alternifolia* (Tea Tree Oil)," *American Journal of Infection Control* 24, no. 3 (June 1996): 186–9.

1531. S. Messager, et al., "Effectiveness of Hand–Cleansing Formulations Containing Tea Tree Oil Assessed Ex Vivo on Human Skin and in Vivo with Volunteers Using European Standard EN 1499," *The Journal of Hospital Infection* 59, no. 3 (March 2005): 220–8.

1532. T. A. Syed, et al., "Treatment of Toenail Onychomycosis with 2% Butenafine and 5% *Melaleuca alternifolia* (Tea Tree) Oil in Cream, *Tropical Medicine & International Health* 4, no. 4 (April 1999): 284–7.

1533. D. S. Buck, et al., "Comparison of Two Topical Preparations for the Treatment of Onychomycosis: *Melaleuca alternifolia* (Tea Tree) Oil and Clotrimazole," *Journal of Family Practice* 38, no. 6 (June 1994): 601–5.

1534. I. B. Bassett, et al., "A Comparative Study of Tea–Tree Oil Versus Benzoylperoxide in the Treatment of Acne," *The Medical Journal of Australia* 153, no. 8 (October 15, 1990): 455–8.

1535. Concha, "Antifungal Activity of *Melaleuca alternifolia*," 489–92.

1536. Pierce, *Practical Guide to Natural Medicines*, 628–630.

1537. M. M. Tong, et al., "Tea Tree Oil in the Treatment of *Tinea pedis*," *The Australasian Journal of Dermatology* 33, no. 3 (1992): 145–9.

1538. Cech, *Making Plant Medicine*, 219.

1539. Scientific Committee on Consumer Products, "Opinion on Tea Tree Oil Adopted by the SCCP during the 2nd plenary meeting of 7 December 2004," European Commission, Health & Consumer Protection Directorate–General: Directorate C. Public Health and Risk Assessment. C7– Risk assessment. SCCP/0843/04.

1540. Johnson, *Pocket Guide to Herbal Remedies*, 94.

1541. Cech, *Making Plant Medicine*, 219.

1542. Johnson, *Pocket Guide to Herbal Remedies*, 94.

1543. D. M. Rubel, et al., "Tea Tree Oil Allergy: What is the Offending Agent? Report of Three Cases of Tea Tree Oil Allergy and Review of the Literature," *The Australasian Journal of Dermatology* 39, no. 4 (November 1998): 244–7.

1544. Skin & Cancer Foundation Australia "Human studies Draize method," *Study No. DT-029* (1997)

1545. D. P. Bruynzeel, "Contact Dermatitis Due to Tea Tree Oil," *Tropical Medicine & International Health* 4, no. 9 (September 1999): 630.

1546. D. Villar, et al., "Toxicity of Melaleuca Oil and Related Essential Oils Applied Topically on Dogs and Cats," *Veterinary and Human Toxicology* 36, no. 2 (April 1994): 139–42.

1547. National Library of Medicine and the National Institutes of Health, "Tea Tree Oil (*Melaleuca alternifolia*)," *MedlinePlus Health Information* http://www.nlm.nih.gov/medlineplus/druginfo/natural/patient–teatreeoil.html.

1548. National Library of Medicine and the National Institutes of Health, "Tea Tree Oil."

1549. Pierce, *Practical Guide to Natural Medicines*, 631–633.

1550. H. A. Seda and G. S. Moram, "Antimicrobial Effect of Some Plant Essential Oils Against Some of Microorganisms," *Annals of Agricultural Science* 38, no. 3 (2000): 1615–1622; H. J. Dorman and S. G. Deans, "Antimicrobial Agents From Plants: Antibacterial Activity of Plant Volatile Oils," *Journal of Applied Microbiology* 88, no. 2 (February 2000): 308–16.

1551. Pierce, *Practical Guide to Natural Medicines*, 631–633.

1552. Grieve, "Thyme," *Botanical.com: A Modern Herbal.*

1553. P. Hersch–Martinez, et al., "Antibacterial Effects of Commercial Essential Oils over Locally Prevalent Pathogenic Strains in Mexico," *Fitoterapia* 76, no. 5 (July 2005): 453–7.

1554. Grieve, "Thyme," *Botanical.com: A Modern Herbal.*

1555. C. O. Van den Broucke, "The Therapeutic Value of *Thymus* Species," *Fitoterapia* 4 (1983): 171–74.

1556. M. H. Boskabady, et al., "Relaxant effect of *Thymus vulgaris* on Guinea–Pig Tracheal Chains and its Possible Mechanism(s)," *Phytotherapy Research* 20, no. 1 (January 2006): 28–33.

1557. E. Vigo, et al., "In–Vitro Anti–Inflammatory Effect of *Eucalyptus globulus* and *Thymus vulgaris*: Nitric Oxide Inhibition in J774A.1 Murine Macrophages," *The Journal of Pharmacy and Pharmacology* 56, no. 2 (February 2004): 257–63.

1558. R. S. Ramsewak, et al., "In Vitro Antagonistic Activity of Monoterpenes and their Mixtures against 'Toe Nail Fungus' Pathogens," *Phytotherapy Research* 17, no. 4 (April 2003): 376–9.

1559. C. Pina-Vaz, et al., "Antifungal Activity of Thymus Oils and their Major Compounds," *Journal of the European Academy of Dermatology and Venereology* 18, no. 1 (January 2004): 73–8; R. Giordani, et al., "Antifungal Effect of Various Essential Oils against *Candida albicans*, Potentiation of Antifungal Action of Amphotericin B by Essential Oil from *Thymus vulgaris*," *Phytotherapy Research* 18, no. 12 (December 2004): 990–5.

1560. Pierce, *Practical Guide to Natural Medicines*, 631–633.

1561. Pierce, *Practical Guide to Natural Medicines*, 631–633.

1562. Pierce, *Practical Guide to Natural Medicines*, 631–633.

1563. Pierce, *Practical Guide to Natural Medicines*, 631–633.

1564. Johnson, *Pocket Guide to Herbal Remedies*, 166.

1565. Pierce, *Practical Guide to Natural Medicines*, 631–633.

1566. Johnson, *Pocket Guide to Herbal Remedies*, 166.

1567. Pierce, *Practical Guide to Natural Medicines*, 631–633.

1568. Pierce, *Practical Guide to Natural Medicines*, 631–633.

1569. Johnson, *Pocket Guide to Herbal Remedies*, 166.

1570. Pierce, *Practical Guide to Natural Medicines*, 631–633.

1571. Pierce, *Practical Guide to Natural Medicines*, 631–633.

1572. M. Benito, et al., "Labiatae Allergy: Systemic Reactions Due to Ingestion of Oregano and Thyme," *Annals of Allergy, Asthma and Immunology* 76, no. 5 (May 1996): 416–8.

1573. Pierce, *Practical Guide to Natural Medicines*, 638–641.

1574. West TCM, "Jiang Huang," *Traditional Chinese Medicine and Acupuncture Health Information Organization* http://tcm.health-info.org/Herbology.Materia.Medica/jianghuang-properties.htm.

1575. M. Tomoda, et al., "A Reticuloendothelial System Activating Glycan from the Rhizomes of *Curcuma longa*," *Phytochemistry* 29 (1990): 1083.

1576. West TCM, "Jiang Huang."

1577. V. Thamlikitkul, et al., "Randomized Double Blind Study of *Curcuma domestica* Val. for Dyspepsia," *Journal of the Medical Association of Thailand* 72, no. 11 (November 1989): 613–20.

1578. C. Prucksunand, et al., "Phase II Clinical Trial on Effect of the Long Turmeric (*Curcuma longa* Linn) on Healing of Peptic Ulcer," *The Southeast Asian Journal of Tropical Medicine and Public Health* 32, no. 1 (March 2001): 208–15.

1579. A. Asai and T. Miyazawa, "Dietary Curcuminoids Prevent High-Fat, Diet-Induced Lipid Accumulation in Rat Livers and Epididymal Adipose Tissue," *Journal of Nutrition* 131, no. 11 (2001): 2932–5.

1580. R. R. Ahmad-Raus, et al., "Lowering of Lipid Composition in Aorta of Guinea Pigs by *Curcuma domestica*," *BMC Complementary and Alternative Medicine* 1 (2001): 6; J. L. Quiles, et al. "*Curcuma longa* Extract Supplementation Reduces Oxidative Stress and Attenuates Aortic Fatty Streak Development in Rabbits," *Arteriosclerosis, Thrombosis, and Vascular Biology* 22, no. 7 (July 1, 2002): 1225–31.

1581. K. B. Soni, R. Kuttan. "Effect of Oral Curcumin Administration on Serum Peroxides and Cholesterol Levels in Human Volunteers," *Indian Journal of Physiology and Pharmacology* 36, no. 4 (October 1992): 273–5.

1582. B. H. Shaw, et al. "Inhibitory Effects of Curcumin, a Food Spice from Turmeric on Platlet Activating Factor and Arachidonic Acid-Mediated Platlet Aggregation through Inhibition of Thromboxane Formation and Ca2+ Signaling," *Biochemical Pharmacology* 58, no. 7 (1999): 1167–72.

1583. T. P. Ng, P. C. Chiam, T. Lee, H. C. Chua, L. Lim, and E. H. Kua. "Curry Consumption and Cognitive Function in the Elderly," *American Journal of Epidemiology* 164 (2006): 898–906.

1584. F. Yang, et al., "Curcumin Inhibits Formation of Amyloid Beta Oligomers and Fibrils, Binds Plaques, and Reduces Amyloid In Vivo," *Journal of Biological Chemistry* 18, no. 7 (February 18, 2005): 5892–901.

1585. L. Li, et al., ["Effects of *Curcuma phaeocaulis* on Learning and Memory and Lipid Peroxide in Mice,"] *Zhong Yao Cai: Journal of Chinese Medicinal Materials* 21, no. 10 (October 1998): 522–3 (Article in Chinese).

1586. Akana, *Hawaiian Herbs of Medicinal Value*, 33.

1587. Pierce, *Practical Guide to Natural Medicines*, 638–641.

1588. "*Curcuma longa* (Turmeric) Monograph," *Alternative Medicine Review* 6 (September 2001): S62–66.

1589. R. R. Satoskar, et al., "Evaluation of Anti–Inflammatory Property of Curcumin (Diferuloyl Methane) in Patients with Postoperative Inflammation," *International Journal of Clinical Pharmacology, Therapy, and Toxicology* 24, no. 12 (December 1986): 651–4.

1590. G. S. Sidhu, et al., "Curcumin Enhances Wound Healing in Streptozotocin Induced Diabetic Rats and Genetically Diabetic Mice," *Wound Repair and Regeneration* 7, no, 5 (September–October 1999): 362–74; H. Mani, et al., "Curcumin Differentially Regulates TGF–beta1, its Receptors and Nitric Oxide Synthase During Impaired Wound Healing," *Biofactors* 16, no. 1–2 (2002): 29–43.

1591. G. C. Jagetia and G. K. Rajanikant. "Role of Curcumin, a Naturally Occurring Phenolic Compound of Turmeric in Accelerating the Repair of Excision Wound, in Mice Whole–Body Exposed to Various Doses of Gamma–Radiation," *Journal of Surgical Research* 120, no. 1 (July 2004): 127–38.

1592. D. Chandra and S. S. Gupta, "Anti-inflammatory and Anti-Arthritic Activity of Volatile Oil of *Curcuma longa* (Haldi)," *Indian Journal of Medical Research* 60 (1972): 138.

1593. J. F. Innes, et al., "Randomised, Double–Blind, Placebo–Controlled Parallel Group Study of P54FP for the Treatment of Dogs with Osteoarthritis," *The Veterinary Record* 152, no. 15 (April 12, 2003): 457–60.

1594. National Library of Medicine and the National Institutes of Health, "Turmeric (*Curcuma longa* Linn.) and Curcumin," *MedlinePlus Health Information* http://www.nlm.nih.gov/medlineplus/druginfo/natural/patient–turmeric.html.

1595. International College of Herbal Medicine, "Turmeric—*Cucuma longa*," *Herb of the Month, February/March 2002* http://www.herbcollege.com/herbofthemonth.asp?id=40.

1596. International College of Herbal Medicine, "Turmeric—*Cucuma longa*."

1597. Commission E, "Turmeric Root," *The Commission E Monographs: IHerb Health Encyclopedia* http://www.herbalgram.org/iherb/commissione/Monographs/Monograph_0361.html; Low Dog and Riley, "Management of Hyperlipidemia," 28–41.

1598. Johnson, *Pocket Guide to Herbal Remedies*, 51.

1599. Wu N. Chainani, "Safety and Anti–Inflammatory Activity of Curcumin: A Component of Turmeric (*Curcuma longa*)," *Journal of Alternative and Complementary Medicine* 9, no. 1 (February 2003): 161–8.

1600. S. Quershi, et al., "Toxicology Studies on *Alpinia galanga* and *Curuma longa*," *Planta Medica* 58 (1992): 124.

1601. Pierce, *Practical Guide to Natural Medicines*, 638–641.

1602. Johnson, *Pocket Guide to Herbal Remedies*, 51.

1603. "Echinacea (*E. angustifolia DC*, *E. pallida*, *E. purpurea*)," *Medlineplus Herb and Supplement* http://www.nlm.nih.gov/medlineplus/druginfo/natural/patient-echinacea.html.

1604. Johnson, *Pocket Guide to Herbal Remedies*, 51.

1605. Johnson, *Pocket Guide to Herbal Remedies*, 51.

1606. N. Arun, et al., "Efficacy of Turmeric on Blood Sugar and Polyol Pathway in Diabetic Albino Rats," *Plant Foods for Human Nutrition* 57, no. 1 (Winter 2002): 41–52.

1607. Johnson, *Pocket Guide to Herbal Remedies*, 51.

1608. Johnson, *Pocket Guide to Herbal Remedies*, 51.

1609. Remington and Woods, *The Dispensatory of the United States of America*.

1610. National Library of Medicine and the National Institutes of Health, "Valerian (*Valeriana officinalis* L.)," *MedlinePlus Health Information* http://www.nlm.nih.gov/medlineplus/druginfo/natural/patient-valerian.html.

1611. National Library of Medicine and the National Institutes of Health, "Valerian."

1612. S. Fernandez, et al., "Sedative and Sleep-Enhancing Properties of Linarin, a Flavonoid-Isolated from *Valeriana officinalis*," *Pharmacology, Biochemistry, and Behavior* 77, no. 2 (February 2004): 399–404.

1613. Tyler, *Herbs Of Choice: The Therapeutic Use of Phytomedicinals*, 209.

1614. H. Schulz, C. Stolz, and J. Muller, "The Effect of Valerian Extract on Sleep Polygraphy in Poor Sleepers: A Pilot Study," *Pharmacopsychiatry* 27 (1994): 147–51.

1615. S. Bent, et al., "Valerian for Sleep: A Systematic Review and Meta-Analysis," *American Journal of Medicine* 119, no. 12 (December 2006): 1005–12.

1616. Grieve, "Valerian," *Botanical.com: A Modern Herbal.*

1617. D. B. Mowrey, "The Scientific Validation of Herbal Medicine," (New Canaan, CT: Keats Publishing, 1986): 316.

1618. R. Kohnen and W. D. Oswald, "The Effects of Valerian, Propranolol, and their Combination on Activation, Performance, and Mood of Healthy Volunteers under Social Stress Conditions," *Pharmacopsychiatry* 21 (1988): 447–8.112.

1619. M. P. Sousa, P. Pacheco, and V. Roldao, "Double-Blind Comparative Study of The Efficacy and Safety of Valdispert vs Clobazapam," *KaliChemie Medical Research and Information* 1992.

1620. N. G. Bissett, *Herbal Drugs and Phytopharmaceuticals* (Stuttgart: MedPharm CRC Press, 1994): 566.

1621. Nancy J. Turner, Laurence C. Thompson, and M. Terry Thompson, et al., *Thompson Ethnobotany: Knowledge and Usage of Plants by the Thompson Indians of British Columbia* (Victoria: Royal British Columbia Museum, 1990): 290; Ralph V. Chamberlin, "The Ethno-Botany of the Gosiute Indians of Utah," *Memoirs of the American Anthropological Association* 2, no. 5 (1911): 349; Huron H. Smith, "Ethnobotany of the Menomini Indians," *Bulletin of the Public Museum of the City of Milwaukee* 4 (1923): 57; Smith, "Ethnobotany of the Meskwaki Indians," 251; F. Perry, "Ethno-Botany of the Indians in the Interior of British Columbia," *Museum and Art Notes* 2, no. 2 (1952): 40.

1622. A. Ebringerova, et al., "Mitogenic and Comitogenic Activities of Polysaccharides from some European Herbaceous Plants," *Fitoterapia* 74, no. 1–2 (February 2003): 52–61.

1623. Pierce, *Practical Guide to Natural Medicines*, 649–652.

1624. Kathi J. Kemper, "Valerian," *Longwood, Duke Herbal Task Force* http://www.mcp.edu/herbal/default.htm.

1625. "Insomnia," *MotherNature.com* http://www.mothernature.com/Library/Bookshelf/Books/15/16.cfm.

1626. M. Goppel and G. Franz, "Stability Control of Valerian Ground Material and Extracts: a New HPLC–Method for the Routine Quantification of Valerenic Acids and Lignans," *Pharmazie* 59, no. 6 (June 2004): 446–52.

1627. R. Bos, et al. "Seasonal Variation of the Essential Oil, Valerenic Acid and Derivatives, and Velopotriates in *Valeriana officinalis* Roots and Rhizomes, and the Selection of Plants Suitable for Phytomedicines," *Planta Medica* 64, no. 2 (March 1998): 143–7.

1628. Johnson, *Pocket Guide to Herbal Remedies*, 179.

1629. Johnson, *Pocket Guide to Herbal Remedies*, 179; Pierce, *Practical Guide to Natural Medicines*, 649–652.

1630. Johnson, *Pocket Guide to Herbal Remedies*, 179.

1631. Grieve, "Valerian," *Botanical.com: A Modern Herbal*

1632. S. Gutierrez, et al. Assessing Subjective and Psychomotor Effects of the Herbal Medication Valerian in Healthy Volunteers," *Pharmacology, Biochemistry, and Behavior* 78, no. 1 (May 2004): 57–64.

1633. Harkness and Bratman, *Handbook of Drug-Herb and Drug-Supplement Interactions*, 204.

1634. "Echinacea," *Medlineplus Herb and Supplement*.

1635. "Ginseng," *Medlineplus Herb and Supplement*.

1636. Johnson, *Pocket Guide to Herbal Remedies*, 179.

1637. Pierce, *Practical Guide to Natural Medicines*, 665–667.

1638. Pierce, *Practical Guide to Natural Medicines*, 665–667.

1639. Pierce, *Practical Guide to Natural Medicines*, 665–667.

1640. Hamel and Chiltoskey, *Cherokee Plants and Their Uses*, 61.

1641. Pierce, *Practical Guide to Natural Medicines*, 665–667.

1642. N. Krivoy, et al., "Effect of *Salicis cortex* Extract on Human Platelet Aggregation," *Planta Medica* 67, no. 3 (April 2001): 209–12.

1643. J. J. Gagnier, "Herbal Medicine for Low Back Pain: A Cochrane Review," *Spine* 32, no. 1 (January 1, 2007): 82–92.

1644. R. Shrivastava, "*Tanacetum parthenium* and *Salix alba* (Mig–RL) Combination in Migraine Prophylaxis: A Prospective, Open–Label Study," *Clinical Drug Investigation* 26, no. 5 (2006): 287–96.

1645. Michael Moore, "Herbs Best Used as a Strong Decoction," *Materia Medica Factsheet* http://www.swsbm.com/ManualsMM/DecoctPrf.txt.

1646. Pierce, *Practical Guide to Natural Medicines*, 665–667.

1647. Johnson, *Pocket Guide to Herbal Remedies*, 141.

1648. Pierce, *Practical Guide to Natural Medicines*, 665–667.

1649. Johnson, *Pocket Guide to Herbal Remedies*, 141.

1650. Johnson, *Pocket Guide to Herbal Remedies*, 141.

1651. Remington and Woods, *The Dispensatory of the United States of America*.

1652. Pierce, *Practical Guide to Natural Medicines*, 670–673.

1653. Pierce, *Practical Guide to Natural Medicines*, 670–673.

1654. Hamel and Chiltoskey, *Cherokee Plants and Their Uses*, 62

1655. Melvin R. Gilmore, *Some Chippewa Uses of Plants* (Ann Arbor: University of Michigan Press, 1933): 131.

1656. Herrick, *Iroquois Medical Botany*, 347.

1657. Steven Foster "Witch Hazel: *Hamamelis virginiana*," *Steven Foster Group* http://www.stevenfoster.com/education/monograph/witchhazel.html.

1658. Steven Foster "Witch Hazel: *Hamamelis virginiana*."

1659. Title 21 Food and Drugs, Chapter I—Food and Drug Administration, Department of Health and Human Services (Continued). Part 347–Skin Protectant Drug Products for Over–the–Counter Human Use. Subpart A—astringent Drug Products. Code of Federal Regulations, Title 21, Volume 5. From the U.S. Government Printing Office via GPO Access. Revised as of April 1, 2002. CITE: 21CFR347. Accessed: March 13, 2007. Page 270–271.

1660. M. Duwiejua, et al., "Anti–Inflammatory Activity of *Polygonum bistorta, Guaiacum officinale* and *Hamamelis virginiana* in rats," *The Journal of Pharmacy and Pharmacology* 46, no. 4 (April 1994): 286–90; H. C. Korting, et al., "Anti–Inflammatory Activity of Hamamelis Distillate Applied Topically to the Skin: Influence of Vehicle and Dose," *European Journal of Clinical Pharmacology* 44, no. 4 (1993): 315–8.

1661. Grieve, "Witch Hazel," *Botanical.com: A Modern Herbal*.

1662. B. J. Hughes Formella, et al., "Anti–Inflammatory Efficacy of Topical Preparations with 10% Hamamelis Distillate in a UV Erythema Test," *Skin Pharmacology and Applied Skin Physiology* 15, no. 2 (March–April 2002): 125–32; B. J. Hughes Formella, et al., "Anti–Inflammatory Effect of Hamamelis Lotion in a UVB Erythema Test," *Dermatology* 196, no. 3 (1998): 316–22.

1663. H. Masaki, et al. "Active–Oxygen Scavenging Activity of Plant Extracts," *Biological and Pharmaceutical Bulletin* 16, no. 1 (January 1995): 162–6; H. Masaki, et al., Hamamelitannin as a New Potent Active Oxygen Scavenger," *Phytochemistry Oxford* 37, no. 2 (September 1994): 337–343.

1664. F. Ellingwood, *Ellingwood's Therapeutist: A Monthly Journal of Direct Therapeutics* (Ann Arbor: University of Michigan, 1908): 197

1665. Pierce, *Practical Guide to Natural Medicines*, 670–673.

1666. Steven Foster "Witch Hazel: *Hamamelis virginiana*."

1667. Michael Moore, "Herbs Best as Cold Infusion," *Materia Medica Factsheet* http://www.swsbm.com/ManualsMM/CldInfus.txt.

1668. Michael Moore, "Herbs Best Used as a Strong Decoction," *Materia Medica Factsheet* http://www.swsbm.com/ManualsMM/DecoctPrf.txt.

1669. Steven Foster "Witch Hazel: *Hamamelis virginiana*."

1670. Pierce, *Practical Guide to Natural Medicines*, 670–673.

1671. Cech, *Making Plant Medicine*, 228.

1672. Remington and Woods, *The Dispensatory of the United States of America*.

1673. Ody, *The Complete Medicinal Herbal*, 30.

1674. Grieve, "Yarrow," *Botanical.com: A Modern Herbal*.

1675. Pierce, *Practical Guide to Natural Medicines*, 679–682.

1676. John C. Hellson, "Ethnobotany of the Blackfoot Indians," *Mercury Series* (Ottawa: National Museums of Canada, 1974): 74; Jeff Hart, *Montana Native Plants and Early Peoples* (Helena: Montana Historical Society Press, 1992): 6.

1677. Nancy J. Turner, "The Ethnobotany of the Bella Coola Indians of British Columbia," *Syesis* 6 (1973): 201; Hart, *Montana Native Plants,* 6; Harlan I. Smith, "Materia Medica of the Bella Coola and Neighboring Tribes of British Columbia," *National Museum of Canada Bulletin* 56 (1929): 65; Ralph V. Chamberlin, "The Ethno–Botany of the Gosiute Indians of Utah," *Memoirs of the American Anthropological Association* 2 no. 5 (1911): 360.

1678. Grieve, "Yarrow," *Botanical.com: A Modern Herbal.*

1679. Kowalchik and Hylton, *Rodale's Illustrated Encyclopedia of Herbs,* 293.

1680. Pierce, *Practical Guide to Natural Medicines,* 679–682.

1681. F. Candan, et al. "Antioxidant and Antimicrobial Activity of the Essential Oil and Methanol Extracts of *Achillea millefolium* subsp. millefolium Afan (*Asteraceae*)," *Journal of Ethnopharmacology* 87 no. 2–3 (August 2003): 215–20; S. Barel, et al. "The Antimicrobial Activity of the Essential Oil from *Achillea fragrantissima*," *Journal of Ethnophamacology* 33 no. 1–2 (May–June 1991): 187–91; K. H. Baser, et al., "Composition and Antimicrobial Activity of the Essential Oil of *Achillea multifida*," *Planta Medica.* 68, no. 10 (October 2002): 941–3.

1682. M. K. Al–Hindawi, et al., "Anti–Inflammatory Activity of Some Iraqi Plants Using Intact Rats," *Journal of Ethnophamacology* 26, no. 2 (September 1989): 163–8.

1683. M. Y. Shapira, et al., "Treatment of Atopic Dermatitis with Herbal Combination of *Eleutherococcus, Achillea millefolium,* and *Lamium album* has no Advantage over Placebo: A Double Blind, Placebo–Controlled, Randomized Trial," *Journal of the American Academy of Dermatology* 52, no. 4 (April 2005): 691–3.

1684. G. A. Van der Weijden, et al., "The Effect of Herbal Extracts in an Experimental Mouthrinse on Established Plaque and Gingivitis," *Journal of Clinical Periodontology* 25, no. 5 (May 1998): 399–403.

1685. Jacques Rousseau, "Ethnobotanique Abenakise," *Archives de Folklore* 11 (1947): 174; Meredith Jean Black, "Algonquin Ethnobotany: An Interpretation of Aboriginal Adaptation in South Western Quebec," *Mercury Series Number* 65 (Ottawa, National Museums of Canada, 1980): 240; Turner, "The Ethnobotany of the Bella Coola Indians of British Columbia," 201; Hellson, *Ethnobotany of the Blackfoot Indians,* 70; Harlan I. Smith, "Materia Medica of the Bella Coola and Neighboring Tribes of British Columbia," *National Museum of Canada Bulletin* 56 (1929): 65; Hamel and Chiltoskey, *Cherokee Plants and Their Uses,* 62; Mark S. Fleisher, "The Ethnobotany of the Clallam Indians of Western Washington," *Northwest Anthropological Research Notes* 14, no. 2 (1980): 199; Hart, *Montana Native Plants,* 6.

1686. Pierce, *Practical Guide to Natural Medicines,* 679–682.

1687. Grieve, "Yarrow," *Botanical.com: A Modern Herbal.*

1688. Remington and Woods, *The Dispensatory of the United States of America.*

1689. Pierce, *Practical Guide to Natural Medicines,* 679–682.

1690. E. Barrie Kavasch and Karen Baar, *American Indian Healing Arts* (New York: Bantam, 1999): 179.

1691. Cech, *Making Plant Medicine,* 232.

1692. Pierce, *Practical Guide to Natural Medicines,* 679–682.

1693. Bown, *Encyclopaedia of Herbs and their Uses.*

1694. Remington and Woods, *The Dispensatory of the United States of America.*

1695. Pierce, *Practical Guide to Natural Medicines,* 679–682.

1696. Johnson, *Pocket Guide to Herbal Remedies,* 1.

1697. Pierce, *Practical Guide to Natural Medicines*, 679–682.

1698. Pierce, *Practical Guide to Natural Medicines*, 679–682.

1699. Johnson, *Pocket Guide to Herbal Remedies*, 1.

1700. Pierce, *Practical Guide to Natural Medicines*, 679–682.

1701. Pierce, *Practical Guide to Natural Medicines*, 679–682.

1702. P. R. Dalsenter, et al., "Reproductive Evaluation of Aqueous Crude Extract of *Achillea millefolium* L. (*Asteraceae*) in Wistar Rats," *Reproductive Toxicology* 18, no. 6 (August–September 2004): 819–23; T. Montanari, et al., "Antispermatogenic Effect of *Achillea millefolium* L. in Mice," *Contraception* 58, no. 5 (November 1998): 309–13.

Chapter Three: Preparing the Herbs

1703. David M. Rollins, "The Control of Microbial Growth," *BSCI 223—General Microbiology, University of Maryland* http://www.life.umd.edu/classroom/bsci424/BSCI223WebSiteFiles/Chapter7.htm.

1704. Henriette Kress, "Troubleshooting Herbal Oils," *Henriette's Herbal Blog* http://www.henriettesherbal.com/blog/?p=162.

1705. Kavasch and Baar, *American Indian Healing Arts*, 179.

1706. Kress, "Troubleshooting Herbal Oils."

1707. Kavasch and Baar, *American Indian Healing Arts*, 232–239.

1708. Cech, *Making Plant Medicine*, 83.

1709. Kress, "Troubleshooting Herbal Oils."

1710. Kress, "Troubleshooting Herbal Oils."

1711. Ody, *The Complete Medicinal Herbal*, 124.

1712. Kavasch and Baar, *American Indian Healing Arts*, 232–239.

1713. T. Futami, ["Actions and Mechanism of Counterirritants on the Muscular Circulation,"] *Nippon Yakurigaku Zasshi* 83, no. 3 (March 1984): 219–26 (Article in Japanese).

Chapter Four: Applications and Uses

1714. "Cayenne," *Whole Health MD*.

1715. "Capsaicin," *Wikipedia* http://en.wikipedia.org/wiki/Capsaicin; A. Dray "Mechanism of Action of Capsaicin-Like Molecules on Sensory Neurons," *Life Sciences* 51, no. 23 (1992): 1759–65.

1716. Ody, *The Complete Medicinal Herbal*, 56.

1717. Ody, *The Complete Medicinal Herbal*, 30.

1718. M. Kucera, et al., "Efficacy and Safety of Topically Applied Symphytum Herb Extract Cream in the Treatment of Ankle Distortion: Results of a Randomized Controlled Clinical Double Blind Study," *Wiener Medizinische Wochenschrift* 154, no. 21–22 (November 2004): 498–507.

1719. Pierce, *Practical Guide to Natural Medicines*, 198.

1720. Pierce, *Practical Guide to Natural Medicines*, 198.

1721. Cech, *Making Plant Medicine*, 93.

1722. Ody, *The Complete Medicinal Herbal*, 130.

1723. Henriette Kress, "Herbs in Salves," *Henriette's Herbal Blog* http://www.henriettesherbal.com/blog/?cat=6.

1724. Pierce, *Practical Guide to Natural Medicines*, 348–50.

1725. Pierce, *Practical Guide to Natural Medicines*, 348–50.

1726. Pierce, *Practical Guide to Natural Medicines*, 348–50.

1727. C. Calabrese and P. Preston, "Report of the Results of a Double–Blind, Randomized, Single–Dose Trial of a Topical 2% Escin Gel versus Placebo in the Acute Treatment of Experimentally–Induced Hematoma in Volunteers," *Planta Medica* 59 (1993): 394–397.

1728. Cech, *Making Plant Medicine*, 83.

1729. Hoffmann, *Herbal Materia Medica*.

1730. Cech, *Making Plant Medicine*, 95.

1731. D. L. Wieder, Treatment of Traumatic Myositis Ossificans with Acetic Acid Iontophoresis," *Physical Therapy* 72, no. 2 (February 1992): 133–7.

1732. Ernestina Parziale, "Agrimony," *Backyard Herbalist* http://earthnotes.tripod.com/agrimony1.htm.

1733. D. MacKay and A. L. Miller, "Nutritional Support for Wound Healing," *Alternative Medicine Review* 8, no. 4 (November 2003): 359–77.

1734. U.S. National Library of Medicine, "Cuts and Puncture Wounds," *Medline Plus* http://www.nlm.nih.gov/medlineplus/ency/article/000043.htm.

1735. Cech, *Making Plant Medicine*, 128.

1736. S. Foster and J. Duke, *Eastern/Central Medicinal Plants* (Boston: Houghton Mifflin Company, 1990).

1737. R. Patzelt–Wenczler, et al., "Proof of Efficacy of Kamillosan(R) Cream in Atopic Eczema," *European Journal of Medical Research* 5, no. 4 (April 19, 2000): 171–5.

1738. S. M. Fuchs, et al., "Protective Effects of Different Marigold (*Calendula officinalis L.*) and Rosemary Cream Preparations Against Sodium–Lauryl–Sulfate–Induced Irritant Contact Dermatitis. *Skin Pharmacology and Physiology* 18, no. 4 (July–August 2005): 195–200.

1739. A. Bjørneboe, E. Søyland, and G. E. Bjørneboe, et al., "Effect of Dietary Supplementation with Eicosapentaenoic Acid in the Treatment of Atopic Dermatitis," *The British Journal of Dermatology* 117 (1987): 463–9; A. Bjørnboe, E. Søyland, and G. E. Bjørnboe, et al. "Effect of n–3 Fatty Acid Supplement to Patients with Atopic Dermatitis," *Journal of Internal Medicine Supplement* 225 (1989): 233–6; E. Søyland, G. Rajka, and A. Bjørneboe, et al. "The Effect of Eicosapentaenoic Acid in the Treatment of Atopic Dermatitis: A Clinical Study," *Acta Dermato-Venereologica* 114 (supplement) (1989): 139; J. Berth–Jones, R. A. C. Graham–Brown, "Placebo–Controlled Trial of Essential Fatty Acid Supplementation in Atopic Dermatitis," *Lancet* 341 (1993): 1557–60.

1740. H. J. Glowania, et al., "The Effect of Chamomile in Healing Wounds: A Clinical, Double–Blind Study," *Zeitschrift für Hautkrankheiten* 17 no. 62 (1987): 1262–1271.

1741. Cech, *Making Plant Medicine*, 138.

1742. Pierce, *Practical Guide to Natural Medicines*, 679–682.

1743. Ody, *The Complete Medicinal Herbal*, 130.

1744. Pierce, *Practical Guide to Natural Medicines*, 24.

1745. J. Leuschner, "Anti–Inflammatory, Spasmolytic and Diuretic Effects of a Commercially Available *Solidago gigantea* Herb Extract," *Arzneimittelforschung* 45, no. 2 (February 1995): 165–8.

1746. Pierce, *Practical Guide to Natural Medicines*, 449–451.

1747. Kathi J. Kemper, "Calendula (*Calendula officinalis*)," *The Longwood Herbal Task Force* http://www.mcp.edu/herbal/default.htm.

1748. Pierce, *Practical Guide to Natural Medicines*, 390–92.

1749. Henriette Kress, "Balms and Liniments," *Henriette's Herbal Blog* http://www.henriettesherbal.com/faqs/medi-4-4-balm.html.

1750. D. MacKay and A. L. Miller, "Nutritional Support for Wound Healing," *Alternative Medicine Review* 8, no. 4 (November 2003): 359–77.

1751. "Plantar Warts," *MayoClinic.com* http://www.mayoclinic.com/health/plantar-warts/DS00509/DSECTION=1.

1752. "Plantar Warts," *MayoClinic.com.*

1753. David Shaw, "Have a Cold or Flu? To Exercise or Not...," *Quantum Health* http://www.quantumhealth.com/news/exercise_with_cold_or_flu.html.

1754. V. Barak, et al., "The Effect Of Sambucol, a Black Elderberry-Based, Natural Product, on the Production of Human Cytokines: I. Inflammatory Cytokines," *European Cytokine Network* 12, no. 2 (April–June 2001): 90–6.

1755. Z. Zakay-Rones, et al., "Inhibition of Several Strains of Influenza Virus In Vitro and Reduction of Symptoms by an Elderberry Extract (*Sambucus nigra* L.) During an Outbreak of Influenza B Panama," *Journal of Alternative and Complementary Medicine* 1, no. 4 (Winter 1995): 361–9; Thom Erling and Therje Wollan, "Randomized Study on The Efficacy and Safety of an Oral Elderberry Extract in the Treatment of Influenza A and B Virus Infections," *The Journal of International Medical Research* 32, no. 2 (2004): 132–140.

1756. L. L. Kulichenko, et al., "A Randomized, Controlled Study of Kan Jang versus Amantadine in the Treatment of Influenza in Volgograd," *Journal of Herbal Pharmacotherapy* 3, no. 1 (2003): 77–93.

1757. A. A. Spasov, et al., "Comparative Controlled Study of *Andrographis paniculata* Fixed Combination, Kan Jang" and an Echinacea Preparation as Adjuvant, in the Treatment of Uncomplicated Respiratory Disease in Children, *Phytotherapy Research* 18, no. 1 (2004): 47–53.

1758. R. Saller, et al., "Dose-Dependancy of Symptomatic Relief of Complaints by Chamomile Steam Inhalation in Patients with Common Cold," *European Journal of Pharmacology* 183 (1990): 728–729.

1759. Ody, *The Complete Medicinal Herbal*, 136–137.

1760. G. Puodziuniene, et al., ["Development of Throat Clearing Herbal Teas,] *Medicina (Kaunas, Lithuania)* 40, no. 8 (2004): 762–7 (Article in Lithuanian).

1761. Ody, *The Complete Medicinal Herbal*, 69.

1762. Ody, *The Complete Medicinal Herbal*, 136–137.

1763. Wardwell, *The Herbal Home Remedy Book*, 108.

1764. Wardwell, *The Herbal Home Remedy Book*, 108.

1765. International College of Herbal Medicine "Chilli: *Capsicum Minimum, C. Fructescens*," *Herb of the Month, January/ February 2004* http://www.herbcollege.com/herbofthemonth.asp?id=61.

1766. "Chamomile," *Whole Health MD.*

1767. Pierce, *Practical Guide to Natural Medicines*, 488–91.

1768. H. Schilcher, *Phytotherapy in Pediatrics—Handbook for Physicians and Pharmacists* (Stuttgart: Medpharm Scientific Publishers, 1997): 61–62.

1769. Ody, *The Complete Medicinal Herbal*, 164–5.

1770. Cech, *Making Plant Medicine*, 182.

1771. Ody, *The Complete Medicinal Herbal*, 164–5.

1772. "Ginger," *Whole Health MD.*

1773. Cech, *Making Plant Medicine*, 123.

1774. Kowalchik and Hylton, *Rodale's Illustrated Encyclopedia of Herbs*, 288.

1775. Grieve, "Arnica," *Botanical.com: A Modern Herbal.*

1776. "Borage Oil," *Whole Health MD.*

1777. Pierce, *Practical Guide to Natural Medicines*, 628–630.

1778. Henriette Kress, "Warming salve," *Henriette's Herbal Blog* http://www.henriettesherbal.com/blog/?p=43.

1779. Z. S. Saify, et al., "Cineole as Skin Penetration Enhancer," *Pakistan Journal of Pharmaceutical Sciences* 13, no. 1 (January 2000): 29–32.

1780. C. E. Ficker, et al., "Inhibition of Human Pathogenic Fungi by Ethnobotanically Selected Plant Extracts," *Mycoses* 46, no. 1–2 (February 2003): 29–37.

1781. R. S. Ramsewak, et al., "In Vitro Antagonistic Activity of Monoterpenes and their Mixtures against 'Toe Nail Fungus' Pathogens," *Phytotherapy Research* 17, no. 4 (April 2003): 376–9.

1782. S. Tunc, et al., "Combined Effect of Volatile Antimicrobial Agents on the Growth of *Penicillium notatum*," *International Journal of Food Microbiology* 113, no. 3 (September 29, 2006): 263–270; M. Valero, et al., "Synergistic Bactericidal Effect of Carvacrol, Cinnamaldehyde or Thymol and Refrigeration to Inhibit *Bacillus cereus* in Carrot Broth," *Food Microbiology* 23, no. 1 (February 2006): 68–73.

1783. "Garlic," *Whole Health MD.*

1784. "Garlic," *Whole Health MD.*

1785. Mountain Rose Herbs, "Athlete's Foot. Simple Herbal Remedies Information," http://www.herbalremediesinfo.com/AthletesFoot.html.

1786. Marianne Wait, ed., *1,801 Home Remedies* (Pleasantville, NY: Reader's Digest, 2004): 261.

1787. Hoffmann, "Caraway."

1788. Hoffmann, "Anise."

Chapter Five: Herbal Contraindications

1789. U.S. National Institutes of Health, "Herbs and Supplements," *Medline Plus* http://www.nlm.nih.gov/medlineplus/druginformation.html.

1790. U.S. National Institutes of Health, "Herbs and supplements."

1791. U.S. National Institutes of Health, "Herbs and supplements."

1792. U.S. National Institutes of Health, "Herbs and supplements."

1793. U.S. National Institutes of Health, "Melatonin," *Medline Plus* http://www.nlm.nih.gov/medlineplus/druginfo/natural/patient-melatonin.html.

1794. "Echinacea," *Medlineplus Herb and Supplement.*

1795. "Devil's Claw," *Medlineplus Herb and Supplement.*

1796. "Creatine," *Medlineplus Herb and Supplement.*

1797. "Ginseng," *Medlineplus Herb and Supplement.*

Chapter Seven: Glossary

1798. Gregory S. Kelly, "*Rhodiola rosea*: A Possible Plant Adaptogen," *Smart Nutrition* http://smart-drugs.net/Rhodiola-rosea.htm.

Bibliography of Frequently Cited Works

American Botanical Council. Herbalgram: *The Journal of the American Botanical Council.* Available on the Internet: http://cms.herbalgram.org/herbalgram/index.html.

Blumenthal, M., et al. *The Complete German Commission E Manuscripts*. Boston: Integrative Medicine Communications, 1998.

Bown, D. *Encyclopedia of Herbs and Their Uses*. New York: DK Publishing, Inc., 1995.

Cech, Richo. *Making Plant Medicine*. Williams, OR: Horizon Herbs, 2000.

Felter, Harvey Wickes. *The Eclectic Materia Medica, Pharmacology and Therapeutics*. Cincinnati: John K. Scudder, 1922. Reprinted and abridged by the Southwest School of Medicine, Bisbee, Arizona, http://www.swsbm.com/FelterMM/Felters_Materia_Medica.pdf

Fyfe, John William. *The Essentials of Modern Materia Medica and Therapeutics*. Cincinnati: The Scudder Brothers Company. 1903.

Grieve, Maud. *A Modern Herbal.* New York: Harcourt, Brace & Company, 1931. Electronic version published by Botanical.com http://www.botanical.com/botanical/mgmh/b/borage66.html.

Harkness, Richard and Steven Bratman. *Handbook of Drug–Herb and Drug-Supplement Interactions*. St. Louis, MO: Mosby, 2003.

Healthways. *Whole Health MD*. Sterling, VA. http://www.wholehealthmd.com

Hoffmann, David L. "Herbal Materia Medica," *Health World*, http://www.healthy.net/scr/MMList.asp?MTId=1.

Kowalchik, Claire and William Hylton, eds. *Rodale's Illustrated Encyclopedia of Herbs*. Emmaus, PA: Rodale Press, 1987.

Moore, Michael. Clinical Herb Manuals. Southwest School of Botanical Medicine. Tucson, AZ, n.d., http://www.swsbm.com/ManualsMM/MansMM.html.

Ody, Penelope. *The Complete Medicinal Herbal.* London: Dorling Kindersley, 1993.

Pierce, Andrea. *American Pharmaceutical Association Practical Guide to Natural Medicines*. New York: Stonesong Press, 1999.

Johnson, Lane P. *Pocket Guide to Herbal Remedies*. Malden, MA: Blackwell Science, 2002.

Remington, Joseph P. and Horatio C. Woods, et al., eds. *The Dispensatory of the United States of America.* 20th ed. Philadelphia: J.B. Lippincott Company, 1918. Digitized by Michael Moore, www.swsbm.com/Dispensatory/USD-1918-complete.pdf.

Scudder, John M. *Specific Medication and Specific Medicines*. Cincinnati: Wilstach, Baldwin & Co., 1870. Scanned and edited by Henriette Kress http://www.henriettesherbal.com/eclectic/spec-med/index.html

Thompson Healthcare. *PDR for Herbal Medicines*, 4th ed. New York: Thompson Reuters, 2007.

Wardwell, Joyce A. *The Herbal Home Remedy Book*. Pownal, VT: Storey Publishing, 1998.

Index

About the Author

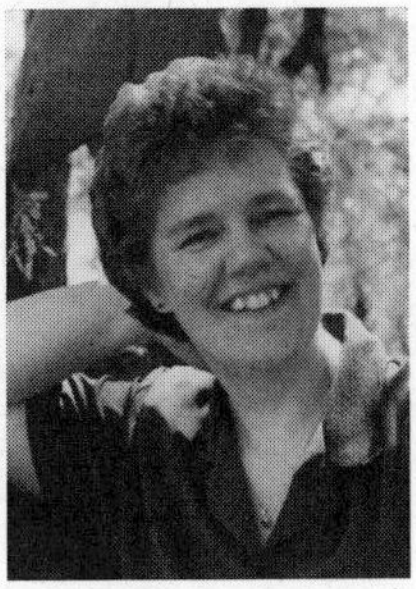

Susan Lynn Peterson has made a career of writing about complex topics in a straightforward entertaining way. Building on a lifetime of interest in health, especially alternative healing practices, she has spent three years and thousands of hours investigating the way herbs have been used in various cultures to treat injuries. *A Martial Artist's Guide to Western Herbs* is her fifth book. Her first three books, published by Tuttle Publishing and Zondervan Publishing House, a subsidiary of Harper Collins, have been translated into five languages. For the first book, she earned a Gold Medallion Book award nomination. She has also contributed to several national magazines including *Black Belt*, *New Body*, *Complete Woman*, and *Fighting Woman News.*

Peterson has been a martial artist for more than twenty years. She holds a fifth-degree black belt in Okinawan Shuri-ryu karate, a second-degree black belt in traditional Okinawan weapons, and has also studied Yang-style Tai Chi Chuan and Martial Kinesiology, a hands-on system of mind-body healing for several years. Her other martial arts experience includes Kenpo, Wing Chun, Aikido, Taekwondo, Jujitsu, Seven Star Qigong, and Shaolin Chuan Fa.

She was a 1995 USA Karate Federation (USAKF) national gold medalist in kobudo (traditional weapons), a USAKF Arizona gold medalist in advanced kata and kobudo, and a 2001 USAKF Pacific League Tournament gold medalist in advanced kata and kobudo, and in 2006 placed fourth in the United States Karate Masters' Division.

Susan Lynn Peterson holds an MA in Linguistics and a Ph.D. in the Humanities, Text Theory. When she is not writing, she teaches karate at KoSho Pantano and runs Alcuin Communications, an Internet and print media communications company. She resides with her family in Tucson, Arizona.

BOOKS FROM YMAA

6 HEALING MOVEMENTS	B906
101 REFLECTIONS ON TAI CHI CHUAN	B868
108 INSIGHTS INTO TAI CHI CHUAN—A STRING OF PEARLS	B582
A WOMAN'S QIGONG GUIDE	B833
A SUDDEN DAWN	B1989
ADVANCING IN TAE KWON DO	B072X
ANCIENT CHINESE WEAPONS	B671
ANALYSIS OF SHAOLIN CHIN NA 2ND ED.	B0002
THE ART OF HOJO UNDO—POWER TRAINING FORTRADITIONAL KARATE	B1361
ARTHRITIS RELIEF—CHINESE QIGONG FOR HEALING & PREVENTION, 3RD ED.	B0339
BACK PAIN RELIEF—CHINESE QIGONG FOR HEALING & PREVENTION, 2ND ED.	B0258
BAGUAZHANG 2ND ED.	B1132
CARDIO KICKBOXING ELITE	B922
CHIN NA IN GROUND FIGHTING	B663
CHINESE FAST WRESTLING—THE ART OF SAN SHOU KUAI JIAO	B493
CHINESE FITNESS—A MIND/BODY APPROACH	B37X
CHINESE TUI NA MASSAGE	B043
COMPLETE CARDIOKICKBOXING	B809
COMPREHENSIVE APPLICATIONS OF SHAOLIN CHIN NA	B36X
CROCODILE AND THE CRANE	B0876
THE CUTTING SEASON (HARD COVER)	B0821
THE CUTTING SEASON (PAPER BACK)	B1309
DR. WU'S HEAD MASSAGE—ANTI-AGING AND HOLISTIC HEALING THERAPY	B0576
EIGHT SIMPLE QIGONG EXERCISES FOR HEALTH, 2ND ED.	B523
ESSENCE OF SHAOLIN WHITE CRANE	B353
ESSENCE OF TAIJI QIGONG, 2ND ED.	B639
EXPLORING TAI CHI	B424
FIGHTING ARTS	B213
INSIDE TAI CHI	B108
KATA AND THE TRANSMISSION OF KNOWLEDGE	B0266
THE LITTLE BLACK BOOK OF VIOLENCE	B1293
LIUHEBAFA FIVE CHARACTER SECRETS	B728
LITLE BLACK BOOK OF VIOLENCE	B1293
MARTIAL ARTS ATHLETE	B655
MARTIAL ARTS INSTRUCTION	B024X
MARTIAL WAY AND ITS VIRTUES	B698
MEDITATIONS ON VIOLENCE	B1187
MIND/BODY FITNESS—A MIND / BODY APPROACH	B876
MUGAI RYU—THE CLASSICAL SAMURAI ART OF DRAWING THE SWORD	B183
NATURAL HEALING WITH QIGONG—THERAPEUTIC QIGONG	B0010
NORTHERN SHAOLIN SWORD, 2ND ED.	B85X
OKINAWA'S COMPLETE KARATE SYSTEM—ISSHIN RYU	B914
POWER BODY	B760
PRINCIPLES OF TRADITIONAL CHINESE MEDICINE	B99X
QIGONG FOR HEALTH & MARTIAL ARTS, 2ND ED.	B574
QIGONG FOR LIVING	B116
QIGONG FOR TREATING COMMON AILMENTS	B701
QIGONG MASSAGE—FUND. TECHNIQUES FOR HEALTH AND RELAXATION, 2ND ED.	B0487
QIGONG MEDITATION—EMBRYONIC BREATHING	B736
QIGONG MEDITATION—SMALL CIRCULATION	B0673
QIGONG, THE SECRET OF YOUTH	B841
QUIET TEACHER	B1262
ROOT OF CHINESE QIGONG, 2ND ED.	B507
SHIHAN TE—THE BUNKAI OF KATA	B884
SIMPLE CHINESE MEDICINE	B1248
SUNRISE TAI CHI	B0838
SURVIVING ARMED ASSAULTS	B0711
TAEKWONDO—ANCIENT WISDOM FOR THE MODERN WARRIOR	B930
TAE KWON DO—THE KOREAN MARTIAL ART	B0869
TAEKWONDO—A PATH TO PERSONAL EXCELLENCE	B1286
TAEKWONDO—SPIRIT AND PRACTICE	B221
TAO OF BIOENERGETICS	B289
TAI CHI BOOK	B647
TAI CHI CHUAN—24 & 48 POSTURES	B337
TAI CHI CHUAN MARTIAL APPLICATIONS, 2ND ED.	B442
TAI CHI CONNECTIONS	B0320
TAI CHI DYNAMICS	B1163
TAI CHI SECRETS OF THE ANCIENT MASTERS	B71X
TAI CHI SECRETS OF THE WU & LI STYLES	B981
TAI CHI SECRETS OF THE WU STYLE	B175
TAI CHI SECRETS OF THE YANG STYLE	B094
TAI CHI THEORY & MARTIAL POWER, 2ND ED.	B434
TAI CHI WALKING	B23X
TAIJI BALL QIGONG	B1996
TAIJI CHIN NA	B378

more products available from...

YMAA Publication Center, Inc. 楊氏東方文化出版中心

1-800-669-8892 • ymaa@aol.com • www.ymaa.com

BOOKS FROM YMAA *(continued)*

TAIJI SWORD, CLASSICAL YANG STYLE	B744
TAIJIQUAN, CLASSICAL YANG STYLE (REVISED)	B2009
TAIJIQUAN THEORY OF DR. YANG, JWING-MING	B432
TENGU—THE MOUNTAIN GOBLIN (HARD COVER)	B1255
TENGU—THE MOUNTAIN GOBLIN (PAPER BACK)	B1231
THE WAY OF KATA—A COMPREHENSIVE GUIDE TO DECIPHERING MARTIAL APPS.	B0584
THE WAY OF KENDO AND KENJITSU	B0029
THE WAY OF SANCHIN KATA	B0845
THE WAY TO BLACK BELT	B0852
TRADITIONAL CHINESE HEALTH SECRETS	B892
TRADITIONAL TAEKWONDO—CORE TECHNIQUES, HISTORY, AND PHILOSOPHY	B0665
WILD GOOSE QIGONG	B787
WISDOM'S WAY	B361
XINGYIQUAN, 2ND ED.	B416
WESTERN HERBS FOR MARTIAL ARTISTS AND CONTACT ATHLETES	B1972

DVDS FROM YMAA

ADVANCED PRACTICAL CHIN NA—IN DEPTH-	D1124
ANALYSIS OF SHAOLIN CHIN NA	D0231
BAGUAZHANG 1, 2, & 3—EMEI BAGUAZHANG	D0649
CHEN STYLE TAIJIQUAN	D0819
CHIN NA IN DEPTH COURSES 1–4	D602
CHIN NA IN DEPTH COURSES 5–8	D610
CHIN NA IN DEPTH COURSES 9–12	D629
EIGHT SIMPLE QIGONG EXERCISES FOR HEALTH	D0037
ESSENCE OF TAIJI QIGONG	D0215
FIVE ANIMAL SPORTS	D1106
KUNG FU FOR KIDS	D1880
NORTHERN SHAOLIN SWORD—SAN CAI JIAN, KUN WU JIAN, QI MEN JIAN	D1194
QIGONG MASSAGE—FUNDAMENTAL TECHNIQUES FOR HEALTH AND RELAXATION	D0592
QIGONG—15 MINUTES TO HEALTH	D2078
SABER FUNDAMENTAL TRAINING	D1088
SANCHIN KATA	D1897
SHAOLIN KUNG FU FUNDAMENTAL TRAINING 1 & 2	D0436
SHAOLIN LONG FIST KUNG FU—BASIC SEQUENCES	D661
SHAOLIN LONG FIST KUNG FU—INTERMEDIATE SEQUENCES	D1071
SHAOLIN LONG FIST KUNG ADVANCED SEQUENCES	D2061
SHAOLIN SABER—BASIC SEQUENCES	D0616
SHAOLIN STAFF—BASIC SEQUENCES	D0920
SHAOLIN WHITE CRANE GONG FU BASIC TRAINING 1 & 2	D599
SHAOLIN WHITE CRANE GONG FU BASIC TRAINING 3 & 4	D0784
SHUAI JIAO KUNG FU WRESTLING	D1149
SIMPLE QIGONG EXERCISES FOR ARTHRITIS RELIEF	D0890
SIMPLE QIGONG EXERCISES FOR BACK PAIN RELIEF	D0883
SIMPLIFIED TAI CHI CHUAN—24 & 48 POSTURES	D0630
SUNRISE TAI CHI	D0274
SUNSET TAI CHI	D0760
SWORD FUNDAMENTAL TRAINING	D1095
TAI CHI CONNECTIONS	D0444
TAI CHI ENERGY PATTERNS	D0525
TAI CHI FIGHTING SET—TWO PERSON MATCHING SET	D0509
TAIJI BALL QIGONG COURSES 1 & 2—16 CIRCLING AND 16 ROTATING PATTERNS	D0517
TAIJI BALL QIGONG COURSES 3 & 4—16 PATTERNS OF WRAP-COILING & APPLICATIONS	D0777
TAIJI CHIN NA — COURSES 1, 2, 3, & 4	D0463
TAIJI MARTIAL APPLICATIONS—37 POSTURES	D1057
TAIJI PUSHING HANDS 1 & 2—YANG STYLE SINGLE AND DOUBLE PUSHING HANDS	D0495
TAIJI PUSHING HANDS 3 & 4—MOVING SINGLE AND DOUBLE PUSHING HANDS	D0681
TAIJI WRESTLING—ADVANCED TAKEDOWN TECHNIQUES	D1064
TAIJI SABER—THE COMPLETE FORM, QIGONG, & APPLICATIONS	D1026
TAIJI & SHAOLIN STAFF—FUNDAMENTAL TRAINING	D0906
TAIJI YIN YANG STICKING HANDS	D1040
TAIJIQUAN CLASSICAL YANG STYLE	D645
TAIJI SWORD, CLASSICAL YANG STYLE	D0452
UNDERSTANDING QIGONG 1—WHAT IS QI? • HUMAN QI CIRCULATORY SYSTEM	D069X
UNDERSTANDING QIGONG 2—KEY POINTS • QIGONG BREATHING	D0418
UNDERSTANDING QIGONG 3—EMBRYONIC BREATHING	D0555
UNDERSTANDING QIGONG 4—FOUR SEASONS QIGONG	D0562
UNDERSTANDING QIGONG 5—SMALL CIRCULATION	D0753
UNDERSTANDING QIGONG 6—MARTIAL QIGONG BREATHING	D0913
WHITE CRANE HARD & SOFT QIGONG	D637
WUDANG KUNG FU FUNDAMENTALS	D1316
WUDANG SWORD FUNDAMENTALS	D1903
WUDANG TAIJIQUAN	D1217
XINGYIQUAN—TWELVE ANIMALS KUNG FU AND APPLICATIONS	D1200
YMAA 25 YEAR ANNIVERSARY DVD	D0708